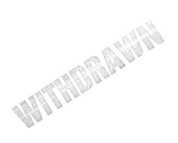

Informed Consent and Clinician Accountability

The Ethics of Report Cards on Surgeon Performance

This timely collection analyses and evaluates ethical and social implications of recent developments in reporting surgeon performance. It contains chapters by leading international specialists in philosophy, bioethics, epidemiology, medical administration, surgery and law, demonstrating the diversity and complexity of debates about this topic, raising considerations of patient autonomy, accountability, justice and the quality and safety of medical services. Performance information on individual cardiac surgeons has been publicly available in parts of the US for over a decade. Survival rates for individual cardiac surgeons in the UK have recently been released to the public. This trend is being driven by various factors, including concerns about accountability, patients' rights, quality and safety of medical care and the need to avoid scandals in medical care. This trend is likely to extend to other countries, to other clinicians, and to professions beyond health care, making this text an essential addition to the literature available.

Dr Steve Clarke is a Senior Research Fellow at the Centre for Applied Philosophy and Public Ethics, Charles Sturt University, Australia, and a Research Fellow with the Programme on the Ethics of the New Biosciences, James Martin 21st Century School, University of Oxford.

Associate Professor **Justin Oakley** is Director of the Centre for Human Bioethics at Monash University, Victoria, Australia.

Informed Consent and Clinician Accountability

The Ethics of Report Cards on Surgeon Performance

Edited by

Steve Clarke

University of Oxford, UK, and Charles Sturt University, New South Wales, Australia

Justin Oakley

Monash University, Victoria, Australia

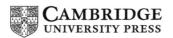

CAMBRIDGE UNIVERSITY PRESS
Cambridge, New York, Melbourne, Madrid, Cape Town, Singapore, São Paulo

Cambridge University Press
The Edinburgh Building, Cambridge CB2 8RU, UK

Published in the United States of America by Cambridge University Press, New York

www.cambridge.org
Information on this title: www.cambridge.org/9780521865074

First published 2007

Printed in the United Kingdom at the University Press, Cambridge

A catalogue record for this publication is available from the British Library

ISBN 978-0-521-86507-4 hardback
ISBN 978-0-521-68778-2 paperback

Cambridge University Press has no responsibility for the persistence or
accuracy of URLs for external or third-party internet websites referred to
in this publication, and does not guarantee that any content on such
websites is, or will remain, accurate or appropriate.

Every effort has been made in preparing this publication to provide accurate and up-to-date
information which is in accord with accepted standards and practice at the time of publication.
Although case histories are drawn from actual cases, every effort has been made to disguise the
identities of the individuals involved. Nevertheless, the authors, editors and publishers can make
no warranties that the information contained herein is totally free from error, not least because
clinical standards are constantly changing through research and regulation. The authors, editors
and publishers therefore disclaim all liability for direct or consequential damages resulting from the
use of material contained in this publication. Readers are strongly advised to pay careful attention
to information provided by the manufacturer of any drugs or equipment that they plan to use.

Contents

Contributors

David A. Asch is Executive Director of the Leonard Davis Institute of Health Economics at the University of Pennsylvania and Director of the Center for Health Equity Research and Promotion at the Philadelphia Veterans Affairs Medical Center.

Paul Aylin is Senior Clinical Lecturer in the Division of Epidemiology, Public Health and Primary Care, and Assistant Director of the Dr Foster Unit, at Imperial College London.

Paul Barach is Professor at the Colleges of Medicine and Public Health, at the University of South Florida. He has written extensively on patient safety and event reporting.

Stephen Bolsin, Melbourne University academic and anaesthetist, exposed the Bristol Royal Infirmary paediatric cardiac surgeons' poor performance and is developing new technologies to enhance clinical performance monitoring and incident reporting.

Michael D. Cantor is a geriatrician and attorney whose scholarly work focuses on ethics, ageing and technology. He is an Assistant Professor of Medicine at Harvard Medical School.

Steve Clarke is Senior Research Fellow in the Centre for Applied Philosophy and Public Ethics, Charles Sturt University, and Research Fellow in the Program on the Ethics of the New Biosciences, James Martin 21st Century School, University of Oxford.

Tony Eyers is a colo-rectal surgeon, and Chair of the clinical ethics advisory committee, at the Royal Prince Alfred Hospital, Sydney.

Ian Freckelton is a barrister in Melbourne, Australia. He is also Professor, Law Faculty, University of Sydney, and Honorary Professor of Law, Psychological Medicine and Forensic Medicine at Monash University.

Liadain Freestone is a specialist anaesthetist at the Royal Hobart Hospital, Tasmania, Australia.

Joseph Ibrahim is a practising consultant physician and professor of geriatric medicine at Monash University. He also works at the State Coroner's Office and the Victorian Institute of Forensic Medicine investigating system failures associated with healthcare deaths.

Neil Levy is Senior Research Fellow in the Centre for Applied Philosophy and Public Ethics, University of Melbourne, and a Researcher at the Program on the Ethics of the New Biosciences, James Martin 21st Century School, University of Oxford.

David Macintosh is Associate Professor, Ethics and Professional Development, at the Medical School, James Cook University, North Queensland. He has a particular interest in trust and professional integrity.

Silvana Marasco is a cardiothoracic surgeon at The Alfred Hospital, Melbourne. She is Head of the Lung Transplant Surgery Service and has research interests in thoracic organ transplantation and bioethics.

Yujin Nagasawa is Lecturer in the Department of Philosophy at the University of Birmingham and Honorary Research Fellow at the Centre for Applied Philosophy and Public Ethics at the Australian National University.

David Neil is a lecturer in philosophy at the University of Wollongong, NSW, Australia.

Justin Oakley is Director of Monash University Centre for Human Bioethics. His books include *Virtue Ethics and Professional Roles* (with Dean Cocking)(Cambridge, 2001), and *Morality and the Emotions* (Routledge, 1993).

Michael Parker is Professor of Bioethics at the University of Oxford and Director of the Ethox Centre. His research interests include multidisciplinarity in bioethics, ethics in clinical genetics, and international genomics.

Tom Sorell is John Ferguson Professor of Global Ethics in the Department of Philosophy at the University of Birmingham. He has published widely in moral theory and applied ethics.

Merle Spriggs is a Bioethicist at the Murdoch Childrens Research Institute, Melbourne, Australia. She is author of *Autonomy and patients' decisions* (Lexington Books, 2005).

Adrian J. Walsh is a Senior Lecturer at the University of New England and a Research Associate with the Centre for Applied Philosophy and Public Ethics. His research is in political philosophy with a particular interest in debates about markets and commodification.

Merrilyn Walton is Associate Professor of Medical Education at the University of Sydney. She was the founding Commissioner for the NSW Health Care Complaints Commission (1993–2000). She teaches students and clinicians about ethical practice and patient safety.

Rachel M. Werner is a general interest and health economist at the University of Pennsylvania. She is also an investigator at the Center for Health Equity Research and Promotion at the Philadelphia Veterans Affairs Medical Center.

Acknowledgements

A proper assessment of the issues raised in this volume requires drawing on expertise in philosophy and bioethics, along with expert knowledge of factors influencing surgical performance, clinical practice, the measurement and reporting of healthcare outcomes, relevant studies in healthcare quality and safety, professional regulation, and practitioner and consumer views on report cards. Accordingly, we have gathered contributions from philosophers and bioethicists, along with surgeons and other health professionals, epidemiologists, regulators and lawyers.

This collection had its origins in a workshop, organized by the editors, entitled 'Publicizing performance data on individual surgeons: the ethical issues'. The workshop was held at the University of Melbourne in November 2004. A report on the workshop appears in the *Academy of the Social Sciences in Australia's* on-line journal *Dialogue* (Clarke and Oakley, 2005). The chapters contained in this volume authored by Silvana Marasco and Joe Ibrahim, Tony Eyers, Yujin Nagasawa, Justin Oakley, Stephe Bolsin and Liadain Freestone, Steve Clarke, Adrian Walsh, Neil Levy, Merrilyn Walton and David Macintosh are all descendants of papers first presented at this workshop. Also present at the workshop, and heavily involved in discussions, were David Neil, Merle Spriggs, Ian Freckelton and Mike Parker, who have contributed chapters. Funding for the initial workshop from which this book developed was generously provided by the Academy of the Social Sciences in Australia and by the Centre for Applied Philosophy and Public Ethics. Thanks to all who participated in the workshop and to Richelle Maclean, Seumas Miller and Mark Pinoli for their help and encouragement. The workshop arose from a 3-year research project funded by National Health and Medical Research Council project grant # 236877, led by Oakley and Clarke, entitled *An ethical analysis of the disclosure of surgeons' performance data to patients within the informed consent process.*

To produce a balanced volume that better reflects the international nature of research on healthcare performance assessment, particularly in relation to issues of accountability, we invited contributions by Tom Sorell, Paul Aylin, Paul Barach and Michael Cantor. Also reproduced here, and the subject of much discussion in this volume, is 'Informed consent and surgeons' perform-ance', by the editors of this volume, Steve Clarke and Justin Oakley, *The Journal of Medicine and Philosophy*, **29**(1) (2005), pp. 11–35. Copyright © *The Journal of Medicine and Philosophy*, Inc., reprinted with permission. Thanks to the editors of this journal for permitting reproduction of this article. The contri-bution by Rachel Werner and David Asch is a slightly revised version of a recent article, 'The unintended consequences of publicly reporting quality information', which first appeared in the *Journal of the American Medical Association*, **293**(10) (2005), pp. 1239–1244. Copyright © 2005, American Medical Association. All rights reserved. Thanks to the editors of this journal for permission to reproduce this article.

All the chapters in the collection, with the exception of the two that were previously published as journal articles, have been anonymously refereed. We wish to thank Richard Barling, who was Executive Director, Science, Technology and Medicine at Cambridge University Press, for his expert guidance, and several anonymous readers for the Press, for their excellent suggestions. We are grateful to Rachael Lazenby and Jeanette Alfoldi for their help with coordi-nating proofreading and their work on the production side of things, and to Mary Sanders, for her diligent copy-editing. Thanks also to Steve Matthews, Steven Coleman, Jeanette Kennett, Ian Olver, David Benatar, Andrew Alexandra, Lewis Wall, Don Ross, Graeme Maclean, Robert Young, Tom Campbell, Daniel Star and Steven Tudor for their assistance in producing this volume. Justin also wishes to acknowledge Toni Hoffman, whistleblower at Bundaberg Base Hospital and Monash Master of Bioethics graduate, for her inspirational efforts, and for her insight into the difficulties that may be encoun-tered in publicizing problems with surgeon performance. Justin would like to give special thanks to his partner Kathryn Bailey, and son, Jordan Oakley, for their support and encouragement with this book.

Steve Clarke
Justin Oakley

Reference

Clarke, S. and Oakley, J. (2005). Publicising performance data on individual surgeons: the ethical issues. *Dialogue (Journal of the Academy of the Social Sciences in Australia)*, http://www.assa.edu.au/publications/dial.asp, **24**, 62–67.

Introduction: Accountability, informed consent and clinician performance information

Justin Oakley

Monash University Centre for Human Bioethics, Australia

Steve Clarke

Centre for Applied Philosophy and Public Ethics, Charles Sturt University and Program on the Ethics of the New Biosciences, James Martin 21st Century School, University of Oxford, UK

Every few years a rogue doctor comes to prominence in the international media. Some, like James Wisheart, the senior paediatric cardiac surgeon at the centre of the Bristol Royal Infirmary Scandal are deemed to be plainly incompetent to perform the operations that they have been undertaking.[1] Others, like Jayant Patel, the surgeon at the centre of the recent scandal at the Bundaberg Base Hospital in Queensland, Australia, appear from the evidence to combine incompetence to perform operations undertaken with a willingness to place their patients in situations of unnecessary risk.[2] The focus of the media on such sensational cases can obscure the fact that there are many less newsworthy, but nevertheless incompetent, physicians practising.[3] According to Atul Gawande, science and technology writer for the *New Yorker*:

In medicine, we all come to know such physicians: the illustrious cardiologist who has slowly gone senile and won't retire; the long-respected obstetrician with a drinking habit; the surgeon who has somehow lost his touch. (2002, p. 89)

When people are faced with the prospect of having to undergo surgery, they invariably like to be reassured that they will receive a high standard of care. There are many variables that contribute to the determination of the standards of care in a surgical operation. One of them is surgeons' performance ability. Surgeons vary considerably in their ability to conduct particular operations. Some are outstanding performers, some are adequate performers and some are inadequate. The performance of surgeons and other medical professionals has become the focus of heightened public scrutiny in recent years. While the work of professionals in healthcare and other areas has long been monitored through peer review, highly systematic measures of performance are now being developed, and there is a growing international trend towards the public release of performance information. Healthcare is in the vanguard of this movement, with the

Informed Consent and Clinician Accountability: The Ethics of Report Cards on Surgeon Performance, Steve Clarke and Justin Oakley (eds.). Published by Cambridge University Press. © Cambridge University Press 2007.

publication in many countries of aggregated information about outcomes in different hospitals for a variety of medical procedures.

There is also an emerging trend towards publishing information about the performance of individual clinicians. This modern trend can be traced back to 1991, when New York State published comparative performance data showing individual cardiac surgeons' mortality rates for coronary artery bypass graft operations. A few other US states, including Pennsylvania and New Jersey, subsequently published similar information about the performance of cardiac surgeons. After lengthy research, the UK Healthcare Commission launched a publicly accessible website in 2006 showing coronary artery bypass graft survival rates for many individual cardiac surgeons in Great Britain, as well as survival rates for aortic valve replacement surgery conducted by particular surgeons. The Commission has described this initiative as ushering in a new era of transparency, and as a step towards publishing similar information on other clinicians and surgical specialties in the future (Healthcare Commission, 2006).

Moves to publish individual surgeon performance information, presented in ways intended to be useful for patients, have been made largely in response to demands by regulators and the public for greater openness and accountability in healthcare. The public reporting of such information has the potential to enable healthcare regulators and the community to better determine the effectiveness of healthcare funding, and can help to protect patients from avoidable medical and surgical errors. The trend towards publishing clinician performance information has been catalysed by a range of factors, including the rise of the evidence-based medicine movement, which originated in Britain in the 1960s (Parker, this volume), the availability of more sophisticated information technology, the increasing importance given to clinical governance and the development of hospital 'open disclosure' policies (Barach and Cantor, this volume).

This collection brings together chapters that examine ethical and social issues concerning the reporting of surgeon performance information. Several of the chapters consider issues of accountability in medicine. Others examine the relation between the publication of surgeon performance information and the doctrine of informed consent. Others look at ethical and social issues raised by the process of reporting surgeon performance information. Public reporting of surgeon performance information is fast becoming an international phenomenon. But there has been a striking lack of sustained analysis and discussion of the *ethical* implications of this phenomenon. The present collection is intended to help redress this imbalance by providing valuable new perspectives on the ethics of reporting surgeon performance information. The richness and complexity of ethical thinking that has been brought to bear on the ethics of reporting surgeon performance information by our contributors are evident in the chapters contained in this collection.

Ethical arguments for reporting clinician performance information

There is a burgeoning literature in medicine and related fields on healthcare quality and safety, clinical governance and audit, adverse event reporting and evidence-based practice.[4] The public release of individual surgeon performance information – instances of which are commonly known as 'surgeon report cards' – is now being discussed and debated by surgeons, professional associations, health administrators, patient support groups and policy makers in a number of countries.[5] A host of complex and interesting ethical questions are raised by the public reporting of healthcare performance information, and particularly, information about individual clinician performance.

Broadly speaking, the publication of performance information about individual surgeons can be supported on three different ethical grounds. First, public reporting of such information enables patients to make better-informed decisions about surgery, and so providing patients with these details can be a way of respecting or enhancing their autonomy, a widely accepted ethical demand in medicine (Beauchamp and Childress, 2001). Second, publishing such information helps fulfil surgeons' professional obligations to be accountable to the community, by giving the community the means to determine whether surgeons are providing services to the requisite standard, under which the community has typically agreed to grant them a monopoly of expertise. And third, the public release of clinician performance information has the potential to improve the overall quality and safety of surgical care, as public scrutiny provides surgeons with further incentives to improve their performance, and makes it more difficult for substandard individual surgical performance to be concealed within the overall results of a surgical unit. This last ethical argument about quality and safety is sometimes supplemented by an economic argument for the conclusion that the overall quality of surgical care will increase, as better-informed consumers seek out better-performing surgeons and avoid surgeons whose performance is relatively poor. It is important to assess the strength of all three arguments along with other rationales for publishing performance information on individual surgeons. Different rationales may have different implications for what sort of information is to be collected and published, what format the information is to be presented in and what uses it is intended to have.

Autonomy-based arguments, for the conclusion that surgeon performance information should be published to help patients make more informed decisions, seem naturally to support providing patients with access to relatively fine-grained information about significant surgical outcomes – such as each surgeon's mortality and/or survival rates for a particular procedure. This is because it seems that such information can help patients gain a clearer understanding of the risks involved in undergoing that procedure with a given surgeon (however, see Clarke, this volume). Providing these sorts of details can also assist patients to make better-informed choices between available surgeons, as well as to make better choices between particular forms of surgery and available non-surgical alternatives.[6]

Autonomy-based arguments for public reporting can be developed through the familiar notion of informed consent. According to the standard account of informed consent, the information patients must be provided with to enable effective informed consent includes information about the significant risks associated with the procedure, along with information that the patient regards as material or relevant to their decision. The risks involved in undergoing a surgical procedure will vary, according to which surgeon performs that procedure. So, providing patients with information about the performance abilities of individual surgeons should be understood as an essential part of the informed consent process (Clarke and Oakley, this volume).

Given the autonomy-based rationale for publishing surgeon performance information, developed through the notion of informed consent, it is particularly important that individual surgeon data are presented accurately and in ways that make such data readily comprehensible by patients. Some patients might regard performance information as relevant to a decision about which surgeon they prefer to carry out a procedure (where a choice of surgeon is available to them), whereas other patients might see this information as material to their decision about whether to have the procedure or to have a non-surgical alternative. In any case, providing this information to patients who value it is clearly part of enabling patients to provide what Faden and Beauchamp (1986, p. 299) call 'autonomous authorization' to the procedure, even in cases where the presence or absence of this information would not lead the patient to change their mind about surgery, or about which surgeon they prefer to undertake the procedure.[7]

The second argument for public reporting of surgeon performance data is based on the ethical obligation professionals have to the public, to be accountable for the standard of their work. It is widely accepted that surgeons have a general obligation to be accountable to the community. This obligation is sometimes claimed to be met by the collection of surgeon performance data for internal purposes and traditional peer review. However, the professional accountability argument emphasizes what is owed to the community in return for the monopoly of expertise on the provision of surgical procedures that the community allows the surgical profession to have. Those who become surgeons are selected from the rest of the community and are given extensive training to carry out procedures which others typically are not allowed to perform. On the professional accountability argument, this monopoly of expertise and service provision that surgeons are entrusted with creates a reciprocal obligation for surgeons to allow, and indeed to assist, the community to determine whether the services provided by surgeons are of the required standard. Public reporting is an indispensable means of meeting this obligation.

On the professional accountability argument for publishing clinician performance information, less fine-grained performance information may suffice for identifying clinicians whose performance is substandard. This argument might therefore support public reporting of clinician performance in terms of broad categories – such as whether a clinician's performance is within or below acceptable standards – rather than in terms of a table comparing each surgeon's mortality rates. Providing patients with opportunities to discuss the surgical outcomes of practitioners whose performance is within acceptable standards could also become less important on this approach than it might be given the autonomy-based rationale.

The third argument for publishing surgeon performance information holds that public reporting improves the overall quality and safety of surgical care. This argument would naturally seem to support the collection and presentation of fine-grained information about clinician performance – such as the mortality and/or survival rates of each surgeon – to the extent that publishing such information, in a manner enabling meaningful comparisons between surgeons, helps provide surgeons with an additional incentive to improve their performance and to avoid poor performance. This rationale might also be thought to justify moves to rethink the distribution of surgeons, in ways that promote the overall improvement of surgical care.

The quality improvement argument for public reporting has a natural affinity with utilitarian approaches to ethics, where right actions or policies are those that maximize overall utility. Proponents of this form of argument can point to evidence from long-standing public reporting schemes, such as that in New York State, that the publication of individual surgeon performance information leads to a long-term increase in the overall quality of surgical care provided to the community (Peterson et al., 1998; Chassin, 2002; Marshall and Brook, 2002; Hannan et al., 2003). While there is evidence to support this contention, the mechanisms through which public reporting may improve clinician performance have yet to be determined. In New York State, some surgeons with below-average performance improved their outcomes after the advent of public reporting, and several surgeons with consistently poor performance had their operating privileges restricted or left the profession altogether.[8]

Whether surgeon performance information is to be published to enable more informed patient decisions, to meet clinicians' professional accountability obligations, to help drive quality improvement by healthcare providers or for some combination of these reasons, bears on how the success or otherwise of publishing such information is to be understood and assessed. Empirical research into the extent to which patients make use of such information, and of the ways that they use it, is crucial to determining the success of public reporting, on both the autonomy-based rationale and the quality improvement argument. However, such studies might be less relevant for the professional accountability rationale, which can be expected to lead to greater emphasis on research into how regulators and healthcare administrators respond to published information on individual clinician performance. Nevertheless, policy makers in this area will typically be guided by more than one of the three goals we have described.

The types of ethical rationale given for public reporting also bear on the relevance or otherwise of various objections to the publication of such information. For instance, the worry that surgeons protect their report cards from negative outcomes by avoiding high-risk patients is directly relevant to evaluating the utilitarian quality improvement rationale for public reporting, as this worry claims that report cards result in worse outcomes for many patients. However, this concern might be less important on an autonomy-based rationale for public reporting, where better-informed patient decision-making is aimed for, quite apart from any resultant improvement in overall surgical care. Should this concern turn out to be well founded, then utilitarian and autonomy-based arguments may give conflicting directives about whether surgeon-specific performance information ought to be published. In that case, reaching an overall assessment of this question will require determination of the plausibility and relative importance of these approaches, in general. There are analogous debates about the principles of autonomy and beneficence in medical ethics, whose directives will sometimes, but not always, converge and so resolving certain ethical problems in patient care may require settling the proper role and relative strength of these considerations.

Many regard disclosures of performance information on cardiac surgeons as the first step towards providing the public with performance information on other types of surgeons, such as orthopaedic and vascular surgeons, and on other medical professionals, such as obstetricians and cardiologists. Public reporting of individual cardiac surgeon performance information is also widely seen as a test case for professionals in fields other than healthcare, such as lawyers and teachers, and so the issues addressed here also have relevance for many professionals outside medicine. If the publicizing of performance information on individual cardiac surgeons is perceived as being a success, then pressure may soon be brought to bear on lawyers, nurses, accountants and members of many other professions to make individual performance information available to the public.

Historical background to surgical outcomes reporting

While the monitoring of surgical outcomes is a topic that has attracted much recent attention, it is also a topic with a rich history. The first person to systematically collect and report data on surgical outcomes is generally agreed to be Florence Nightingale, who is better known as a pioneer of nursing. Nightingale, who was Britain's chief military nurse during the Crimean war, instituted a series of reforms in the sanitary conditions of military hospitals and barracks that dramatically reduced mortality rates in the British military.[9] In 1855, 6 months after arriving in Scutari, the main British hospital in the Crimean war, Nightingale's efforts resulted in a reduction of military hospital mortality rates from 42.7 per cent to just 2.2 per cent (Cohen, 1984, p. 101). As part of her programme of reform of military hospitals in the field and at home, Nightingale employed 'coxcomb' diagrams[10] and tables of comparative data to record and publicize mortality rates as well as other outcome measures. Following the success of these reforms, Nightingale started an ambitious campaign for the collection of uniform hospital and surgical statistics in civil hospitals. As a result of her efforts, comparative statistics for hospitals in London and for some British provincial hospitals for the years 1861–1865 were collected and published in the *Journal of the Statistical Society of London* (Spiegelhalter, 1999, p. 49).

Whereas Nightingale initiated what might be termed an 'epidemiological' approach to surgical audit, the US physician Ernest Avery Codman initiated a 'clinical' approach to audit (Spiegelhalter, 1999, p. 45). From 1900 onwards, Codman promoted the 'end-result idea' (Kaska and Weinstein, 1998). This is:

The common-sense notion that every hospital should follow every patient it treats, long enough to determine whether or not the treatment has been successful, and then to inquire 'if not, why not?' with a view to preventing similar failures in the future. (Codman, 1934, pp. v–xl)

Although this idea seems commonsensical today, at the beginning of the twentieth century it was highly controversial, and Codman drew attention to its controversial implications by resigning from the Massachusetts General Hospital in protest at the seniority system of promotion, which he held to be incompatible with the end-result idea (Kaska and Weinstein, 1998).

In 1911 Codman founded the private Codman Hospital to develop and promote the end-result idea, bypassing the Massachusetts medical system (Kaska and Weinstein, 1998). Unlike Nightingale, who preferred to work behind the scenes, Codman courted controversy. In 1915 he unveiled an 8-foot high cartoon at a public meeting, satirizing the Boston medical establishment as using unproven techniques to acquire golden eggs (large fees) from residents of the Back Bay area in Boston, who are depicted as an ostrich with its head in the sand, ignorant of the quality of available physicians and the efficacy of their techniques. Codman was subsequently sacked as a Harvard instructor and in 1918 his hospital closed (Spiegelhalter, 1999, p. 53). Today, Codman's ideas find a more receptive audience and his reputation has been much restored. Since 1997 the US Joint Commission on Accreditation of Health Care Organizations (2006) has awarded annual Ernest Amory Codman Awards for '. . . achievement by organizations and individuals in the use of process and outcomes measures to improve organization performance and quality of care'.

Modern developments

The efforts made by Nightingale and Codman, in collecting and publicizing healthcare performance information, were exceptional in a long era in which performance information was not systematically collected or disseminated. It is only in the last 15 years that we have seen the emergence of a new trend in which performance information is increasingly collected and reported to the public (particularly in the United States and the United Kingdom). In the opinion of Marshall *et al.* (2003), it is inevitable that this trend will continue.

In the United States there is a plethora of performance information that has recently been made available, produced by state governments, employers, consumer advocacy groups, the media and private enterprise. Perhaps the most characteristic feature of contemporary performance measurement in the United States is its diversity. Information is now available about the comparative performance of hospitals, health insurance plans and individual physicians (Marshall *et al.*, 2003). Examples include *Healthscope*, a service provided by the Pacific Business Group on Health, a consortium of Californian employers who aim to improve the quality of health care for their employees and Californian residents in general (www.healthscope.org), and *Healthgrades*, a private company that sells comparative information on hospitals (www.healthgrades.com). Perhaps, however, the best known and most widely discussed initiative in American performance measurement is the New York State Department of Health (2005a) 'report cards' on coronary artery bypass graft operations. These reports, which have been issued since 1991, compare the risk-adjusted mortality rates of individual surgeons in New York State who conduct this form of heart surgery.

Cardiac surgeons' mortality rates for coronary artery graft surgery (CABG) have been at the forefront of individual clinician performance reporting, in part because this operation is one of the most commonly performed operative procedures in the Western world today (Marasco and Ibrahim, this volume). Extensive clinical databases have been created that monitor patient outcomes for CABG in different hospitals. These databases concentrated on mortality rates, because mortality is an outcome that can be accurately defined and verified, which helps with making reliable comparisons between different healthcare providers.[11] These clinical databases provided the foundation for the development of more sophisticated databases for the monitoring and public reporting of individual cardiac surgeons' outcomes for this procedure.

There have also been developments in public reporting of healthcare outcomes in Canada. For example, a comprehensive report showing hospital-specific outcomes for various cardiac procedures (including CABG surgery) in Ontario was published in 1999 by the Institute for Clinical Evaluative Sciences, Toronto,[12] and some Canadian hospitals have websites reporting their outcomes for various procedures. These initiatives are aimed primarily at improving the accountability of Canada's national health system by making the use of public funds more transparent, and so less emphasis is placed by these reports on facilitating patient choice between different hospitals. Nevertheless, there is evidence that some healthcare providers have responded to public reporting of hospital outcomes by developing various quality improvement activities (Tu and Cameron, 2003; Morris and Zelmer, 2005).

In the United Kingdom, performance measurement has been developed in a much more centralized and coordinated way than in the United States. Unlike the *laissez-faire* United States experience, major developments in performance measurement in Britain have resulted mostly from shifts in government policy.[13] Smith (2005) identifies three phases in the recent history of healthcare performance measurement in the United Kingdom, the 'command-and-control era', the 'market era' and the 'regulatory era'. In the command-and-control era of the 1980s, the modest amount of performance information collected was gathered for the purposes of enabling decision-making in a centralized National Health Service (NHS). In the early 1990s, the prevailing government ideology of centralized command was replaced by one of attempting to emulate the private sector. Performance indicators were developed that were intended to further the functioning of an ersatz market, in which competition between health authorities was engendered in order to enable market mechanisms to function so as to improve the quality and efficiency of health services.

Following the election of the Blair Labour Government in 1997, a new emphasis on establishing formal mechanisms to ensure the accountability of health authorities brought performance measurement to centre stage in healthcare policy. Currently, every NHS organization is rated on a scale between zero and three stars on the basis of a number of performance measures (Smith, 2005, p. 216). A huge impetus for this turn to accountability in medicine was provided by the paediatric cardiac surgery scandal at Bristol Royal Infirmary from the late 1980s to the mid-1990s, and the subsequent government Inquiry chaired by Sir Ian Kennedy.[14] During this period, two paediatric cardiac surgeons at Bristol Royal Infirmary had particularly high mortality rates for certain surgical procedures carried out on infants with congenital heart defects, with the mortality rates for these surgeons at one stage being five to six times the UK average for those procedures. These problems were not widely known (and the children's parents were unaware of them), until anaesthetist Dr Stephen Bolsin, who had been collecting outcome data on procedures performed by these surgeons, presented these data to hospital management. However, faced with a lack of intervention by the hospital Chief Executive, Dr Bolsin took his concerns to the Department of Health, and then to the UK General Medical Council (GMC), who initiated an Inquiry. The GMC inquiry found the surgeons guilty of serious professional misconduct, and one of them was consequently deregistered (see Bolsin, 1998; Bolsin and Freestone, this volume). Sir Ian Kennedy's 2001 Report from the subsequent government inquiry located the source of the Bristol tragedy in the insular and conformist 'club culture' of the NHS and argued for a sea change in the culture of medicine in the United Kingdom (Neil *et al.*, 2004, p. 266).

Although the main trend in British performance measurement has been the development of performance indicators at the institutional level, there have been some recent initiatives in the dissemination of individual level performance measurement. The Bristol Inquiry did not specifically recommend the publication of surgeon-specific performance information, but this Inquiry undoubtedly accelerated moves to make such information available to patients (see Smith, 1998). In January 2002 the then Secretary of Health, Alan Milburn, announced an agreement with the Society of Cardiothoracic Surgeons (SCTS) to publish mortality rates for all British cardiothoracic surgeons. He also indicated that more information regarding individual consultant outcomes would be made available over time (Neil *et al.*, 2004, p. 266). In March 2005, *The Guardian* used Freedom of Information legislation to obtain surgeon-specific data on CABG mortality rates (not all of which were risk adjusted) for many UK cardiac surgeons, which the newspaper published during that month. In 2006 we saw the launch of the UK Healthcare Commission website (which they jointly developed with the SCTS) showing surgeon-specific survival rates for CABG and aortic valve replacements, for UK cardiac surgeons. The Commission envisages broadening this initiative to other surgical specialties in the future. Also, the NHS has announced an internal reporting system to identify surgeons who spend too long on certain procedures,[15] and the UK Royal College of General Practitioners is proposing to introduce a scheme whereby clinics are rated by an expert panel on a three-star scale, according to the level of service they provide for patients, and clinics will be encouraged to publicize their ratings.[16]

So far, in Australia, there have been only tentative steps in the development of clinician performance measurement and reporting. In 2003, the Victorian Department of Human Services began to publish annual reports on public hospital cardiac units (in which unit-level data are de-identified) (Reid *et al.*, 2005). In Western Australia a state-wide audit of surgical mortality has been established (based on a modified version of an established Scottish model) (Reid *et al.*, 2005). Surgeon-specific mortality rates are to be published, but individual surgeons will not be identified. Participation in this audit is voluntary, but high (96%). The Royal Australasian College of Surgeons has endorsed the Western Australian audit as a model for future surgical mortality audit in Australia and New Zealand (Thompson *et al.*, 2005), and this model has now been adopted in South Australia, Tasmania, Queensland and New South Wales. Also, the Australian Commission for Safety and Quality in Health Care is developing a National Cardiac Procedures Register, to record de-identified, risk-adjusted information on the outcomes of a number of procedures, including coronary artery bypass graft surgery (Neil *et al.*, 2004, p. 267). And, a report by the Australian Government's Regulation Taskforce has recently recommended that the government allow public reporting of hospital-specific outcome data for a variety of treatments (Banks et al., 2006).

There have been calls to publish surgeon-specific performance data in response to the recent scandal involving surgeon Dr Jayant Patel – mentioned earlier – at Queensland's Bundaberg Base Hospital, between 2003 and 2005.[17] Dr Patel had very high mortality and complication rates for many surgical procedures during this period, and the subsequent Queensland Government Inquiry into his activities has recommended that Dr Patel's conduct be investigated by the police in relation to several offences, including manslaughter (Davies, 2005, p. 191). The associated Forster Review into administrative, management and performance systems at the Queensland Health Department recommended that quality reports on surgical and other outcomes in Queensland hospitals be published annually (Forster, 2005, p. 338), and Queensland Health is establishing a process for the development and regular publication of such reports. This process is being overseen by the Health Public Reporting Advisory Panel, an independent committee set up in February 2006 by the Queensland Minister for Health, and this committee is also investigating how such reports might best be presented to the public (Scott and Ward, 2006).

These public reporting initiatives in cardiac surgery have prompted moves to publish performance information on other surgeons. For example, vascular surgeons[18] and colo-rectal surgeons[19] in the UK are investigating the publication of the surgeon-specific performance data that is currently collected. Clinician-specific performance information is now being published in non-surgical specialties. The New York State Department of Health (2005b) has been publishing individual cardiologists' risk-adjusted mortality rates for angioplasty since 2001, and the UK Association of Cardiothoracic Anaesthetists are developing a surgical outcomes database suitable for producing performance information on individual anaesthetists (Marasco et al., 2005, p. 1001). Australian and New Zealand obstetricians have also discussed the feasibility and desirability of collecting and publishing performance information on individual obstetricians.[20] Many of the above groups have developed databases monitoring patient outcomes, not always clinician specific, but there are moves towards the latter. Indeed, some practitioner performance information is starting to appear in professions other than healthcare. For example, disciplinary findings against individual lawyers are published in NSW[21] and in Florida.[22]

Further issues in reporting surgeon performance information

While many regard informed patient decision-making, accountability in healthcare, and quality improvement as worthy ideals, there is much debate about how these values might be justifiably promoted. And so, the reporting of performance information raises a cluster of interrelated issues. Most of these issues are discussed in the chapters of this volume. The issues to be introduced here are (1) what data to report, (2) considerations of justice, (3) public vs. institutional reporting, (4) level of information, (5) understanding of risk information, (6) defensive surgery, (7) trainee surgeons, (8) the doctor–patient relationship and (9) the public's use of performance information. This is by no means an exhaustive list of issues that are relevant to the implementation of performance measurement regimes. Issues not taken up here, but which are worthy of consideration, include whether or not reporting should be mandatory, what sorts of incentives should be provided to encourage better performance,[23] and whether or not professional organisations have a duty to encourage public reporting.

A primary issue is the question of (1) what data to report. In the case of cardiac operations such as the coronary artery bypass graft, there is usually a not insignificant chance of mortality, and, given that prospective patients are almost invariably concerned about mortality, this is a measure of performance that there are good grounds to report. There are other aspects of surgery that might seem less worthy of reporting, even if they are easily measured. For example, Clarke and Oakley (this volume) consider whether or not the average chest scar width after healing, following a coronary artery bypass graft, should be reported. Undoubtedly, some prospective patients would consider this information relevant to their decision to have surgery, or their choosing one surgeon over another, but many patients would not. Many other pieces of information that could be considered relevant to some patients' decision making might also be collected. Because coronary artery bypass grafts are a reasonably common form of surgery, sufficient comparative information about the performance of coronary artery bypass grafts can be collected to provide statistically significant information to patients. Other operations are less common. Should information be provided to patients regarding the performance of uncommon operations, where the inferences that can be drawn from such information can only be speculative?

One reason to think that the state should not always collect and provide performance information, wherever and whenever it is requested, is that we should be sensitive to (2) considerations of justice. It would be very costly to attempt to accommodate each and every request for information about the performance of a given class of physicians, and we have to consider whether or not the cost of collecting such information is justifiable, when available funds might be better spent seeking to achieve other ends. However, in a reasonably well-funded medical system, it may be justifiable to collect and provide at least some performance information.

It might be argued that concerns about accountability to the public can be addressed without the (3) *public* reporting of performance information. Performance information can be used internally to ensure accountability within hospitals, and within larger systems of medical administration such as the NHS in the United Kingdom. While this is a possibility, it is one which works best in circumstances where the public has a high degree of trust in such institutions. In situations such as that in which Britain has found itself following the Bristol Royal Infirmary scandal, and in which Australia has found itself following the recent scandal in surgery at Bundaberg Base Hospital, public confidence in medical governance is eroded, and it is not plausible to think that accountability may be ensured unless the mechanisms to ensure accountability are made transparent to the general public. In a recent study, Hibbard *et al.* (2005) provide evidence for the importance of public reporting of hospital performance information. Hibbard *et al.* (2005) argue that public reporting promotes better-informed consumer choice, that concern for institutional reputation is an effective stimulator of quality improvement, and that public reporting stimulates efforts to improve quality because of the existence of professional norms regarding standards of service provision and of effective governance.

A hotly contested issue, which is unlikely to be resolved in the near future, is that of the appropriate level of information to be collected and reported (4). Performance information may be collected at the state level, the district level, the hospital level, the unit level and the individual level. Undoubtedly, the most contentious issue here is whether or not performance information on individual clinicians should be made public. Those who oppose the publicizing of individual-level information such as Levy (this volume) are concerned that this may result in adverse health consequences for patients who may become less able to access the best-performing surgeons. A second concern is that such information is potentially misleading, as surgical outcomes are the result of teamwork, and the reporting of individual level-information could mislead patients into thinking that surgical outcomes are solely the result of the skill of a surgeon. Proponents of publishing individual level information argue that consumers are entitled to suitably fine-grained information, and that unit-level data can also be misleading in cases where a very poorly performing surgeon's performance data is 'washed out' by the performance data of other members of a unit. Acknowledging the extent to which surgical outcomes are a result of teamwork is important, however, surgeons are an especially important part of operating teams, so it seems that information about surgical performance is information that may be useful to prospective patients, even if it needs to be acknowledged that the performance of surgeons is modified by the ability of the teams that are available to them. One way in which the teamwork dimension of individual surgeon performance is implicitly acknowledged, in the New York State Department of Health (2005a, b) report cards, is by breaking down information about the performance of particular surgeons into information about their performance at different hospitals in which they may operate.

Another issue that has inspired much debate is the way in which performance information is to be presented (Walton, this volume). Opponents of the publicizing of performance information often argue that the public cannot be expected to understand complicated displays of comparative performance information (5), and may be liable to make bad decisions as a result of their misunderstandings. For example, patients may infer that, because one surgeon has a higher mortality rate for an operation than another surgeon, the former surgeon is therefore inferior to the latter, at least in respect of ability to conduct the operation in question. However, the former surgeon may have a higher mortality rate than the latter because he or she takes on riskier patients than the former. A solution to this problem is to provide risk-adjusted information. Whether or not performance information has been, or can be, properly risk-adjusted is a matter of debate. Matters are further complicated when we consider psychological evidence, which suggests that all of us are prone to a variety of interpretive errors when it comes to interpreting statistical information (Clarke, this volume). One way of addressing such worries, at least to some extent, is to provide less fine-grained information. The British 'three-star system' of rating NHS units (and the similar approach used to rate some surgeons between 2004 and 2006) on a scale of between zero and three stars is one example of a coarse-grained system of presenting comparative performance information.

Arguments about the efficacy of risk adjustment loom large in debates about what has come to be referred to as the 'defensive surgery objection' (6) (Oakley, this volume; Nagasawa, this volume). Proponents of this line of objection argue that publishing of surgeon performance information leads surgeons to avoid taking on risky patients. Opponents of the defensive surgery objection respond that, if risk-adjustment is properly undertaken and properly understood, then there is no reason to believe that defensive surgery will occur. Some proponents of the defensive surgery objection are sceptical about whether surgeon performance information can be risk-adjusted accurately. Undoubtedly, the publicizing of surgeon performance information could lead to the practice of defensive surgery, but whether it actually has done this is unclear (Oakley, this volume). And, nor does it seem that it will do this under all possible risk-adjustment regimes. We might imagine some circumstances in which surgeons were highly rewarded for taking on risky patients and in which surgeons might be tempted to practice the opposite of defensive surgery, i.e. 'offensive surgery'.

Another line of objection to public reporting of surgeon-specific performance information is that it may impact negatively on the training of new surgeons (Eyers, this volume) (7). The disclosure of performance information on trainees is problematic in several ways. Firstly, there may not be sufficient information on trainees, or indeed on newly qualified practitioners, to yield reliable data. Secondly, if patients are aware of the fact that trainees are often less able to perform certain operations than experienced surgeons, then it may be hard to find patients willing to be operated on by trainees. Thirdly, if prospective surgeons form the view that a report cards system is likely to disadvantage them, then they may be deterred from entering the profession, and the standard of available surgeons may drop in the long run. These lines of objection could be met, at least to some extent, by providing economic incentives to those who do agree to be operated on by trainee surgeons (Clarke and Oakley, this volume).

Another issue raised by performance measurement and reporting is the effect that it may have on the doctor–patient relationship (8). One question here is whether or not the trust of patients in their doctors is enhanced or diminished by the publishing of performance information (Macintosh, this volume). A related issue is whether or not doctors themselves should be expected to reveal performance information to patients. In standard conceptions of the informed consent process (e.g. Wear, 1998), it is a doctor's duty to disclose relevant information to patients before a decision to undergo surgery is made, and it is a doctor's duty to ensure that such information is contextualised in such a way that it is comprehensible. However, it may not be realistic to expect that a surgeon with poor performance indicators, or one who works in a unit or a hospital with poor performance indicators, will provide patients with a fair contextualization of such performance information. They may be motivated to attempt to provide spurious explanations for apparently poor performance statistics, instead of contextualizing these in an unbiased way. To the extent that we are worried about this possibility, we should consider ways of involving third parties in the informed consent process.

A final issue worth mentioning is the question of whether or not the public will make use of performance information (9). To date, available empirical evidence suggests that prospective patients do not often make use of performance information. Nevertheless, patients typically report that they are pleased that performance information is available (Walton, this volume). This may suggest that they value public reporting of performance information as a means of ensuring accountability, rather than as useful information when deciding whether or not to undergo a particular operation with a particular surgeon. It may be that, as the influence of the ethos of medical paternalism wanes and as patients become more used to making informed decisions about medical procedures, more patients will attempt to incorporate performance information into their decision-making procedures.

Further discussion of all the above issues will be found in the chapters contained in this collection. The collection is divided into three sections. Part I concentrates on issues of clinician accountability. It includes chapters by Michael Parker, Neil Levy, Tom Sorell, Merrilyn Walton, Paul Barach and Michael Cantor, and Stephen Bolsin and Liadain Freestone. Part II contains chapters considering the nature and moral significance of informed consent, in light of new demands for performance information on institutions and clinicians. It includes chapters by Steve Clarke and Justin Oakley, Merle Spriggs,

David Neil, David Macintosh, Steve Clarke, and Adrian Walsh. Part III comprises chapters focusing specifically on the disclosure of individual surgeon and hospital performance information. It contains contributions by Silvana Marasco and Joseph Ibrahim, Rachel Werner and David Asch, Paul Aylin, Justin Oakley, Yujin Nagasawa, Tony Eyers and Ian Freckelton.[24]

Notes

1. Mr Wisheart's mortality rate for paediatric atrioventricular canal surgery was recorded as being six times the UK average in an audit in 1993 (Bolsin, 1998, p. 370). He was struck off the medical register following an inquiry conducted by the UK General Medical Council Professional Conduct Committee (Bolsin, 1998, p. 372).
2. The Queensland Public Hospitals Commission of Inquiry (Davies, 2005) was prompted by allegations made regarding Dr Patel's conduct at the Bundaberg Base Hospital. It found that Dr Patel conducted surgical procedures that ' ... were beyond his competence, skill and expertise' and that 'As a result of negligence on the part of Dr Patel, 13 patients at the Base died and many others suffered adverse outcomes' (Davies, 2005, p. 190). A victim of a botched operation conducted by Patel, commenting on the reckless attitude of Patel towards his patients, described him as a sociopath who became a psychopath when he came to Australia (Sandall, 2005, p. 12).
3. According to Gawande, between three and five per cent of practising physicians are unfit to see patients (2002, p. 94).
4. For example, see: Corrigan et al. (2001); Epstein (1995); Schneider and Lieberman (2001); Kohn, Corrigan and Donaldson (2000); Leape and Berwick (2005); Mohammed et al. (2001); Sharpe and Faden (1998); Rubin and Zoloth (2000); Goodman (2002); Ashcroft and ter Meulen (2004).
5. For example, see Bridgewater et al. (2003); Hughes and Bearham (2005); Keogh et al. (2004); Chassin, Hannan and DeBuono (1996); Chassin (2002); Kennedy (2004); Marshall et al. (2000).
6. The goal of helping patients with such choices also provides a rationale for enabling patients to discuss surgeon performance information with a practitioner who is independent of the surgeon who may conduct a particular operation.
7. The autonomy-based rationale might appear to entail that there is no ethical case for publishing surgeon-specific performance information in countries with national health schemes like those of the UK, Canada, and Australia, where choice of surgeon is usually not available to patients lacking private health insurance. Alternatively, this rationale might be thought to support the provision of such performance information, but only to privately insured patients in those countries. However, the importance of patients autonomously authorizing a procedure to be performed on them indicates that there is still a plausible autonomy-based rationale for making surgeon-specific performance information available to patients in countries with national health schemes, whether or not those patients have private health insurance and choice of surgeon.
8. One clear way in which performance statistics can be improved is by increasing the volume of operations conducted. High volume hospitals have consistently demonstrated lower than average mortality rates for a variety of different surgical

procedures (Begg and Scardino, 2003). Patients improve their chances of surviving an operation by making sure that it is conducted at a hospital that conducts many such operations. They improve their chances of survival even further by choosing to be operated on by a surgeon who performs the operation in question frequently (Birkmeyer *et al.*, 2003). Hu *et al.* (2003) argue for a more extreme conclusion than Birkmeyer *et al.* (2003). Their study of radical prostatectomy outcomes suggests that, after we adjust for physician volume, hospital volume is not significantly associated with patient outcomes.

9. Hungarian physician Ignaz Semmelweis also used systematic data collection to reduce the mortality rate of infants from puerperal fever at the Vienna General Hospital in the late 1840s. Semmelweis's careful observations revealed a correlation between unhygienic practices like inadequate hand-washing and the transmission of puerperal fever. The more hygienic policies he instituted reduced the ward's mortality rate from 12 per cent to 2 per cent (see Nuland, 2003).

10. Also known as 'polar area diagrams', these are an early form of the now much more common pie chart.

11. There is some dispute about how and when to attribute the occurrence of death to an operation, as when a patient dies several months after the operation, and where there may be further medical complications. The mortality rates shown in the New York State cardiac surgeon report cards reflect deaths up to 30 days following CABG surgery.

12. See Naylor and Slaughter (1999). The 2nd edition of this report was published in May 2006 (see Tu, Pinfold, McColgan and Laupacis, 2006).

13. One notable private initiative in Britain is 'Dr Foster'. See www.drfoster.co.uk.

14. See Bristol Royal Infirmary Inquiry. Learning from Bristol: the report of the public inquiry into children's heart surgery at the Bristol Royal Infirmary 1984–1995. 2001. Command Paper: CM 5207. Available from: http://www.bristol-inquiry.org.uk/index.htm.

15. *The Sunday Times*, 2 July 2006.

16. *The Times*, 6 June 2006.

17. See Clarke, Oakley, Neil, Ibrahim (2005), and further discussion in Hughes and Mackay (2006).

18. See The Vascular Society of Great Britain and Ireland, National Vascular Database 2002, available at: http://www.vascularsociety.org.uk/NVD2002.pdf; and Fourth National Vascular Database Report 2004 (published February 2005). Available at: http://www.vascularsociety.org.uk/nvdr2004.pdf.

19. See Thompson (2004).

20. Discussions of the possibility of developing a report cards system for obstetricians took place, in the context of a general debate about the possibility of report cards systems being introduced in Australia, during the Royal Australian and New Zealand College of Obstetricians and Gynaecologists, Annual Congress, 2005, following a presentation on the use of individual surgeons' report cards in the US and the UK by one of the editors of this volume (Steve Clarke). See Konkes (2005).

21. See NSW Office of the Legal Services Commissioner, Disciplinary Register. http://www.lawlink.nsw.gov.au/olsc/nswdr.nsf/pages/index.

22. See The Florida Bar, Lawyer Regulation. http://www.floridabar.org/tfb/TFBLaw Reg.nsf/E0F40AF2C23904C785256709006A3713/12E6C80E88BA08FD85256B2F 006C9D15?OpenDocument.

23. The most commonly considered incentive is, unsurprisingly, a financial one. In the US there is currently much debate regarding the possible implementation of 'pay for performance' (or 'P4P') schemes. See, for example, Glastris (2005).
24. The editors wish to thank Tom Campbell, Steve Matthews and Daniel Star for their helpful comments on this Introduction.

References

Ashcroft, R. and ter Meulen, R. (2004). Ethics, philosophy and evidence-based medicine. *Journal of Medical Ethics*, **30**, 119.

Banks, G., Halstead, R., Humphry, R. and MacRae, A. (2006). Rethinking regulation, Australian Government, Canberra. Available at: http://www.regulationtaskforce. gov.au/finalreport/index.html.

Beauchamp, T. L. and Childress, J. F. (2001). *Principles of Biomedical Ethics*. New York: Oxford University Press.

Begg, C. B. and Scardino, P. T. (2003). Taking stock of volume-outcome studies. *Journal of Clinical Oncology*, **21**, 393–4.

Birkmeyer, J. D., Stukel, T. A., Siewers, A. E., Goodney, P. P., Wennberg, D. E. and Lucas, F. L. (2003). Surgeon volume and operative mortality in the United States. *New England Journal of Medicine*, **349**, 2117–27.

Bolsin, S. N. (1998). Professional misconduct: the Bristol case. *Medical Journal of Australia*, **169**, 369–72.

Bridgewater, B., Grayson, A. D., Jackson, M. *et al.* (2003). Surgeon specific mortality in adult cardiac surgery: comparison between crude and risk stratified data. *British Medical Journal*, **327**, 13–17.

Chassin, M. R. (2002). Achieving and sustaining improved quality: Lessons from New York State and cardiac surgery. *Health Affairs*, **21**, 40–51.

Chassin, M. R., Hannan, E. L. and DeBuono, B. A. (1996). Benefits and Hazards of Reporting Medical Outcomes Publicly. *New England Journal of Medicine*, **334**, 394–8.

Clarke, S., Oakley, J. G., Neil, D. A. and Ibrahim, J. E. (2005). Public reporting of individual surgeon performance. [Letter] *Medical Journal of Australia*, **183**, 543.

Codman, E. A. (1934). *The Shoulder: Rupture of the Supraspinatus Tendon and other Lesions in or about the Subacromial Bursa*. Boston: Todd.

Cohen, I. B. (1984). Florence Nightingale. *Scientific American*, **250**, 98–107.

Corrigan, J. M., Donaldson, M. S., Kohn, L. T., Maguire, S. K. and Pike, K. C. (2001). *Crossing the Quality Chasm: A New Health System for the 21st Century*. Washington: Institute of Medicine, National Academy of Sciences.

Davies, G. (2005). Queensland public hospitals Commission of Inquiry – report, Brisbane: Queensland State Government. Also at: www.qphci.qld.gov.au.

Epstein, A. (1995). Performance reports on quality – prototypes, problems and prospects. *New England Journal of Medicine*, **333**, 57–61.

Faden, R. R. and Beauchamp, T. L. (1986). *A History and Theory of Informed Consent*. New York: Oxford University Press.

Forster, P. (2005). Queensland health systems review – final report, Brisbane, Queensland State Government. Also at: http://www.health.qld.gov.au/health_sys_review/ final/default.asp.

Gawande, A. (2002). *Complications: A Surgeon's Notes on an Imperfect Science*. London: Profile Books.

Glastris, P. (2005). Pay for Performance Medicine, *Washington Monthly*, March 13: http://www.washingtonmonthly.com/archives/individual/2005_03/005834.php.

Goodman, K. W. (2002). *Ethics and Evidence-Based Medicine: Fallibility and Responsibility in Clinical Science*. Cambridge: Cambridge University Press.

Hannan, E. L., Vaughn Sarrazin, M. S., Doran, D. R. and Rosenthal, G. E. (2003). Provider profiling and quality improvement efforts in coronary artery bypass graft surgery: the effect on short-term mortality among Medicare beneficiaries. *Medical Care*, **41**, 1164–72.

Healthcare Commission (2006). Press Release, 'Patients now have access to rates of survival for health surgery for the first time', available at: www.healthcarecommission. org.uk (published 27 April 2006).

Hibbard, J. H., Stockard, J. and Tusler, M. (2005). Hospital performance reports: impact on quality, market share and reputation. *Health Affairs*, **24**, 1150–60.

Hu, J. C., Gold, K. F., Pashos, C. L., Mehta, S. S. and Litwin, M. S. (2003). Role of surgeon volume in radical prostatectomy outcomes. *Journal of Clinical Oncology*, **21**, 401–5.

Hughes, C. F. and Bearham, G. (2005). Surgeon-specific report cards. *Australian and New Zealand Journal of Surgery*, **75**, 927–8.

Hughes, C. F and Mackay, P. (2006). Sea change: public reporting and the safety and quality of the Australian health care system. *Medical Journal of Australia*, **184**, S44–7.

Joint Commission on Accreditation of Health Care Organizations (2006). Ernest Amory Codman Award: http://www.jointcommission.org/Codman/.

Kaska, S. C. and Weinstein, J. (1998). Ernest Avery Codman, 1869–1940: a pioneer of evidence-based medicine: the end result idea. *Spine*, **23**, 629–33.

Kennedy, I. (2004). Setting of clinical standards. *The Lancet*, **364**, 1399.

Keogh, B., Spiegelhalter, D., Bailey, A., Roxburgh, J., Magee, P. and Hilton, C. (2004). The legacy of Bristol: Public disclosure of individual surgeons' results. *British Medical Journal*, **329**, 450–4.

Kohn, L. T., Corrigan, J. M. and Donaldson, M. S. (2000). *To Err is Human: Building a Safer Health System*. Washington: Institute of Medicine, National Academy Press.

Konkes, C. (2005). Rating plan for doctors a bitter pill. *The Hobart Mercury*, April 13.

Leape, L. L. and Berwick, D. M. (2005). Five years after *To err is human*: What have we learned? *Journal of the American Medical Association*, **293**, 2384–90.

Marasco, S. F., Ibrahim, J. E. and Oakley, J. (2005). Public disclosure of surgeon specific report cards – current status of the debate. *Australian and New Zealand Journal of Surgery*, **75**, 1000–4.

Marshall, M. N., Shekelle, P. G., Brook, R. H. and Leatherman, S. (2000). *Dying to Know: Public Release of Information about Quality of Health Care*. Santa Monica CA: RAND Corporation/Nuffield Trust, 2000. Available at: www.rand.org/publications/MR/ MR1255/.

Marshall, M. N. and Brook, R. H. (2002). Public reporting of comparative information about quality of healthcare. *Medical Journal of Australia*, **176**, 205–6.

Marshall, M. N., Shekelle, P. G., Davies, H. T. O. and Smith, P. C. (2003). Public reporting on quality in the United States and the United Kingdom. *Health Affairs*, **23**, 134–48.

Mohammed, M., Cheng, K., Riyse, A. and Marshall, T. (2001). Bristol, Shipman, and clinical governance: Shewhart's forgotten lessons. *The Lancet*, **357**, 463–7.

Morris, K. and Zelmer, J. (2005). Public Reporting of Performance Measures in Health Care, Canadian Policy Research Networks, Health Care Accountability Papers no. 14, Ottawa: http://www.cprn.com/documents/34864_en.pdf.

Naylor, C. D. and Slaughter, P. (eds.) (1999). *Cardiovascular Health and Services in Ontario: An ICES Atlas*. Toronto: Institute for Clinical Evaluative Sciences.

Neil, D. A., Clarke, S. and Oakley, J. G. (2004). Public reporting of individual surgeon performance information: United Kingdom developments and Australian issues. *Medical Journal of Australia*, **181**, 266–8.

New York State Department of Health (2005a). *Adult Cardiac Surgery in New York State 2001–2003*: http://www.health.state.ny.us/nysdoh/heart/pdf/2001-2003_cabg.pdf.

New York State Department of Health (2005b). *Percutaneous Coronary Interventions (Angioplasty) in New York State, 2001–2003:* http://www.health.state.ny.us/nysdoh/heart/pdf/pci_2001-2003.pdf.

Nuland, S. B. (2003). *The Doctor's Plague: Germs, Childbed fever and the Strange Story of Ignac Semmelweis*. New York: Norton.

Peterson, E. D., De Long, E. R., Jollis, J. G., Muhlbaier, L. H. and Mark, D. B. (1998). The effects of New York's bypass surgery provider profiling on access to care and patient outcomes in the elderly. *Journal of the American College of Cardiology*, **32**, 993–9.

Reid, C. M., Davern, P., Birrell, S., Billah, B., Skillington, P. and Shardey, G. (2005). Cardiac surgery in Victorian public hospitals 2003–04: report to the public: http://www.health.vic.gov.au/specialtysurgery/downloads/cardiac-surgery-report04.pdf.

Rubin, S. B. and Zoloth, L. (2000). *Margin of Error: The Ethics of Mistakes in the Practice of Medicine*. Hagerstown: University Publishing Group.

Sandall, R. (2005). Doctor Death in Bundaberg. *Quadrant*, **422**(12), 11–20.

Schneider, E. C. and Lieberman, T. (2001). Publicly disclosed information about the quality of health care: response of the US public. *Quality Health Care*, **10**, 96–103.

Scott, I. A. and Ward, M. (2006). Public reporting of hospital outcomes based on administrative data: risks and opportunities. *Medical Journal of Australia*, **184**, 571–5.

Semmens, J. B., Aitken, R. J., Sanfilippo, F. M., Mukhtar, S. A., Haynes, N. S. and Mountain, J. A. (2005). The Western Australian audit of surgical mortality: advancing surgical accountability. *Medical Journal of Australia*, **183**, 504–8.

Sharpe, V. A. and Faden, A. I. (1998). *Medical Harm: Historical, Conceptual, and Ethical Dimensions of Iatrogenic Illness*. Cambridge: Cambridge University Press.

Smith, P. C. (2005). Performance measurement in health care: history, challenges and prospects. *Public Money and Management*, **25**, 213–20.

Smith, R. (1998). All changed, changed utterly. British medicine will be transformed by the Bristol case. *British Medical Journal*, **316**, 1917–18.

Spiegelhalter, D. J. (1999). Surgical audit: statistical lessons from Nightingale and Codman. *Journal of the Royal Statistical Society, Series A*, **162**, Part 1, 45–58.

Thompson, A., Stonebridge, P. A. and Spigelman, A. D. (2005). Surgical accountability: a framework for trust and change. *Medical Journal of Australia*, **183**, 500.

Thompson, M. R. (2004). ACPGBI – letter from the President. *ColoRectal Disease*, **6**, 295–6.

Tu, J. V. and Cameron, C. (2003). Impact of an acute myocardial infarction report card in Ontario, Canada. *International Journal for Quality in Health Care*, **15**, 131–7.

Tu, J. V., Pinfold, S. P., McColgan, P. and Laupacis, A. (eds.) (2006). Access to Health Services in Ontario: ICES Atlas, 2nd edn., Toronto: Institute for Clinical Evaluative Sciences. http://www.ices.on.ca/file/ICESAccess_atlas_2nd_ed_Prelim.pdf.

Wear, S. (1998). *Informed Consent: Patient Autonomy and Clinician Beneficence within Health Care*. Second edition, Washington: Georgetown University Press.

Part I

Accountability

Part introduction

Accountability

In the United Kingdom a key driver of reforms in healthcare has been the public perception that there has been a failure of regulatory mechanisms in healthcare. These concerns were particularly focused on the Bristol Royal Infirmary scandal. The 'Kennedy Report' from the subsequent national inquiry into this scandal concluded that the culture of medicine required systematic change. In particular, the Report recommended that the conformist 'club culture' of the British National Health Service be transformed into a 'patient-centred' culture in which the quality and safety of medical services becomes of paramount concern and the potential for substandard service to be provided and for attempts to hide evidence of substandard service is minimised (Bristol Royal Infirmary Inquiry, 2001). The broad thrust of the Kennedy Report was that this transformation is to be achieved by the use of mechanisms designed to ensure accountability. Although the Kennedy Report did not specifically recommend that surgeon-specific performance data be publicly released, it recommended (among other things) the publication of performance indicators that would enable evidence of underperformance to be identified early on, and would help improve healthcare safety and quality by discouraging underperformance in the medical system (Bristol Royal Infirmary Inquiry, 2001). The key recommendations of the Kennedy report were taken up enthusiastically by the Blair government, which has generally been in favour of establishing formal mechanisms to ensure accountability in the public sector (Smith, 2005).

The first three chapters in this initial section of this book can be understood as reactions to this new era of accountability. Our first chapter is by Michael Parker, who considers the connection between patient-centredness and the movement towards evidence-based medicine. He supports the provision of performance information, including performance information on individual surgeons to patients, but argues that there is a danger of becoming fixated on patient choice. He reminds us that a public medical system should be developed with due regard to considerations of justice and fairness. Neil Levy is also concerned with the just distribution of health resources. He worries that the publicizing of individual surgeons' performance information may lead to the exacerbation of injustices in the distribution of healthcare resources, and argues that we should have report cards on institutions but not on individual surgeons. Our next contributor, Tom Sorell, has a different reaction to the development of a patient-centred culture. In his view the Kennedy report is much too sanguine about the capacity of unified mechanisms of accountability to address problems in healthcare delivery. He distinguishes between safety and egalitarian ideals as goals of new accountability measures, and argues that accountability initiatives should place improving patient safety ahead of redressing power imbalances, where these goals conflict.

Merrilyn Walton identifies ways in which current 'report cards' on surgeons fail to enable genuine patient choice. She argues for systemic changes in the ways in which patients are enabled to participate more effectively in decision-making about their healthcare outcomes, which she sees as a means to enhancing patient trust in doctors and in hospitals. Paul Barach and Michael Cantor's chapter focuses on the detail of mechanisms of accountability. They consider the process of reporting adverse events in medicine, where the focus has sometimes been on faulty healthcare systems, rather than on the performance of individual clinicians. They discuss a variety of benefits and drawbacks for both doctor and patient that result from the disclosure of adverse events, and argue that disclosure can help to mitigate the damage caused by such events. Stephen Bolsin and Liadain Freestone also consider the process of monitoring performance in healthcare. They argue that mechanisms of performance monitoring should be extended to all health care workers. They further argue that developing a culture of transparency in healthcare must include creating a culture in which healthcare workers are trusted to regularly report 'local data'.

References

Bristol Royal Infirmary Inquiry (2001). Learning from Bristol: the report of the public inquiry into children's heart surgery at the Bristol Royal Infirmary 1984–1995. Command Paper: CM 5207. Available from: http://www.bristol-inquiry.org.uk/index.htm.

Smith, P. C. (2005). Performance measurement in health care: history, challenges and prospects. *Public Money and Management*, **25**, 213–20.

Clinician report cards and the limits of evidence-based patient choice

Michael Parker
University of Oxford, UK

Evidence-based patient choice

The concept of 'evidence-based patient choice' brings together two developments of ethical importance in contemporary medicine: evidence-based medicine and the growth of patient-centredness (Parker, 2001). The concept of evidence-based medicine, whilst problematic in many respects, encapsulates the belief that decision-making in medicine should be justified on the basis of good-quality evidence for the effectiveness of the intervention rather than on the basis of tradition, established models of practice, clinician preference and authority or other grounds. Patient-centred medicine too has arisen out of a concern with, and a critical response to, traditional medical practice and in particular to its over-emphasis on the authority of the health care professional. To some extent, this latter development has been driven by broader social changes outside medicine including a greater willingness to challenge the decisions of professionals including those of health professionals and to require such decisions to be both accountable and transparent. It is also related to relatively rapid developments in medical science and technology, which have created, along with social changes, an ever-increasing range of ethical questions with regard to which patient values vary significantly. Thirdly, and related to the other two, the move to patient centredness, and indeed to evidence-based medicine, has also been driven by increased media attention on developments in medical technology and by public and media discussion of scandals in medicine and in medical research. Advocates of patient-centred medicine argue that the best protection for patients from excessive paternalism is to be gained by emphasizing the central role of patients in decision-making about their clinical care. The concept of patient-centred medicine complements that of evidence-based medicine therefore, by requiring that healthcare decisions are not made on the basis of tradition or clinician preference but on the basis of the patient's own values.

Taken together, these two ideas which have a natural affinity, mark a significant shift in thinking about the relationship between health professionals and

Informed Consent and Clinician Accountability: The Ethics of Report Cards on Surgeon Performance. Steve Clarke and Justin Oakley (eds.). Published by Cambridge University Press. © Cambridge University Press 2007.

their patients (Hope, 1997, p. 1). Evidence-based patient choice requires that patients are informed about the various courses of action available to them and about the evidence for and against these options, and are supported in the making of choices on the basis of their own values and beliefs. An interesting aspect of this combination of movements is that it brings to the fore the importance in the doctor–patient relationship of the complementary roles of ethics and communication. The requirement that clinicians be both able and willing to justify their suggestions and recommendations, the requirement to support patients in their decision-making and the recognition that such decisions involve the making of value-judgements bring with them an implicit claim that the doctor–patient encounter should be deliberative (Emanuel and Emanuel, 1992). Taken seriously, evidence-based patient choice has the potential to enhance the power of patients and aid the development of an increasingly informed patient-centred healthcare (Elwyn and Edwards, 2001).

The widening circle of evidence

Until recently, the implications of the move to evidence-based patient choice had largely been conceptualized in terms of the combination of an emphasis on the importance of patients being at the centre of decision-making, with a requirement that, in the making of such decisions, patients be informed in ways that they can understand about the nature of the proposed intervention. This has been taken to mean that patients should be informed about the details of the diagnosis and prognosis and the likely prognosis if the condition is left untreated, options for treatment or management, including the option not to treat, the purpose and details of the treatment itself including common and serious side effects, the likely benefits of treatment and so on (General Medical Council, 2000).

Recently, however, driven to some extent at least in the United Kingdom by official reports such as that of the Bristol Inquiry (Bristol Royal Infirmary Inquiry, 2001), the circle of evidence considered to be potentially relevant to evidence-based decision-making has begun to widen to include evidence of other kinds, such as information about the overall quality of care provided by a particular institution and, more controversially, information about the specific skills, experience and training of individual health professionals, i.e. about the particular clinician available to carry out a proposed procedure. One manifestation of this has been the growing use of clinician report cards on the performance of individual surgeons, particularly in cardiac care (Neil, Clarke and Oakley, 2004). In the United States for example, data on the risk-adjusted mortality rates of individual cardiac surgeons has been available to the public in New York State and Pennsylvania for the past 15 years and in New Jersey for 10 years. In the United Kingdom, until recently, a more limited, star-based, form of information about the performance of cardiac surgeons using coronary artery bypass graft, as an index procedure, had been in place since 2004. This star-based system categorized surgeons into those who 'failed', 'met' or 'exceeded' the standards of the Society of Cardiothoracic Surgeons. In April 2006, however, the UK Healthcare Commission published surgeon-specific report cards listing the risk-adjusted survival rate, using coronary artery bypass graft as an index procedure, for each surgeon. This new system is currently voluntary (Healthcare Commission, 2006). In other countries too, initiatives of this kind are in place or are being considered.

The call for the widening of the circle of evidence to be provided to patients has been supported by many practitioners (Bolsin and Freestone, this volume) and bioethicists (Clarke and Oakley, 2004). Clarke and Oakley have argued that, as the risks associated with a procedure vary significantly depending upon which surgeon is carrying it out, such information ought to be made available to patients who are making decisions about whether, and where, to undergo surgery. Despite the fact that the risks associated with a procedure depend significantly upon the experience, training, and skills of the clinician performing it, patients are for the most part, with the notable exceptions described above, only provided with information about the generalized, population risk associated with procedures, based on average mortality and success rates across clinical and healthcare settings and not on the risks associated with actual procedure-practitioner combinations. This averaged risk information will, in virtually all cases, be a significant over-or underestimate of the likely success or failure of the procedure when carried out by particular practitioners and will therefore, Clarke and Oakley claim, distort rather than inform patient choices. If policy makers and health professionals are serious about patient choice and about the claim that such choice should be 'evidence-based', Clarke and Oakley argue, they should ensure that all relevant evidence is collected and made available to those at the centre of decision-making, i.e. patients themselves. Information about the skills, experience and success rates of the practitioner who would carry out the procedure is relevant in just this way and should therefore, they argue, be made available to patients.

Ethical justifications for the widening circle of evidence-based patient choice

The ethical justifications for widening the circle of evidence available to patients fall into three main categories. The first of these comprises arguments based, as we have seen above, on the importance of respect for patients' values and for their interest in making informed decisions about important events in their own lives, such as whether or not to undergo major surgery based on these values. This brings with it an obligation on health professionals to ensure that patients are provided with, and helped to understand, information material to the decision at hand (Clarke and Oakley, 2004). This means, it is argued, that such patients should not only be provided with information about the generalized risks associated with a treatment but also provided with specific information about the evidence regarding the risk of undergoing a particular treatment with a particular health professional in a particular institution. That is, they should be provided with accurate information, or as close to accurate as possible, about the risks that they will in fact face. As risks can vary significantly between practitioners, such information is highly relevant to the decision at hand and should be both collected and made available. This suggests that respect for patient choice brings with it a responsibility on the part of those who offer and provide healthcare to collect such information in a systematic fashion and to make it available in a form understandable and accessible to those who need to make such decisions. The decision about what information is material should moreover, it is argued, be made by those most likely to be affected by the decision at hand and not by healthcare institutions or doctors themselves. This implies a responsibility to provide a reasonably inclusive range of information.

The second category of ethical argument in favour of the widening circle of evidence comprises those suggesting that the collection and availability of information about the performance of health professionals will have the effect of improving performance, avoiding significant harms, and improving the care of patients. Such arguments will sometimes draw upon evidence such as that provided by the Bristol Report suggesting that the collection of performance data leads to better standards of practice, greater efficiency, improved safety and better patient care (Bristol Royal Infirmary Inquiry, 2001). These improvements will, it is argued, accrue because: surgeons will be better placed and motivated to monitor their own performance; healthcare institutions such as hospitals will be better able to monitor the performance of their employees where necessary intervening to improve standards by, for example, providing training; and because of the combined influences of greater competition between health providers and increasing patient pressure for improvements in care and access to better experienced health professionals. These arguments are different to those based on the importance of choice and might even on occasion conflict with them. Were it, for example, to turn out that collecting and using such statistics improved practice only when combined with limited patient choice, i.e. where the choices of individual patients were restricted in order to obtain a greater public benefit, e.g. through weighting access to the best surgeons to benefit the most vulnerable patients, this would imply a tension between arguments for the use of report cards based on choice and those based on the achievement of benefits.

The third category of ethical arguments in favour of report cards and hence of the widening circle of evidence, arises neither out of the importance of respect for patient choice nor out of concern to improve standards of care but rather out of commitments grounded in procedural considerations such as the importance of openness, transparency and democratic accountability in the management of public institutions. Whilst such arguments might in practice be closely allied to a belief that greater openness and accountability would enhance patient choice and lead to improved standards of care, they cannot be fully identified with them as these three sets of considerations may well on occasion all come into conflict. It might, hypothetically, for example, be possible for an institution to be both transparent and accountable in its decision-making and yet, for its decisions, whilst made on the basis of information collected on report cards, to lead to reduced rather than increased choice for individual patients. This might happen if, for example, as I suggested above, a policy was developed that ruled out certain choices to individuals on the grounds of *justice* or *fairness*, or on the basis of *need*. What is more, whilst such decisions might be made openly, transparently and accountably, they might hypothetically lead to an overall *reduction* in the standard of care or the provision of less than optimal care for similar reasons, e.g. a particular health care system might come to the conclusion that moral principles such as *fairness*, on the basis of the high-quality information about expertise and performance provided by report cards, are more important, within certain limits, than the total health benefit of an intervention. Arguments for report cards based on claims about the importance of openness, transparency and accountability are therefore different to those in the other two categories in important respects.

Whilst these three types of argument are different, they need not, in practice, come into conflict. Indeed, advocates of report cards argue that their introduction will enhance choice, improve practice, and increase accountability.

Main arguments against the use of report cards

A number of potential practical difficulties with the use of report cards have been identified (Marasco and Ibrahim, this volume). These difficulties have important moral implications. Perhaps the most important of these, particularly with regard to arguments based on the importance of report cards to the enhancement of informed patient choice, arises out of a concern with the possibility that the data collected and made available in the form of report cards might be misinterpreted by patients and or by their family practitioners, and have the potential for patient decision-making to be less rather than more evidence-based as a result. This might be because of the difficulties of making

proposal for something of this kind is the call for a combination of fair processes and a threshold guarantee.

Threshold guarantees

The three main arguments in favour of the introduction of report cards, i.e. that this will increase choice, improve standards of care and constitute fair process, are vulnerable to empirical and ethical challenge. In response to these challenges, some have argued in favour of what has come to be known as the 'threshold' approach to professional competence (Clarke and Oakley, 2004, p. 20). What is argued here is that, whilst people who need or wish to access a clinical service have a right to know that those who will treat them practise above a certain agreed threshold of expertise and competence, and that the allocation of surgeons to patients is fair, they have no right to be told any further details about the particular skills and expertise of individual practitioners (Davis, cited in Clarke and Oakley, 2004, p. 20). The merit of the threshold approach is that it acknowledges that, whilst the provision of individual information about practitioners might be problematic, patients do have a legitimate interest in information about the competence of those who treat them. In much the same way that a patient should know the risks, side effects and alternative treatments, etc., they should also be in a position to feel confident that such information relates to the provision of competent care and that they will, in fact, receive such care.

The advantages of this approach, and to some extent the UK's star-based system, which lay midway between the threshold approach and the use of full league tables, also has these benefits, which are that it guarantees patients access to competent care and provides them with sufficient information about these standards of care to enable them to make a decision about whether or not to proceed. Whilst they may well end up with a clinician practising at a very high level of competence, they can be confident that they will not be treated by someone who does not meet agreed standards. In the application of the threshold in practice a certain degree of fairness is imported and, whilst the threshold approach reduces the scope of patient choice to some extent, it does so against a background guarantee of competent care for all.

For those in favour of the use of report cards in patient decision-making, however, the threshold argument (particularly when the threshold is simply one of 'competence') pays inadequate attention to the importance of evidence-based patient choice. Clarke and Oakley, for example,

...find implausible the general suggestion that our rights to know details about the performance of individual professionals extend only as far as the information necessary to establish that they meet some threshold of basic competence. (Clarke and Oakley, 2004, p. 21)

When we choose a surgeon to carry out an operation on us, information about that surgeon's experience and skills is highly significant, they argue. Patients should not be denied such information, simply on the basis of a public interest in solidarity or as a result of an overriding concern with maximizing the overall standard of healthcare across the population.

One possible response to this criticism of the threshold approach would be to say that, to some extent, it simply begs the question. For it is what patients or potential patients can reasonably expect to know that is precisely the question under discussion. Do patients have the right to know the exact level of competence of the person who will be treating them or do they simply have the right to know that this practitioner is capable of practising above a professionally acceptable standard? If one accepts at least the possibility of the detrimental effects of a completely transparent and accessible system of surgeon report cards, particularly when this is combined with a free market in healthcare, then the decision about whether or not to introduce report cards cannot be answered without making a value judgement about the relative strengths of the principles of respect for informed patient choice and the importance of healthcare benefits, justice, equality and non-discrimination. It seems unlikely that anyone of these is going to trump the others in all cases. What the threshold approach brings out nicely, in conjunction with the above critiques of the use of report cards, is that, whilst all patients have an interest in the availability of health professionals practising to a high standard, and in being informed about the standard of treatment available in order to make an informed choice about whether to proceed, this need not imply either unlimited choice or unlimited information. A judgement may in some cases need to be made between competing moral principles and these are judgements that will, at least in part, have to be made at the level of public policy. Interestingly, Clarke and Oakley suggest that they would be less concerned about an approach based on thresholds, were this standard a high one, rather than one simply of 'competence' and this implies that they too agree that a judgement is to be made here between different demands.

The training of health professionals: a test case

In what has preceded, I have explored the arguments in favour and against the use of clinician report cards and the most often cited alternative, the use of a threshold, in relation to the clinical relevance of the variations in ability and experience of fully qualified clinicians.

An important test case for those on all sides of this argument is the question of whether patients should know about, and be free to choose for or against, the fact that they are going to be operated on by someone who is training to be a surgeon or other clinician, and perhaps performing this operation for the first time. This is an interesting test case because, on the one hand, the information that one is going to be operated on by a trainee is material in the sense used by Clarke and Oakley. Information that a person has never performed an operation like this before is at least as significant as any other information discussed thus far and probably much more important when it comes to the risks associated with an intervention. Many, if not most, patients would choose to avoid being treated by such a person if they had the chance, unless there was no other option. Nevertheless, the fact is that those who would wish not to be treated by a trainee are able to make that choice only because their doctor trained on others and this suggests that those who are in favour of freedom of choice ought to be willing to participate in the conditions which make such freedom possible.

On the other hand, however, just as the patient choice approach to report cards faces problems dealing with trainees, this question is not resolved by the adoption of the threshold approach either because trainees will frequently not be capable of meeting the requirements of the threshold if it is set sufficiently high to reassure patients. This implies that, even if in general a high threshold of practice should be maintained, there is a broader public interest in there being at least some patients treated by those who do not meet such standards. Whilst it is in most patients' individual interest to avoid being treated by inexperienced surgeons, and whilst such trainees may not reach any publicly acceptable threshold of good practice, it is in everyone's interest that some patients are treated by them. It is here the demands of solidarity, justice and reciprocity are the strongest.

Conclusions

I began this chapter by introducing the twin concepts of 'patient-centred medicine' and 'evidence-based medicine', arguing that, taken together, these concepts, which have a natural affinity, mark a significant shift in thinking about the doctor–patient relationship which is captured in the concept of 'evidence-based patient choice'. Most arguments in favour of the widespread introduction of clinician report cards draw in great measure upon something like the idea of evidence-based patient choice, combined with a claim that the gathering of data on the success rates of clinicians and its distribution to patients will, in addition to respecting and promoting choice, lead to significant improvements in standards of available care. In this chapter I have argued amongst other things that the ethical dimensions of the decision whether or not to introduce clinician report cards are not exhausted by the combined consideration of the concepts of patient choice, evidence-based medicine and beneficence.

We have very strong individual and public interests, other things being equal, in increasing the standards of care in surgery and clinical practice more widely. The evidence of the Bristol Inquiry and from elsewhere suggests that the collection of good-quality data about the success rates of surgeons, and its subsequent feedback, along with other data, to clinicians for use in their training and appraisal improves practice significantly. Where the costs associated with the collection and use of this data are not so significant as to themselves undermine practice, the arguments in favour of this kind of use of report cards seem convincing.

Furthermore, where patients are considering whether or not to consent to treatment or refuse it, they should in my view be provided, as Clarke and Oakley suggest, with all information material to that decision. Following the General Medical Council's lead, it seems reasonable to expect that this will include information about all relevant common or serious side effects and risks associated with the intervention and that this ought to include information about the risks, as far as these are calculable, of undergoing a particular treatment, with a particular clinician in a particular hospital. This is not, of course to suggest that health professionals have an obligation to provide patients with limitless amounts of information but it does suggest that they have an obligation to provide the kinds of information that a reasonable person in this position would want in order to make their decision about whether or not to proceed. Information about the skills, experiences and success rates of the surgeon proposing to treat them, is in my view information of this type.

Having accepted that patients should be informed about the risks associated with being treated by particular clinicians, and also that clinician report cards should be used in the training and appraisal of clinicians, does not imply, it seems to me, that patients should necessarily be provided with a high degree of choice about by whom they will be treated. Patients should only have as much choice as is compatible with the just and fair provision of healthcare and with the maintenance of acceptably high standards of care generally. This implies that patients cannot be coherently said to have rights to either unlimited information or unlimited choice (Neil, Clarke and Oakley, 2004). And, the need to train new clinicians implies too that patients can also have no absolute threshold guarantee, provided that appropriate supervision and oversight are in place.

Patients in their decisions about whether or not to proceed with a treatment should in my view be given full and frank information about the risks associated with the actual treatment they are going to receive (related to the actual abilities and experiences of the clinician at hand, including trainees) and information about the real alternatives, including no treatment. Despite this, the choices available may on occasion be legitimately constrained on moral grounds, e.g. because of concerns about justice. Where this is the case, these grounds should be made explicit to patients. Patients, both as individuals and as members of a community within which healthcare is provided have, in addition to their own healthcare interests, an interest in the moral principles

a goal more important than enhancing the autonomy of those whose resources already give them a wide range of significant options.

Adverse consequences of the Clarke–Oakley proposal

Let's turn, first, to the question of why we might want report cards at all. Clarke and Oakley highlight a number of failings in recent medical history which, they suggest, could have been avoided if a report card system had been in place (2004, pp. 16–17). Consider the scandal surrounding the elevated death rates for paediatric cardiac operations at the Bristol Royal Infirmary (Kennedy, 2002). The elevated death rates were due, in significant part, to the incompetence of two surgeons working at the hospital. The report into the case concluded that Bristol had between 30 and 35 extra deaths between 1991 and 1995 than would have been the case in a 'typical' unit. Now, it seems likely that reports on the incompetent surgeons would have prevented at least some deaths. Many parents would have chosen to have the operation performed elsewhere, or by other surgeons at Bristol, and needless deaths would have been prevented.

But all that shows is that in one (very important) respect, having individual report cards would be an improvement on the situation that prevailed at Bristol. It does not show that such a system is the best conceivable, or even a very good system. The failings at Bristol were not due solely to the incompetence of the two surgeons involved. Instead, there were failures at almost every level of the institution as well as outside it. Individual report cards would have identified some of those failings, but left too many unaddressed, and patient outcomes might well have suffered, at least relative to what is achievable.

Suppose that the UK had a system of report cards in the early 1990s, such as the one Clarke and Oakley recommend. If the system worked as planned, then the incompetent surgeons would have been identified as poor performers. Parents would have chosen to go elsewhere, when they could. In that event, what would have happened? One possibility is that once the hospital identified the problem, the surgeons involved might have received adequate training, which would have allowed their standards to improve (though there is a problem with this approach: what parent is going to place their child's life in the hands of a surgeon with a poor record, even one who has taken steps to improve her performance? Surgeons who have been identified as in need of further training may find it difficult to reintegrate into the surgical community). That's one, rather happy, outcome (though I shall soon have cause to raise questions about just how happy it would be). Here's another: suppose hospitals compete with one another for patients (a reasonable supposition). Then they might respond to the identification of a poorly performing surgeon simply by sacking her, and hiring one with a better report card.

Suppose that had happened at Bristol. In that case, the results would have been suboptimal, both for the patients at Bristol and for those elsewhere in the UK. Consider, first, Bristol. Though the report of the Bristol Inquiry found that the surgeons at the centre of the scandal were culpable, nevertheless it also found that 'to a very great extent, the flaws and failures of Bristol were within the hospital, its organisation and culture, and within the wider NHS as it was at the time' (Department of Health, 2002, p. 9). It added that 'poor teamwork [. . .] had implications for performance and outcome' (Department of Health, 2002, p. 4). If Bristol had sacked the relevant surgeons (or if the senior surgeon, who was also an administrator, had retired from surgery, as he did shortly afterwards), these systematic institutional problems would have gone unaddressed. Effectively, the surgeons would have been scapegoated, for poor outcomes for which they were partially, but only partially, to blame. The unacceptably high mortality rates for paediatric open-heart surgery at Bristol would probably have fallen, but the wider problems, both within the hospital and in the NHS, would have gone unaddressed. These problems might well have continued to lead to excess deaths, at Bristol and beyond.

Now consider the wider impact of a report card system if this kind of response were repeated across the country. It might have the effect of identifying incompetent doctors, forcing them to improve or leave the profession. But report cards do not identify incompetence, *per se*; they give a score, and even when all doctors are good enough to count as competent, some will do better than others. One possibility, then, is that a pattern will rapidly emerge: the better-resourced hospital will hire the better performing doctors, and the rest will go to poorer hospitals. We might see a two (or more)-tier hospital system emerging. The wealthy will go to the best hospitals, which will also have the best surgeons – and the highest prices. A report card system could have the effect, in a healthcare environment like that of Australia or the UK, of siphoning the best performing surgeons out of the public system and into the private. The poor will be left with the dregs: operated upon by the worst surgeons in the worst conditions.

As Clarke and Oakley point out, it is already the case that the poor bear a disproportionate amount of the burdens associated with surgical training (2004, p. 33, n. 29). But the hierarchical health system that might emerge under a regime of report cards threatens to exacerbate the inequality. We should be reducing the extent to which money can buy health, not increasing it (so long as such reductions do not lower the average standard of care available). Already the wealthy have access to better primary healthcare, better advice, better nutrition, decreased exposure to risks of death or injury through accidents. We ought not give them the further advantage of the best surgeons in the best hospitals as well. Instead, there is a strong argument that, as a matter of justice, the best surgeons should be encouraged to work at worse performing hospitals: so that risks are borne more equitably, and so that under-resourced hospitals have advocates who are articulate and whose opinions carry weight. Allow the concentration of medical capital envisaged, and we risk setting in motion two circular processes, one which rapidly ratchets up the quality of the best hospitals and one that will lower the worst. Worse resources leads to concentration of poorer performing surgeons, which makes the hospital unattractive to patients, which leads to worse resources, on the one hand; on the other, the same pressures work in reverse to concentrate medical capital.

In this context, it is worth remarking on a perverse incentive, which might result from instituting individual report cards for surgeons. The better surgeons might be discouraged from working at poorer hospitals, since the lack of resources would almost certainly translate into poorer success rates for them. To be fair, Clarke and Oakley discuss perverse incentives which might arise from their proposal, and have a number of suggestions designed to avoid them (2004, pp. 24–5). For instance, they suggest that, rather than making raw mortality figures available to the public, which might discourage surgeons from taking on harder cases, we provide adjusted scores. These scores might be adjusted to give a measure of the competence of the surgeon, based on their mortality rate adjusted for the degree of difficulty of their operations. It might be that the kind of consideration I have just adduced can be dealt with in the same kind of way: weighting surgical success in poorer hospitals more heavily than similar success in better-resourced institutions. However, I shall shortly adduce some doubts about this kind of weighting.

Even if the danger of a hierarchical medical system can be avoided, there remain significant problems with the proposal. What the focus on the hospital environment and resources should remind us is that patient outcomes are never due to the performance of any one person, no matter how skilled he or she may be. Instead, a happy surgical outcome is the product of a team effort, involving the collaboration of the doctors and nurses involved in the operation itself, the pre- and post-operative care delivered, very often, by other medical staff, the institutional structures, even the administrative arrangements. To take an example that is obvious once it is pointed out, but is often overlooked, even cleaning staff have an important impact upon health outcomes, since a dirty hospital is a breeding ground for infections.

Suppose, now, that all the dangers just mentioned had been avoided. Suppose, to return to the beginning of our scenario, the hospital had not reacted by firing its comparatively poorly performing surgeons, but instead offered them further training. That, I said above, would be a happy outcome, at least compared to the dangers which I have just sketched. But how happy would it be, compared to other feasible alternatives? I suggest that the focus on the individual surgeon, which would be the upshot in this kind of circumstance, would not serve the patient all that well. We do better to focus on institutions and whole health systems than individual doctors if our primary aim is to improve patient outcomes.

As I previously mentioned, the report of the Bristol Inquiry identified widespread and systematic failings at the hospital. Apart from the worse performance of the two surgeons, the report noted that the arrangements for caring for very ill infants were 'not safe', that there was a significant doubt whether the hospital should have been designated a centre for paediatric cardiac surgery (Department of Health, 2002, pp. 226–7), that there was a lack of leadership and teamwork at the hospital (Department of Health, 2002, p. 1.) and that the culture of the unit was too closed (Department of Health, 2002, p. 2). Many of these systematic problems, the report noted, were not confined to Bristol. In addition, problems with the National Health system itself, and its management of acutely ill infants, were identified.

It should now be apparent why a focus on the performance of individual surgeons carries risks. In particular, it risks taking attention away from systemic failures which might be as, or more, significant. The focus on individual surgeons might lead even well-motivated administrators, health systems and the general public to look in the wrong place, or at least to overlook some of the right places, when it comes to improving health systems. It is also potentially unfair to focus exclusively on surgeons' performance. If we take mortality, for instance, as a measure of surgeons' success, we may unfairly apportion praise and blame. High mortality rates could be the consequence of faults down the line which do not reflect badly on surgical skill; on the other hand, low mortality rates are always the product of many people doing their jobs well, and do not reflect well on just the surgeon. To ensure the best possible healthcare, surgeons' performances must be situated in the wider context of the institutions and structures, which are essential components of well-functioning health systems. It may be better, all things considered, to take the focus off individual doctors, and instead place it squarely on the institutions of which they are one, but only one, essential part.[1]

An institution-focused alternative

Suppose that, rather than providing data upon the performance of individual surgeons, we provide data on the performance of institutions as a whole. This data should be quite fine-grained; since institutions may be good in some areas and not in others, we will want to provide data which is divided up appropriately (I don't pretend to the expertise to suggest just how this should be done). In that case, the outcomes will better reflect the contribution of the teams who are genuinely responsible for successes and failures (where the team consists of all the personnel who are directly or indirectly responsible for patient outcomes – not just the surgical team, but nursing staff, administrators, and so on). If an institution performs badly, relative to others, the data will not be able to provide an explanation of the failure, but that is a good thing. It will serve as a spur to administrators or government to seek the causes, rather than leading to the scapegoating of people who may not be the cause of the problem at all.

An adverse report on a hospital's performance, say in a particular speciality, will prove an effective spur to administrators. There is already evidence that publication of this kind of information leads to an improvement in performance, as hospitals seek to restore their reputation and their market share (Hibbard *et al.*, 2005). Of course, an adverse report will not identify the source of the problem, which may lie with organizational culture, procedures, or individual medical personnel (or, as in Bristol, a combination of all these and other factors). As we have seen, however, individualized reports do not necessarily identify the source of problems either, since whole teams are always responsible for surgical outcomes. Having received an adverse report, the hospital will need to investigate further to locate the problem or problems. But that's a good thing, not a bad. Individualized reporting gives hospitals a sometimes false sense of where problems lie, and how they can be fixed. Institution-based reporting serves as a spur to further investigation, and the discovery of problems that might otherwise be overlooked.

Of course, in locating the source of the problem, it might be necessary for the hospital to examine the performance of individual surgeons. To that extent, institution-based reporting is not incompatible with individualized reporting. Two points must be borne in mind, however. Firstly, the emphasis ought to be on institution-based reporting, in order to reflect the fact that health outcomes are the product of teams and not individuals, and to better identify problems that may extend well beyond teams. Secondly, though public reporting of institutional performance might be necessary to improve health outcomes, there seems little need for *public* reporting of the performance of individuals. Training and maintenance of the skills of surgeons ought to be routine activities in hospitals, and this activity might require or entail monitoring of their performance. But there seems little need for this data to be publicized – so long as institutional performance data is public. It is, after all, this information that is most pertinent to the decision patients face: the aggregated performance rate of the institution for their procedure is the relevant statistic, not the success of their surgeon.

To the extent to which this information is the most pertinent to patient decisions, institution-based reporting might enhance autonomy at least as effectively as the Clarke–Oakley proposal (since outcomes are the product of teams and not individuals). More importantly, they are likely to lead to a better health system for everyone. Firstly, they will not lead to the concentration of medical capital which is a probable consequence of the individually focused system. Surgeons will not be penalized for going to worse performing hospitals, since everyone will recognize that poor results do not reflect badly upon particular individuals. Secondly, rather than focusing blame upon individuals, institutional reporting is likely to lead to improvements in the institutions.

Sometimes, poor performance is the result of factors over which the institution has little or no control. Now, as a matter of fact, we respond quite differently to the information that X is a poorly performing *hospital* than to the proposition that X is a poorly performing *surgeon*. We blame the poor surgeon, but we look for explanations of the poor performance of the institution. We shall find them, more often than not, in poor resourcing. If we had discovered that *Bristol* was performing poorly, the faults in the NHS the report identified might have been brought to light much earlier, to the benefit of all patients. Reporting on the performance of institutions can therefore play an important role in increasing the justice of the health system, by placing pressure upon governments to increase funding to relatively impoverished hospitals.

An institution-focused approach can therefore simultaneously avoid the worst problems with the Clarke–Oakley proposal, while playing a role in improving the equity of the system. Whereas report cards for individuals risk making the health system more unjust, report cards for institutions might help make it more just than it is at present.

The patient–surgeon relationship

Finally, some somewhat speculative comments on the effects of the Clarke–Oakley proposal upon the relationship between doctor and patient. The proposal seems to have a certain view on this question implicit within it. They seem to envisage the relationship as essentially commercial. Patients are customers, who should shop around for the best 'deal'. What weight they give to surgeon's performance in this comparison shopping is presumably up to them; we enhance patient autonomy simply by giving them the information they need to make informed choices. If they then choose, as Clarke and Oakley think they might, to trade off performances for other goods, that is their prerogative. Thus, surgeons can compete, with some offering the best mortality figures, and others offering lower cost operations, or reduced waiting times for non-emergency procedures. However, the relationship between a doctor and a (potential) patient might be better conceptualized as a fiduciary relationship; and to that extent we ought to be promoting structures which make it rational for the patient to trust her doctor.

Here I want to contrast two approaches to trust. Firstly, there is the model implicit in the Clarke–Oakley view. On this model, trust is an individual relationship. Patients are consumers who seek out physicians who can best serve their interests as they, the patients, see them. If we adopt this model, then we need to put in place systems which enhance the capacity of patients to shop well – for instance, by providing them with as much information as possible as to the specifications of the product they're buying. Now, patient autonomy, the value which lies at the foundation of this view, is certainly a good worth fighting for, and medical ethicists are right to highlight the dangers of a return to the days of paternalism, in which physicians made all the significant decisions for their patients in the light of their conception of what the patient's best interests were, rather than what patients took them to be. Nevertheless, the alternatives that confront us do not boil down to maximal patient autonomy versus paternalism. There are other models available, which trade off some degree of patient autonomy for other goods.

On the model I advocate, patients are seen as having special but not certain knowledge of their own interests. Clarke and Oakley seem to think that generally patients are very good at assessing the subjective value of surgical outcomes; at least, so their example of Clarke's knee operation suggests. In discussing this case, they claim that 'it is reasonable to think that someone can estimate the magnitude of this subjective value, roughly at least' (2004, p. 31, n. 4.); in the absence of particular reasons to think that knees are somehow special, it seems that they are committed to generalizing this claim to other surgical outcomes. In fact, this tempting view (whether it is appropriately attributed to Clarke and Oakley or not) is quite wrong: patient estimates of the subjective value of surgical outcomes can be completely off-base. Consider, for instance, the phenomenon of hedonic adaptation. A number of studies have shown that people systematically overestimate the hedonic impact of events on their lives; that is, they think that certain classes of events will lead them to be much more unhappy than is in fact the case. In coming to their view of the impact of the event on their life, they fail to take into account the way in which people adapt to alterations in their life situation. Thus, for instance, most able-bodied people say that if they were to become disabled, they would be extremely unhappy; perhaps they would no longer think their lives worth living. But, after actually becoming disabled, people adapt; they return to their 'set point', which is the baseline level of well-being they experienced before disability. The same phenomenon can be detected in the experience of the recently disabled: one week after the disability, negative emotions outweigh positive, but as soon as the eighth week, the subjects report a preponderance of positive emotions.[2] The application to surgical outcomes is obvious: patients may reject the option of amputation, for instance, in the belief that the loss of the limb would be experienced as devastating for them, whereas in fact they would not merely have a life worth living after the operation; they would actually experience no diminution in well-being.

Secondly, consider gender reassignment surgery. People who opt for this surgery do so because they believe it will repair a mismatch between their actual body and their body as they experience it. But much of the research suggests that gender reassignment surgery just doesn't deliver what is hoped for from it. A review of more than 100 studies of post-operative transsexuals reveals that it does little to improve their subjective well-being (Batty, 2004).

Now, I am not arguing that these cases give us grounds for simply ignoring or overriding the clearly expressed preferences of patients. In fact, while I think there's no entirely satisfactory way to respond to these cases, there are some clearly unsatisfactory ways, and simply ignoring patient wishes is one of them. Nevertheless, it is also unsatisfactory simply to ignore these kinds of findings, and watch patients make decisions on the basis of false assessments of the impact of surgical outcomes on the quality of their lives. Fortunately, there are options besides ignoring the expressed wishes of patients or blindly implementing them. We can, for instance, be directive in counselling them (there is evidence that drawing the attention of subjects to the phenomenon of adaptation is effective in making estimates of the hedonic impact of life events more realistic).[3] Patients should have the final say over the surgery to which they are subjected, but it is permissible to attempt to change their mind with rational pressure.

It would be uncharitable to attribute to Clarke and Oakley a view of autonomy, which is unable to make room for this kind of worry. No doubt they would insist that we can best deal with the problem by informing patients of the existence of hedonic adaptation (for instance) and asking them to take it into consideration in their decision-making. The worry is more subtle: it is that the kind of relationship between physician and patient that Clarke and Oakley advocate is unconducive to the kind of directive counselling which is sometimes appropriate. 'The customer is always right' is not just a maxim that salespeople abide by in order to create the kind of atmosphere that promotes sales, but is in fact expressive of the psychology of the commercial transaction. If I am considering buying some goods from you, and I have the choice of several vendors, then I have a significant amount of power in our relationship. To the extent to which doing business matters to you, you are under pressure to cater for my needs as I perceive them. If you attempt to steer me in a direction I don't want to go, you risk losing my custom, and you know it. When it is in my interest not to have an operation that I want, you may not make every effort to dissuade me. When it is in my interest to have an operation, I shall take a jaundiced view of your attempt to persuade me, since I know your remuneration is tied to your success at swaying me.

It would be best, in fact, if those who can gain directly from transactions such as these are not involved in counselling at all. Surgery is, in any case, a specialty, and it would be burdensome to expect surgeons to keep up with psychological findings like set point theory. Instead, specialist counsellors ought to play this role. Systems ought to be in place to ensure that counsellors are not penalized, financially or in any other ways, if they dissuade patients from having expensive procedures. And it ought to be public knowledge that counsellors are independent in these ways.

On the Clarke–Oakley proposal, patients choose surgeons on the basis of their performance. On the model I propose, patients choose *hospitals* on the basis of their performance. They therefore have confidence not just in the surgeon, but in the whole team. To that extent, they will be more receptive to directive counselling, where it is appropriate. They do not deal directly with a surgeon (not a great deal, in any case) from whom they buy a service; they enter into a relationship with a medical team, in whose performance they have confidence and whose advice they have every reason to trust. The Clarke-Oakley proposal does not directly conflict with this kind of relationship, but to the extent to which it is imbued with the logic of the market, it is inhospitable to it.

There are, therefore, many reasons to prefer reporting to target institutions, and not individuals. Such a system is fairer, since it reflects the genuine contribution of entire teams to outcomes, good or bad. It also avoids the likely inequities that might result from the Clarke–Oakley proposal, and might in fact increase justice in healthcare. And, it would help establish a more appropriate relationship, of justified trust, between patients and medical staff. For all these reasons, I suggest, we do better to implement a system of report cards for institutions, and not individuals.[4]

Notes

1. More recently, Neil, Clarke and Oakley (2004) have examined and positively assessed a somewhat different proposal that avoids some of the above problems by implementing a flatter reporting system. Since surgeons are, on this proposal, sorted into a mere three categories, there seems less risk of a concentration of medical resources. However, this proposal still risks some of the dangers of focusing attention on individuals, rather than on the institutions responsible for patient outcomes.
2. See Silver, R. L. (1982).
3. See Ubel *et al.* (2005).
4. I would like to thank the participants in the workshop on surgeons' performance report cards held at the University of Melbourne, and especially Steve Clarke and Justin Oakley for helpful comments on this chapter.

References

Batty, D. (2004). Sex changes are not effective, say researchers. *The Guardian*, July 20.
Clarke, S. and Oakley, J. (2004). Informed consent and surgeons' performance. *Journal of Medicine and Philosophy*, **29**, 11–35.
Department of Health (2002). *Learning from Bristol*. London: HMSO.
Hibbard, J. H., Stockard, J. and Tusler, M. (2005). Hospital performance reports: impact on quality, market share, and reputation. *Health Affairs*, **24**, 1150–61.
Kennedy, I. (2002). Report of the Bristol Royal Infirmary Inquiry. London: HMSO. See: http://www.bristol-inquiry.org.uk/final_report/index.htm.

Neil, D., Clarke, S. and Oakley, J. (2004). Public reporting of individual surgeon performance information: United Kingdom developments and Australian issues. *Medical Journal of Australia*, **181**, 266–8.

Silver, R. L. (1982). Coping with an undesirable life event: a study of early reactions to physical disability. Unpublished doctoral dissertation, Northwestern University.

Ubel, P. A., Loewenstein, G. and Jepson, C. (2005). Disability and sunshine: can predictions be improved by drawing attention to focusing illusions or emotional adaptation? *Journal of Experimental Psychology – Applied*, **11**, 111–23.

3

Safety, accountability, and 'choice' after the Bristol Inquiry

Tom Sorell

University of Birmingham, UK

Ever since the Inquiry into paediatric mortality rates at the Royal Bristol Infirmary, there has been strong pressure in the UK for greater monitoring and reporting of the performance of surgeons. The inquiry, chaired by Sir Ian Kennedy, was asked not only to investigate the disproportionate number of deaths among infants operated upon in Bristol in the 1980s and early 1990s, but to make recommendations that might be acted upon throughout the National Health Service (NHS). Kennedy reported in 2002. Some of the recommendations went far beyond the question of how best to ensure the safety of paediatric surgery, or even of surgery in general. They called for a 'patient-centred' NHS. This theme was enthusiastically taken up in the government response to Kennedy, and there are noticeable affinities between the idea of patient-centredness and the idea of 'patient choice', which is at the heart of UK government health policy.

Patient-centredness in Kennedy's sense is broader than patient safety: it extends to public involvement in national policy-making, and public and patient involvement in decision-making structures of local NHS trusts. In my view, both of these ways of involving patients and the public are at best loosely connected to the problems in Bristol that prompted the inquiry. Nevertheless, they were accepted by the UK government in its response to Kennedy, and in subsequent policy documents. Partly as a result, Department of Health (DoH) policy now runs together, or comes close to running together, the answers to four distinct questions:

1. How can surgeons who are not equal to the kinds of operations they are attempting – whose patients avoidably die or suffer complications – be identified and retrained?
2. What can be done to encourage innovation and higher levels of skill in surgeons who have secure employment and who may be complacent about their performance?
3. How can patients or their advocates be informed of the risks of a certain kind of surgery carried out by a certain surgeon in such a way that informed consent is possible?

   and

Informed Consent and Clinician Accountability: The Ethics of Report Cards on Surgeon Performance. Steve Clarke and Justin Oakley (eds.). Published by Cambridge University Press. © Cambridge University Press 2007.

4. What can be done to democratize a hierarchical hospital medicine in which consultants, in particular surgeons, are at the top, and lots of others, including patients, are lower down or at the bottom of the pile?

The illusion that a system of accountability to patients is the answer to all of these questions is widespread and not easy to dispel.

The most urgent of the four questions, morally speaking, is (1). Unless it is answered, surgeons who are the biggest danger to patients will continue to do serious harm, and, if Bristol is any guide, will add to already unacceptable mortality rates. Doing something about this depends on identifying a range of acceptable results for different surgical procedures, on recording different surgeons' results regularly and accurately, and on having surgeons retrained routinely, or when their results fall below the acceptable. It is possible that routine retraining is also the answer to (2). Neither of these answers involves accountability to the public or to patients; it involves accountability to the custodians of the standards: for example, surgical specialists such as those that advised the Kennedy inquiry itself, or surgeon members of standards bodies like the UK National Institute for Clinical Excellence (NICE), who are able to keep track of and encourage promising innovation in surgery. Accountability to these bodies, though it is not accountability *to* the public, is accountability to a body acting *on behalf of* the public.

Answers to questions (3) and (4) arguably *do* involve some sort of account-ability to the public, at any rate those members of the public who are being offered surgical treatment. If patients or their guardians are to give informed consent to surgery, they need to be advised about the past performance of the relevant consultants when judged by standards imposed by experts. If the surgeon's performance in a particular case turns out to diverge for the worse from past performance, that can be a matter for reasonable misgiving or even investigation and disciplinary action. The knowledge that patients who are advised to do so can refuse surgery; the exposure of a surgeon's record to public gaze; the vulnerability of surgeons' performance to complaint and even legal action; all of these things can work to undo the inflated status of some consultants. But when the surgeons are brought down a peg or two by the exposure of a patchy record of performance, or when they are humbled by patients demanding to be treated by another consultant with a better record, this is not a case of arrogance or undue concentration of power in surgeons being combated for its own sake; a concern with safety is driving accountability. Accountability for the sake of safety and accountability for the sake of correcting imbalances of power in medicine march in step only to a limited extent. They are two quite distinct goals of accountability. Or so I shall argue.

I shall also argue that, in many medical settings, and in surgical settings like Bristol, accountability promotes, and *ought* to promote, the goal of safety (and perhaps also safe innovation) *ahead* of other goals. Accountability in this context is not primarily concerned with promoting democracy or in redistributing power, though that may be a by-product of whatever procedures are justified by safety. Accountability in medicine does not always mean, and should not always mean, a preparedness to justify what one is doing to anyone interested, or to the widest group possible of those who are interested, or even in all cases to those who will be the first to suffer if medical mistakes are made. Instead, it *can* mean, and *ought* sometimes to mean, a preparedness to justify what one is doing to those with an appropriate expertise in the relevant medical practice, acting as protectors of the interests of those who may be harmed.

I shall argue against running together the safety and democratizing or egalitarian goals of accountability, and I shall express scepticism about the value of some of the consumerism that, in the case of UK policy, egalitarian or democratic language sometimes expresses. Both the democratizing and consumerist goals of accountability are less weighty, morally, than the goals of safety and safe innovation, and the safety goals are often independent of the others. In the course of indicating how these goals are confused in the findings and recommendations of the Kennedy Report, and in UK government policy inspired by Kennedy, I shall try to distinguish cases where a major role for patients is highly desirable, and cases where it matters less.

I

The Kennedy Inquiry was ostensibly concerned with the causes and implications of a failure in paediatric surgery in a single hospital in England in the 1980s and 1990s. Yet its terms of reference call for nothing less than recommendations for improving the NHS as a whole – not just surgery in acute hospitals, or the whole range of services given by acute hospitals, not just the part of the NHS consisting of acute and non-acute hospitals, but the *whole* NHS: from GP services to hospitals, from clinical staff and technicians to management, and across the UK. These terms of reference are puzzling, unless the events at the Bristol Royal Infirmary were typical of what was going on in the NHS at the time, or typical of all NHS institutions, and this is highly implausible. There are references in the report to a number of phenomena that were widespread in the NHS in the 1980s and early 1990s – underfunding, and an organization and set of priorities that put healthcare providers' interests before those of patients – but these do not seem to have produced abnormally high mortality rates elsewhere, and they seem to have contributed much less to what went wrong at Bristol than surgical and managerial incompetence combined. In any case, how the problems in paediatric surgery at Bristol could have been taken to typify the problems of the NHS *before* an Inquiry had shown as much is hard to understand. In the same way, it is hard to understand how an inquiry into open-heart surgery on children under 1 year old is the basis for any general conclusions about the role of parents in the delivery of NHS services, or the kinds of services that should be delivered to children in general in the NHS, still less the way patients in *general* should be involved, or the public. Yet, the Kennedy report is not short of recommendations on all of these matters.

The Bristol case does raise a *few* quite general issues about the way patients should be the focal point of activity in the NHS, but when these issues are thought through, the idea of patient-centredness in Kennedy and DoH policy seems neither as unitary nor as effective a remedy for all the ills it is prescribed for, as its proponents suggest.

A good starting point is §17 from the Summary of the Kennedy Report:

Standards of care: Parents taking their children to be treated in Bristol assumed that the level of care provided would be good ... Few had any idea that there were no agreed standards of care for [Paediatric Cardiac Surgery] or for any other specialty. For the future, there must be two developments. There must be agreed and published standards of clinical care for health care professionals to follow, so that patients and the public know what to expect. There must also be standards for hospitals as a whole. Hospitals which do not meet these standards should not be able to offer services within the NHS. (Kennedy, 2002, p. 3)

I take it to be uncontroversial that there should be agreed standards. I take it even that there *were* agreed standards for paediatric cardiac surgery among professional surgeons as a whole in the 1980s and 1990s in England. Otherwise, training in paediatric cardiac surgery could not have gone on; otherwise, peer-reviewed publication on innovative surgical techniques would not have proceeded in the normal way. Otherwise, a *prima facie* case for underperformance in Bristol could not have been made by Dr Stephen Bolsin, the anaesthetist whose doubts were for so long ignored.

Trust was misplaced in the Bristol case not because there were no agreed standards – comparative and average mortality rates for different procedures afforded one measuring stick – but because performance fell well below them, because there was no mechanism for giving early warning of this, and because, when the whistle was blown in the absence of the mechanism, no one acted to stop operations being carried out by dangerous surgeons. Had monitoring and intervention mechanisms been in place, and had someone in the management of the Bristol Royal Infirmary sent underperforming surgeons for retraining, would trust have been misplaced? In particular, would trust have been misplaced if monitoring systems did not involve published standards for paediatric cardiac surgery? Again, my inclination is to say 'No'. It is not the *publication* of the standards but the *enforcement* of the standards that matters to whether trust is well placed.

It is sometimes thought that, in the absence of published standards, patients, or, in the case of Bristol, parents, cannot be properly approached for consent to surgery (Clarke and Oakley, 2004). Here we need to distinguish 'standards of care for paediatric cardiac surgery' from mortality rates, and we have to distinguish acute from elective surgery. It is obviously relevant to a parental decision to agree to surgery on a child under 1 year old that the chances of death under the prospective surgeon are well above the average. It is less urgent to know what the whole range of standards of care are, that the surgeon in question is so far from meeting. Again, if surgery has to be carried out quickly if it is to have any effect, if it is one of a very small range of possible treatments, and if a patient is not able at the time to make an unrushed and informed judgement, then, if the surgery goes ahead with an inferior sort of consent, that is not necessarily wronging the parent or the patient. There are limits to informed consent that no one is to blame for, and the availability of published standards for the patient or parent to read, as opposed to standards that will be monitored and enforced independently, may not help. The supposed ideal of being able to make an informed choice about having surgery and of being able to make an informed choice among surgeons may be an ideal reserved for knees and hips or cataracts, rather than baby's hearts in an acute hospital.

It is true that, in the absence of published standards, the threshold for informed consent may not have been reached in some cases, but this again seems a secondary matter in relation to misplaced trust. Had surgeons been competent at carrying out heart operations but bad or casual communicators of the risks of surgery, that, too would have prevented the threshold for informed consent from being reached, but it would not have rendered misplaced the trust of parents who assumed that standards were high or high enough. It may be true that trust placed in the absence of a process of getting consent or of doing research of one's own for oneself as patient or one's child as patient is sometimes *blind* trust. But blind trust is not necessarily misplaced. It can be placed in someone who is in fact trustworthy. Again, trust need not be entirely blind, even if one is a relatively badly informed patient or parent. This can be because the relatively uninformed can know that there are experts making some of the relevant checks, and ensuring that the general level of treatment offered in a hospital or by surgeons in particular does not fall below a certain level. This is the kind of division of labour that the parents in the Bristol case wrongly assumed was in operation, and that, had it been in operation, might have saved children's lives.

Does the division of labour give undue power to experts, so that it can be criticized as undemocratic? Consider the (in my view) comparable case of airline safety experts in relation to the flying public. No one, to my knowledge, has ever complained that their role gives them too much power, or that the public should be more involved in their monitoring and standard-setting processes. Just as the pilots and engineers who certify air safety are judging other pilots and engineers in ways that maintain high standards of safety, so medical experts are in principle able to hold other practitioners to high standards.

And, this is to say nothing about expert medical witnesses called by medical lawyers in suits for negligence. Although experts know more than most patients and the general public, and justifiably have judgements that are weightier than those of the general public in maintaining standards, this greater authority is not a kind of unfairness or the product of favouritism.

II

Even if we could agree with Kennedy about the specific ways in which parents or patients should have been informed or consulted in Bristol, is there any reason to think that this would be a blueprint, or suggest a blueprint, for the treatment of patients in the rest of the NHS? I think the answer must be 'No', because a vast number of interactions between patients and doctors take place outside the acute hospital sector, with GPs. Yet the description of the 'NHS culture' that Kennedy sometimes thinks aggravated the problems at Bristol is largely based on hospital medicine, and acute hospital medicine at that.

In the Kennedy Report chapter on 'The culture of the NHS', there is the following passage on hierarchy, first among healthcare workers in general, and then among doctors.

> ... the continued existence of a hierarchical approach within and between the health care professions is a significant cultural weakness. While the situation has changed somewhat over the last decade or so, the problem remains. Even today, in some places, it is assumed that the doctor's view is inevitably superior and that nurses are there to carry out doctor's orders. This continues despite the very great efforts made by the nursing profession to create a relationship of mutual respect between doctors and nurses. Many nurses in hospitals and elsewhere still do not feel valued by their medical colleagues or by managers. A sense of hierarchy also persists within medicine. The role of a hospital consultant, for example, is regarded as of higher status than the role of a general practitioner ... [T]he resonance of these assumptions about ranks within medicine persist. More persistent still, perhaps, is the sense of hierarchy between different medical specialties within hospital medicine, such that, for example, as the evidence in Phase One[1] indicated, if a surgeon is in the room, it is he, at least in his eyes, who 'is in charge'. Of course, if he is the person with the most appropriate skills to be in charge this is not a problem. It becomes a problem if status or title can be used automatically to supersede the authority of another more qualified to be in charge. Clearly, these aspects of the current culture of the NHS are simply inappropriate. (Kennedy, 2002, pp. 268–9)

The report goes on to suggest how a culture of hierarchy – combined with a strong claim to 'clinical freedom' on the part of doctors – prevents criticism from below or from others at the same level in the hierarchy.

The point about lack of channels of criticism has a clear bearing on the Bristol case, but not always because a strict hierarchy was in place. As the summary of Kennedy makes clear (Kennedy, 2002, p. 6), management at the highest level of the Trust to which the Bristol Royal Infirmary belonged let it be known that it did not want problems brought to it for discussion. It was not a matter of someone at the top of a hierarchy being beyond criticism. Criticisms addressed by clinicians to colleagues at the same level or by Board members to Trust executives could be ineffective, too.

Hierarchy among professionals is criticizable to the extent that it interferes with efficient co-operation and also with the exposure of clinical incompetence. But it is not like the social class system, in which rank is tied to the sort of family or income group one is born into, rather than to, e.g. knowledge or effort. The hospital hierarchy Kennedy describes reflects, among other things, different levels and lengths of training. In general, the conditions for entry to and successful exit from a medical education are more exacting than those for a nursing education. There is a perfectly clear sense in which, other things being equal, a trained doctor is expected to know more than a trained nurse,[2] and the area in which decision-making is allowed to the two professions reflects this, and reflects it justifiably if the doctor *does* know more.

When it comes to patients, deference to medical opinion can once again be justified by the difference between what the doctor knows or can understand about a certain condition, and what the typical patient knows or can understand.[3] People can reasonably bow to greater knowledge without being servile and without losing self-respect. Deference to knowledge need not be deference to social position or professional rank or some other sort of undemocratic deference. It can co-exist within a wider culture that is highly egalitarian and even unpaternalistic. Indeed, the specialized knowledge that sometimes makes deference appropriate can co-exist with egalitarianism just because the specialized knowledge can be acquired even by the unaristocratic or the unmonied. Again, the consultant whom everyone defers to in the hospital may himself have to defer to the car mechanic when his car goes wrong in ways he cannot understand, or to the electrician if his understanding does not extend to wiring.

Although the greater knowledge of doctors sometimes justifies deference by patients to doctors' view of how treatment should proceed, and sometimes excuses upto a point doctors' condescension, greater knowledge does not rule out an effort by doctors to involve patients in treatment decisions, or an effort by patients to get better informed themselves about what is medically wrong with them. Both of these possibilities reduce the scope for paternalism or condescension, but they do not necessarily undo the inequalities of knowledge that may make some sort of hierarchy inevitable.

Paternalism or condescension is much less excusable, and has worse consequences, in General Practice than in acute services. In the UK, the patient has, or until recently has had, a long-term relationship with an individual GP that endures through medically good and medically bad times. The more routine the visit or the ailment, the less unequal patient and doctor are on account of the difference in their background knowledge. The less of a basis, then, for either deference *or* condescension. Again, because the relationship between a GP or GP practice and a patient is long term, there is a compelling reason for both to work at developing co-operation and honesty, which paternalism and condescension may work against.[4] Finally, because the patient gets access to specialized services via GP referrals, mistrust or difficulty in the relationship with the GP may delay effective specialized treatment further on in the system. It is in this relationship,[5] as opposed to all relationships between patients and NHS professionals, that the ideal of a partnership between patient and doctor seems both well justified and not in the least utopian.[6] Paternalism or condescension seems less excusable in the GP–patient relationship than in a one-off transaction with a specialist. It seems more excusable in a transaction between a specialist and a patient where the condition needs urgent treatment, than in a transaction where there is time to consult. Therefore, condescension or abruptness seems excusable, other things being equal, in a transaction with a specialist in an acute hospital setting. A good GP–patient relationship need *not* be the model for good relationships between patients and NHS professionals generally. Yet that appears to be the drift of the Kennedy report when it comes to undoing the NHS culture.[7]

III

A way of summarizing my doubts about Kennedy is by saying that the idea of *patient-centredness* strikes the wrong note, not only in the setting of Bristol, but also when it comes to stating the overarching goal of the NHS. *Treatment*-centred or even *effective-treatment-centred* is better, because it captures what was wrong with Bristol and yet avoids the lumping together of safety and democratizing issues that I have just been reviewing. It also avoids, as now will become clear, the consumerist connotations that attach themselves to 'patient-centredness'.

Compare the idea that the NHS ought to be centred on the patient with the vaguely similar idea that a particular business or business in general should be *customer centred*. In commercial settings there is something perverse about a manufacturing or service industry which is organized for the convenience of employees or management *as opposed* to customers. After all, it is the customers who provide the money that pays the salaries of management and employees, and if they take their business elsewhere, that can mean commercial ruin. This is the sort of consideration that motivates the phrase 'The customer is always right'. It is a way of summarizing the dependence of a business upon, and so the necessity of achieving and maintaining, customer satisfaction.

Now in the 'NHS culture' we have just seen being described, there are elements of perversity as well. For example, the hierarchical organization made so much of by Kennedy may well suit those at the top, but if it interferes with treating patients effectively, and Kennedy is sure it does, that is perverse. It is perverse not because, as in the commercial case, it will lead to patients voting with their feet or with their money and taking their medical problems from unsatisfactory hospitals to better-performing ones. It is perverse because it runs counter to the main purpose of medicine, which is not to provide a comfortable life for surgeons or Trust managers, but to reduce as far as possible pain and disease. If oversight and audit advance these goals on balance, then, even when they are a nuisance to doctors and managers, oversight and audit mechanisms need to be in place. If more extensive consultation with patients advances these goals, then, even when it is felt to be a burden by doctors, there ought to be more extensive consultation. In this way, the thinking that leads to 'the customer is always right' has a counterpart, but only a loose counterpart, in a thought about patients in the NHS.

Now in Kennedy, the argument for patient-centredness does not start with the goals of medicine, but with Labour government policy for the NHS,[8] and the results of consultation with Bristol parents and other sections of the public. The connection between the problems of infant mortality after surgery in Bristol and the recommendation of patient-centredness in the NHS lies in the claim that there was something wrong with NHS culture, and that this culture was partly to blame for Bristol. I have already queried the crucial connecting reasoning. NHS culture pervaded even NHS institutions with low rates of death from paediatric surgery, and there is no necessary connection between safety and a sense on the patient's part of involvement in decision-making. It is true that a lack of responsiveness was central to the problems of Bristol, and that in the 1980s and 1990s there was a background of unresponsiveness to patients. But the crucial unresponsiveness in the Bristol case was the unresponsiveness to reports of disturbing mortality rates from Dr Bolsin to the Trust Management – *not* general unresponsiveness to patients on the part of doctors or healthcare staff.

Since Kennedy reported, there has been both an official UK government response to the Bristol Inquiry (D.O.H. 2002), and many policy initiatives chiming in with that response. These take patient-centredness even further from the safety and effectiveness issues that, according to me, should have been the focal point of Kennedy, and further in the direction of an unapologetic consumerism. Kennedy had proposed greater patient involvement in decisions about their treatment and representation of patients in various decision-making bodies connected to a reformed NHS; the government response reiterated its pre-existing policy of involving the public in local NHS priority-setting, and involving independent expert bodies in clinical standard-setting. Otherwise, the government response changed the subject: instead of addressing the question of more patient participation in treatment, the response gives patients (or the public) a role in choosing where and when a service is provided: a choice *between* hospitals rather than a bigger or major say in what happens to some-one once they are being treated.

This may not *seem* like changing the subject: after all, wouldn't increased patient involvement and increased 'patient choice' be two signs of increased NHS *responsiveness* to patients, and isn't responsiveness to patients a suitable lowest common denominator when it comes to stating the value to be pursued in a post-Bristol NHS? It may be *too* low a lowest common denominator. It covers improving hospital food as much as improving the accreditation and training of surgeons. It extends from modernizing ambulances to eradicating the hospital superbugs. And there are *moral* arguments only for some kinds of responsiveness, not for all. It was seriously morally wrong for the high mortal-ity rates at Bristol to have been tolerated for so long, since the value of lost infant lives was not being reflected in an attempt to change surgical practice, and nothing less than that might have been expected, given the value of life. On the other hand, the alleged need for patients to be able to choose between treatment centres is not morally urgent at all: it does not seem to be wrong for the NHS to offer treatment to each patient in a single hospital, so long as the treatment is safe, effective, and timely. Responsiveness that consists in offering a choice of hospitals is not to be compared to responsiveness that consists in measures to raise levels of surgical competence.

What about responsiveness in the form of increased consultation of patients in the treatment process? Does this have a purely moral justification, or does it belong in a spectrum of morally neutral 'responsive' measures that also include improving hospital menus, giving a choice of hospitals, and offering private rooms? This is a bigger question than it looks, because of the scope there is for connecting the values promoted or presupposed by consumerism with values that are thought to be central to morality, such as autonomy.

In a recent report entitled *Health Literacy* (NCC, 2004), partly paid for by the UK DoH, the National Consumer Council devotes a whole chapter to shared decision-making between patients and healthcare professionals, focusing on the discrepancy between patient preferences about consultation and the character of the consultation patients actually receive. It focuses on the discrepancy, but never pauses to consider whether the preferences of patients themselves are reasonable or morally defensible in the first place. Moral appraisal attaches to preferences as much as to actions, and some consumer preferences outside medicine, e.g. for bullfights, or polluting cars or pornography, *can* be questioned. Within medicine, too, patient prefer-ences and parent preferences for child patients, can sometimes be unrea-sonable. Thus, a growing preference for caesarian births over vaginal deliveries in the UK is probably not clinically justified, and is a matter of concern to NICE (http://www.healthypages.net/news.asp?newsid=4244). Refusal to take up the MMR vaccine is another case in point (See Sorell, 2003; Sorell, 2007).

This brings us to a fundamental difficulty with consumerist treatments of measures for which moral arguments are sometimes made: namely that consumerist treatments do not criticise criticizable consumer preferences, and are partisan in favour of consumers when consumer interests are considered alongside those of sellers or providers. Like some of the free market theorists, consumerists suppose either that the customer is always right, or that consumer preferences, whatever they are, ought to be more precisely and less expensively satisfied, never suppressed or ignored. Consumerism does not ask *whether* the preferences should be satisfied, only *how* (see O'Neill, 2002, p. 44ff).

The Consumers' Association in the UK has claimed that 'regarding people as consumers rather than patients sets them in a more autonomous position that is less passive and more participative' (Consumers' Association, 2003). Patients, by contrast, 'are more associated with paternalist models of healthcare'.[9] But the concept of autonomy being used here is compatible with people being slaves to their consumer preferences, and having morally criticizable preferences they refuse to revise.

IV

It is time to sum up. Although I have expressed doubts about some of the measures that, according to Kennedy and the UK government, improve things for patients, and though I think that some kinds of accountability do not improve things at all, I am not arguing against effective means of combating incompetence. I am not even arguing against means of measuring competence that are designed to enter into patients' decisions about treatment. When the context of decision allows for it, there is nothing wrong with introducing measures of competence into patients' practical reasoning about treatment. But, both when the context does allow for this and when it doesn't, there should be mechanisms in place that trigger the suspension of medical staff if evidence of incompetence accumulates. These measures do not have to involve the practical reasoning of patients, and often cannot, if they are to be effective. In other words, safety has to be pursued *anyway*, independently of how informed consent is pursued.

I am not arguing that the ideal of patient–doctor partnership does not make sense in the NHS. On the contrary, it is a pursuable and even an achievable ideal in General Practice, where relationships are long term, where they go through long phases of health and minor illness, rather than acute conditions requiring immediate intervention, and where there is often time for things to be explained appropriately. Patients' exposure to doctors in acute settings is often one-off and unsuited to unhurried practical deliberation informed by calm give and take. These one-off relationships, if they involve quick intervention, do not permit the ideal of partnership to be realised, or realised in the same way as in the GP relationship. The patient may be too ill to think clearly or receive information relevant to his condition, and there may be little time to act. In these circumstances, what matters most is the safety and effectiveness of the treatment. Safety and effectiveness excuse a lot of condescension and brusqueness, and the patient helped through a serious accident or illness can always bring what is unsatisfactory to the notice of a GP, who is very well placed to act as patient advocate or as a channel for complaint.

Do the possibilities of the GP–patient relationship generalize to all relationships between patients and healthcare workers? I should have thought not. One way of putting my disagreement with the kind of partnership recommended in Kennedy is by saying that it surreptitiously forces all healthcare providers into the mould of the GP, and surreptitiously models the NHS relationship with patients on that sometimes explicably afforded by the unique features of the GP–patient relationship. The GP–patient relationship may not generalize.[10]

Notes

1. The Bristol Royal Infirmary Inquiry was divided into two Phases: the first, beginning in 1998, dealt with events in Bristol; the second with how the lessons of Bristol could be applied to the rest of the NHS.
2. The 'in general' and 'other things being equal' are necessary here. Nurses can have expertise that doctors lack.
3. I do not deny that some patients can be better informed than some of their doctors about their condition. When this is so, deference is out of order.
4. The same argument holds for long-term working relationships involving consultants, GPs and nurses. Condescension is more out of place, and does more damage, the longer term the relationship, and the more co-operative the relationship.
5. I mean the relationship between the patient and a particular GP rather than, as is more usual nowadays, a relationship between a patient and a GP practice.
6. But partnership can impose moral requirements on *patients* as well as GPs, moral requirements that are not often recognized. See Draper and Sorell (2002).
7. See Executive Summary §62: 'Partnership between patient and healthcare professional is the way forward . . .' (Kennedy, 2002, p. 13).
8. Particularly the patient-centredness of *The NHS Plan*. See Kennedy (2002, p. 401).
9. Ibid., p. 1.
10. I am grateful to Heather Draper, Andrew Warsop and the editors of this volume for comments on earlier versions.

References

Clarke, S. and Oakley, J. (2004). Informed consent and surgeons' performance. *Journal of Medicine and Philosophy*, **29**, 11–35.

Consumers' Association (2003). Can patients ever be consumers? Patient choice in healthcare. Paper delivered by the Consumers' Association to the Patients' Association as part of the 2003 United Kingdom Labour Party Conference.

Department of Health (2002). *Learning from Bristol*. London: HMSO.

Draper, H. and Sorell, T. (2002). Patients' responsibilities in medical ethics. *Bioethics*, **16**, 335–52.

Kennedy, I. (2002). *Report of the Bristol Royal Infirmary Inquiry*. London: HMSO.

National Consumer Council. (2004). *Health*. Literacy London. National Consumer Council.

O'Neill, O. (2002). *Autonomy and Trust in Bioethics*. Cambridge: Cambridge University Press.

Sorell, T. (2003). Health care provision and public morality. In *Equity in Health and Health Care*, ed. A. Oliver. London: Nuffield Trust, pp. 10–18.

Sorell, T. (2007). Parental choice and expert knowledge in the debate about MMR and autism. In *Ethics, Prevention, and Public Health*, ed. A. Dawson and M. Verweij. Oxford: Oxford University Press.

4

Public reports: putting patients in the picture requires a new relationship between doctors and patients

Merrilyn Walton

University of Sydney, Australia

Should report cards on surgeon performance be publicly available? Yes, but only if the information is presented in ways that can be easily understood by consumers and patients. The merits of public reports or provider profiles have been constantly debated since their first appearance in the public domain in the early 1990s. Some of the arguments against reporting include the potential to misinterpret data, the lack of clarity about what is counted and the potential the information may have in lowering staff morale. Better consumer choice, greater clinical accountability and improved quality are arguments in support of public reporting. But missing in this debate is the need to prepare and enable patients to make real choices about their doctors or hospitals.

A system not designed for patient choice

Many patients lack genuine choices in healthcare either because of the nature of their disease or because the health system is yet to recognize the scope of the informational needs of patients and their obligations to provide it. A redesigned health system is required if patients are to have genuine choice in their healthcare. The way the health system is currently structured and organized relies on patients being passive receivers of their healthcare.

Report cards about surgeons' performance have been available to patients for more than a decade,[1] yet the evidence is that patients rarely use them to choose their surgeons or hospitals (Marshall, 2001; Schneider and Lieberman, 2001). Reasons offered for the poor use include limited relevance to consumers of the items being measured (Hibbard and Jewitt, 1997), the complex format for displaying the results and insufficient use of quality results by healthcare organizations (Schneider and Epstein, 1998). Part of the problem is that public reports appear to be designed for multiple users, not just patients. Patients', clinicians' and organizations' data needs are a mixture of information and

Informed Consent and Clinician Accountability: The Ethics of Report Cards on Surgeon Performance.
Steve Clarke and Justin Oakley (eds.). Published by Cambridge University Press. © Cambridge University Press 2007.

evaluation. Patients' interests centre on short-term mortality and long-term morbidity and survival prospects (Spiegelhalter *et al.*, 2000). Clinicians want to compare their results with their peers so that they may maintain clinical standards. Organizations use them to measure workforce performance. Policy and clinical researchers use them to gain understanding of the nature of variation and the impact on patient outcomes.

But the poor design of public reports only partly explains why consumers do not use them. Understanding the patient's role in healthcare delivery generally may further explain why public reports of individual surgeon performance have been underutilized.

Adverse events reported in the media tend to identify injured patients rather than analyse systemic problems. The media interest in the patient's narrative, what happened and who was responsible, is the bedrock for community views about adverse events. Injured patients are the main characters in these medical dramas. But in the day-to-day healthcare environment, patients are not at the centre; professionals are in control.

Most hospital organizations and health services are not patient-centred and are not designed to take patient perspectives into account. Over the last century, hospitals have become better organized, more professionalized (Starr, 1982) and more complex, yet the structure of hospitals and the role of patients have remained relatively unchanged. Patients are admitted to wards in much the same way they were 100 years ago; they are usually told what is wrong with them, how, where and when their condition will be treated and by whom. Patients are not expected to make decisions other than whether they will have the treatment or not. If we encouraged all patients being admitted to hospitals to make inquiries about the rate of hospital infection, current peer review requirements and credentialling, hospital staff would not be able to cope with the increased demand on their time. The system is just not designed for questioning patients.

Presentation of data

How information is presented, distributed and understood determines the usefulness of report cards, but these factors alone do not fully explain why patients are not using the information. Why is it that patients who report they would change their surgeons if they were told of the surgeon's higher than expected mortality rate also report they do not seek out reports on surgical outcomes (Schneider and Epstein, 1998)? Those who support public reporting argue that consumers will use such reports to help them make decisions about who treats them. Underlying this assumption is the belief that market forces will lead to improved choices for patients. But this is yet to be proven. The Health Care Financing Administration in the United States stopped publicizing mortality reports, not because consumers were using it to select hospitals but because they were not (Mennemyer *et al.*, 1997). Public reports cannot be a catalyst for change unless consumers not only value the information but also find the information useful.

A closed system

A significant barrier to improved consumer choice is that much information, including surgical outcome data, is routinely kept out of the public arena. Public Inquiries in Australia (King Edward Hospital Inquiry (WA) and Campbelltown and Camden Inquiry (NSW)) and England (Bristol and Shipman Inquiries) provide the public with an extraordinary amount of information – much more than that normally available to the public. In such inquiries, statistics on patient deaths, patient injuries, workforce problems, structure and organization of hospitals become an end in themselves rather than a means to understanding the complexity of healthcare. Information-poor consumers have little experience in making sense of this information other than expressing alarm when something appears to go seriously wrong. They are not able to make sense of health care data including outcome data because they have never been equipped to do so. Nor has the health sector educated the media or consumers about the complexity of the health environment (Mennemyer *et al.*, 1997; Millenson, 2002; Romano, 2003).

Health economists and policy makers believe that patients who have information about surgeons' performance will choose the best performing surgeons (Duckett and Hunter, 1999). In response, surgeons with poor results will either lift their performance or be forced out of practice. But, unlike consumers in the commercial market, people in fiduciary relationships tend to play more passive roles. The choices they make are often limited to the recommended treatments preferred by the providers rather than a genuine selection from a range of options. The patient as active participant in their healthcare is a relatively new concept for patients and doctors alike.

Evidence about harm

For nearly a decade the community has been aware of the extent of harm caused to patients resulting from the course of their healthcare. Studies in the United States (Brennan *et al.*, 1991; Brennan *et al.*, 1996; Gawande, 1999), Australia (Wilson *et al.*, 1995), Denmark (Secker-Walker and Taylor-Adams, 2001), the United Kingdom (Vincent *et al.*, 2001) and New Zealand (Davis *et al.*, 2001) show that a significant number of patients are seriously injured or die each year from unnecessary or inappropriate treatments or mistakes.

The Quality in Australian Healthcare Study (Wilson *et al.*, 1995) revealed that 17 per cent of admissions were associated with an adverse event of which 51 per cent (8.3% of admissions) were assessed as preventable. The authors estimated that about 470 000 Australian patients annually experience an adverse event. Patients undergoing surgical procedures comprised about half the adverse events in the Australian and American studies (Weingart *et al.*, 2000).

Despite this evidence, health workers, patients and the community have been slow to act. The extent of injuries caused by healthcare treatments (iatrogenic illness) rather than the underlying diseases has long been recognized (Barr, 1956; Schimmel, 1964; McLamb and Huntley 1967; US Congress House Sub Committee on Oversight and Investigation 1976; Couch *et al.*, 1981; Steel *et al.*, 1981; Friedman, 1982; Dubois and Brook, 1988), but the degree to which the health system acknowledges them varies greatly across the system. The fact that many healthcare workers are ignorant of the extent of injury and that most errors do not cause harm may partly explain this. Medical mistakes affect one patient at a time, not all at the same time, or in the same place. This can camouflage the extent of errors in the system.

Role of regulation

I recently accompanied a resourceful and information-rich friend to his appointment with a surgeon. The surgeon's communication skills and his preparedness to answer questions about outcomes for competing treatments were important to my friend. He asked the surgeon how many times he had performed the procedure and was not put off when the surgeon said his results were not as good as others for one of the treatments. My friend was more interested in the effectiveness of the treatments than the surgeon's skills. He also appreciated the honesty of the surgeon and the fact that he kept records. His starting point like most patients was to presume his surgeon competent.

Public confidence of surgeons is underpinned by regulation and registration through the exclusion of doctors who are either not competent or fit to practice. Magee *et al.*'s (2003) study of consumers in the UK found that most expected a high standard irrespective of where they lived or what problem they had; they did not like the idea of 'shopping around'. At a minimum, patients expect surgeons to have the necessary knowledge, skills and experience for their condition. Licensing boards are trusted to set and maintain standards and patients believe their general practitioner would not refer them to an incompetent surgeon.

Patients who wish to choose their surgeon do not have a lot of information available to help them make a decision apart from the ability to verify qualifications. Medical registration authorities publish the names of doctors on the register and any restrictions applying to them, but there is great variation among these bodies in relation to other details they provide to the public. Typically, only the worst cases reach the public arena and then not until disciplinary action is completed. This means unsuspecting patients may seek and receive treatment even after serious concerns have been raised about a clinician's competence. Fears of innocent doctors suffering unfair publicity (Liptak, 2004) is often stated as a factor for delayed publicity. Another factor is the length of time it takes to adjudicate on these matters.

Complex environment

Medicine has changed greatly in the last 20 years. Technology, the size of the profession, specialization, sub-specialization and commercialization has intruded causing some unintended consequences. New procedures are being performed before evidence showing their benefits are available and surgeons sometimes perform procedures before they have been judged proficient (Topol, 1991; Topol and Califf, 1994). One of the dimensions of quality healthcare is 'effectiveness'. Patients should only be offered treatments that have been proved to be effective, and performed by doctors who have the knowledge, experience and skills necessary to treat them.

Historically, the medical profession has strongly resisted registration boards' attempts to either review or limit medical practice but new public demands for greater accountability have prompted registration authorities to establish programmes that authenticate current competence. New Zealand issues annual practising certificates to doctors. Canada has been conducting a comprehensive competence programme since 1988. The General Medical Council in the United Kingdom now requires doctors to 'revalidate' their credentials. An Australian state, New South Wales, conducts performance reviews for practitioners.

Technology has revolutionized medicine, and there are now many more treatment options available. Keeping up to date with all new information is very difficult and most patients do not expect their doctors to know everything about a particular disease or condition. But patients do expect the doctors who claim expertise in a particular area to have the skills and knowledge to make the claim. Many doctors embrace new technology but some of them are performing the procedures without sufficient training. Laws are inadequate in this area; once it was acceptable within medicine for surgeons to attend a weekend conference, observe a procedure and then perform it on patients. The market place may be important for setting price but it has no place for setting and maintaining standards of healthcare.

Expecting patients to choose a surgeon based on public report cards ignores the position of the patient in the doctor–patient relationship. How many patients ever choose their surgeon? Most patients trust their primary care physician or general practitioner's judgement and will accept a surgeon nominated by them without question or explanation. There is a lack of evidence that referring clinicians use public reports to make referrals. Instead, subjective factors such as familiarity, friendship, shared schooling experience or shared club memberships may be the reason for a referral.

Many hospitals collect de-identified outcome data on surgeons. While Western Australia has reported surgical outcome data for that state, there is yet no national standardized reporting or standardized reporting within hospitals. Some individual surgeons voluntarily maintain a complication and adverse event log which they may show their peer group but they do not routinely share their results with the broader community of surgeons, referring doctors or patients.

Role of healthcare teams

Public report cards also ignore the relationship between good surgical outcomes and contributions made by the healthcare team. Nurses, ward staff, assisting surgeons and anaesthetists all contribute their knowledge and skills; all are crucial for achieving a good post-operative outcome for the patient. In addition, hospital-wide systems for minimizing infection, timely consultations and appropriate discharge also contribute to good outcomes. Similarly suboptimal outcomes may involve more than the performance of the individual clinician; delayed referrals or delays in treatment may also be factors.

In principle, patients should be able to access any information about individual surgeons and hospitals that would assist them to make a decision but statistical data are difficult to understand (Valana and McGlynn, 2002). The type and format of information provided to patients and consumers is often determined by health professionals and managers. Consequently, much information is irrelevant to patients who may want different information reported in a variety of ways.

A new role for patients

The influential Institute of Medicine report *Crossing the Quality Chasm* (Institute of Medicine, 2001) recommended that patients should have access to scientific and personal information without restriction, delay or the need for anyone's permission. Applying this principle to surgery would require the exchange of information between the surgeon and the patient to be considered as important as discussions about the actual surgery or treatment plan: a relationship in which patients feel comfortable to discuss the surgeon's qualifications and training, skills and knowledge, performance and surgical results as well as the risks and benefits of the proposed treatment. Information would be interactive, available in real time, and be prospective as well as retrospective.

Patients as well as doctors need to change. But we do not know if patients are ready for such an active role. Even though we know that younger patients want higher levels of engagement and decision-making than older patients (Guadagnoli and Ward, 1998), this does not include them shopping around for the best surgeon. Surgeons have a leadership role and many are adapting new partnerships with patients and proactively discussing their level of experience, evidence supporting competing treatments and alternatives.

An important first step is for surgeons to measure what they do so that standardized reporting of surgical results can be provided. There is growing consensus on this issue but as yet no consensus on how best to measure results. Patients are not typically asked what it is that they want measured. What constitutes a 'good surgical outcome' for them? What types of performance data do patients need to help them make a decision? Excluding patients or making assumptions about their informational needs risks measuring components that patients find unhelpful.

Public reports of clinician performance have been shown to improve quality of health care (Peterson et al., 1998; Marshall, 2001). Doctors are known to be responsive to adverse reviews by their peers and will make the necessary practice adjustments. Poor reputation can impact on professional standing and referrals. Just as peer feedback can improve safety, patient feedback can improve quality of service and information.

There is growing recognition of the complexities associated with communicating treatment risks to patients. The range of treatments and the potential for complications and side effects necessitates open, two-way exchange of information and opinions about the risks between surgeons and their patients (Edwards and Elwyn, 2001). However, the process of providing accurate and complete information is complex. Firstly, patients vary in their perceptions of the level of risk associated with treatments and, secondly, clinicians have varied levels of knowledge and skills to provide such information to patients.

One of the reasons making it difficult for patients to make decisions rests with the nature of scientific uncertainties and the trade-offs they must consider between the positives and negatives of the treatment options. Lack of knowledge, unclear values and inadequate support from doctors, other health professionals and carers are also factors (O'Connor et al., 2003). Many clinicians do not know how to convey risk to patients in ways they understand; many use confusing explanations of risk such as talking about absolute and relative risk. The few standardized risk communication tools available mean patients are informed about risk in a variety of ways with variable effect. How risk information is framed is also known to influence patients' decisions (Wragg et al.,

2000). When doctors are trained in methods to assist patients to better understand risks, patients will have a greater understanding of the decisions they make (Thornton, 2003).

Conclusions

The medico-legal environment influences how doctors manage mistakes (Applegate, 1986; Kapp, 1997; Vincent *et al.*, 1999). Studies (Novack *et al.*, 1989; Kapp, 1997; Sweet and Bernat, 1997; Green *et al.*, 2000) of the disclosure of medical errors by physicians show a variety of reasons for not telling patients. Fear of litigation (Kapp, 1997; Bayliss, 1997) is the most common for not disclosing while a concern for the patient's right to know the truth of their condition (Sweet and Bernat, 1997) was the main reason for disclosing. The extent to which medico-legal fears influence surgeons' reports of adverse events is unknown.

Patients with genuine choice can only decide after being giving all the relevant information about the treatment, the provider and the facility. Respect for autonomy translates into surgeons anticipating situations where patients will sometimes make an apparently irrational decision, such as refusal of treatment. Genuine choice also anticipates genuine refusal.

Much health activity is obscured from public view. Information about peer review, morbidity and mortality meetings, quality assurance audits and medical record reviews is not yet available. Fear of litigation, misunderstanding of confidentiality, legal instructions and professional sovereignty have compromised open communication. Until patients and doctors are genuine partners, public reports will have limited success.

The evidence shows that micro-activities impact on consumers choices more than macro-level data. The neighbour's experience, the quality of the last encounter and current stories in the media are known to influence patients' decisions. Changes in practice at the doctor–patient level are required before consumers can make sense of information at the macro-level. Sharing information with patients and encouraging them to be active participants will help bring about partnerships. Only after patients feel comfortable questioning their surgeons face-to-face will they be ready to trust and use public reports.[2]

Notes

1. New York State (1991), Pennsylvania (1992), and New Jersey (1994) have public reporting of individual cardiac surgeons' performance.
2. Thanks to Asssociate Professor Jill Gordon for her comments.

References

Applegate, W. (1986). Physician management of patients with adverse outcomes. *Archives of Internal Medicine*, 2294–52.

Barr, D. (1956). Hazards of modern diagnosis and therapy – the price we pay. *Journal of the American Medical Association*, **159**, 1452–6.

Baylis, F. (1997). Errors in medicine: nurturing truthfulness. *The Journal of Clinical Ethics*, **8**, 336–41.

Brennan, T. A., Leape, L. L., Laird, N. M. *et al.* (1991). Incidence of adverse events and negligence in hospitalized patients: results of the Harvard Medical Practice Study I. *New England Journal of Medicine*, **324**, 370–6.

Brennan, T. A., Sox, C. M. and Burstin, H. R. (1996). Relation between negligent adverse events and the outcomes of medical-malpractice litigation. *New England Journal of Medicine*, **335**, 1963.

Couch, N. P., Tilney, N. L., Rayner, A. A. and Moore, F. D. (1981). The high cost of low-frequency events: the anatomy and economics of surgical mishaps. *New England Journal of Medicine*, **304**, 634–7.

Davis, P., Lay Yee, R., Briant, R., Ah, W., Scott, A. and Schug, S. (2001). Adverse events in New Zealand public hospitals: principal findings from a national survey. Occasional Paper 3, Wellington: New Zealand Ministry of Health.

Dubois, R. and Brook, R. (1988). Preventable deaths: who, how often, and why? *Annals of Internal Medicine*, **109**, 582–9.

Duckett, S. and Hunter, L. (1999). *Health services policy review: final report*. Melbourne: Victorian Department of Human Services. http://www.dhs.vic.gov.au/ahs/archive/servrev/servrev.pdf. Accessed 6th October 2004.

Edwards, A. G. and Elwyn, G. (2001). *Evidence-based Patient Choice – Inevitable or Impossible?* Oxford: Oxford University Press.

Friedman, M. (1982). Iatrogenic disease: addressing a growing epidemic. *Post Graduate Medicine*, **71**, 123–9.

Gawande, A. T., Zinner, M. J. and Brennan, T. A. (1999). The incidence and nature of surgical adverse events in Colorado and Utah in 1992. *Surgery*, **126**, 66–75.

Green, M., Farber, N. J. and Ubel, P. A. (2000). Lying to each other: when internal medicine residents use deception with their colleagues. *Archives of Internal Medicine*, **160**, 2317–23.

Guadagnoli, E. and Ward, P. (1998). Patient participation in decision-making. *Social Science Medicine*, **47**, 329–39.

Hibbard, J. H. and Jewitt, J. J. (1997). Will quality report cards help consumers? *Health Affairs*, **16**, 218–28.

Institute of Medicine (2001). *Crossing the Quality Chasm: A New Health System for the 21st Century*. Washington DC: National Academy Press.

Kapp, M. (1997). Legal anxieties and medical mistakes. *Journal of General Internal Medicine*, **12**, 787–8.

Liptak, A. (2004). Death puts spotlight on a doctor and regulators. *The New York Times*. New York.

Magee, H., Davis, L. and Coulter, A. (2003). Public views on healthcare performance indicators and patient choices. *Journal of the Royal Society of Medicine*, **96**, 338–42.

Marshall, M. N. (2001). Accountability and quality improvement: the role of report cards. *Quality and Safety in Health Care*, **10**, 67–8.

McLamb, J. and Huntley, R. (1967). The hazards of hospitalization. *Southern Medical Association Journal*, **60**, 469–72.

Mennemyer, S. T., Morrisey, M. A. and Howard, L. Z. (1997). Death and reputation: how consumers acted upon HCFA mortality information. *Inquiry*, **34**, 117–28.

Millenson, M. L. (2002). Breaking bad news. *Quality and Safety in Health Care*, **11**, 206–7.

Novack, D. H., Detering, B. J., Arnold, R., Forrow, L., Ladinsky, M. and Pezzullo, J. C. (1989). Physicians' attitudes towards using deception to resolve ethical problems. *Journal of the American Medical Association*, **26**, 2980–6.

O'Connor, A. M., Legare, F. and Stacey, D. (2003). Risk communication in practice: the contribution of decision aids. *British Medical Journal*, **327**, 736–40.

Peterson, E. D., DeLong, E. R., Jollis, J. E., Muhlbaier, L. H. and Mark, D. B. (1998). The effect of New York's bypass surgery provider profiling on access to care and patient outcomes in the elderly. *Journal of the American College of Cardiology*, **32**, 993–9.

Romano, P. (2003). *Outcomes of Hospital Outcomes Study*. Springfield VA: National Technical Information Service.

Schimmel, E. (1964). The hazards of hospitalization. *Annals of Internal Medicine*, **60**, 100–10.

Schneider, E. C. and Epstein, A. M. (1998). Use of public performance reports. *Journal of the American Medical Association*, **279**, 1638–42.

Secker-Walker, J. and Taylor-Adams, S. (2001). *Clinical Incident Reporting. Clinical Risk Management*, ed. C. Vincent. London: British Medical Journal Books.

Spiegelhalter, D., Murray, G. and McPherson, K. (2000). *Monitoring Clinical Performance: A Statistical Perspective*. Bristol: Bristol Royal Infirmary Inquiry.

Starr, P. (1982). *The Social Transformation of American Medicine*. New York: Basic Books.

Steel, K., Gertman, P. M., Crescenzi, C. and Anderson, J. (1981). Iatrogenic illness on a general medical practice service at a university hospital. *New England Journal of Medicine*, **304**, 638–42.

Sweet, M. P. and Bernat, J. L. (1997). A study of the ethical duty of physicians to disclose errors. *Journal of Clinical Ethics*, **8**, 341–8.

Thornton, H. (2003). Patients' understanding of risk. *British Medical Journal*, **327**, 693–4.

Topol, E. J. (1991). Promises and pitfalls of new devices for coronary artery disease. *Circulation*, **83**, 689–94.

Topol, E. J. and Califf, R. M. (1994). Scorecard cardiovascular medicine: its impact and future directions. *Annals of Internal Medicine*, **120**, 65–70.

US Congress House Sub Committee on Oversight and Investigation (1976). *Cost and Quality of Health Care: Unnecessary Surgery*, Washington DC: USGPO.

Valana, M. E. and McGlynn, E. A. (2002). What cognitive science tells us about the design of reports for consumers. *Medical Care Research Reviews*, **59**, 3–35.

Vincent, C., Stanhope, N. and Crowley-Murphy, M. (1999). Reasons for not reporting adverse incidents: an empirical study. *Journal of Evaluation in Clinical Practice*, **5**, 13–21.

Vincent, C., Neale, G. and Woloshynowych, M. (2001). Adverse events in British hospitals: preliminary retrospective record review. *British Medical Journal*, **322**, 517–19.

Weingart, S. N., Wilson, R. M., Gibberd, R. W. and Harrison, B. (2000). Epidemiology of medical error. *British Medical Journal*, **320**, 774–7.

Wilson, R. M., Runciman, W. B., Gibberd, R. W., Harrison, B. T., Newby, L. and Hamilton, J. D. (1995). The quality in Australian health care study. *Medical Journal of Australia*, **163**, 458–71.

Wragg, J. A., Robinson, E. J. and Liliford, R. J. (2000). Information presentation and decision to enter clinical trials: a hypothetical trial of hormone replacement therapy. *Social Science and Medicine*, **51**, 453–62.

5

Adverse event disclosure: benefits and drawbacks for patients and clinicians

Paul Barach

University of South Florida, USA

Michael D. Cantor

Harvard Medical School, USA

Introduction

Since the Institute of Medicine (1999) published *To Err is Human* in 1999, many publications have discussed the need for different approaches to disclosing adverse events to patients, and the need to create a culture of safety within the healthcare system. Many of these articles begin with a clinician discussing an adverse event in which they were involved (Richards, 2000; Wu, 2001; Payne, 2002). Each individual story provides the medical and policy communities with an isolated view of an adverse event and the disclosure or non-disclosure of that event to the patient. There have also been research papers in the legal and medical literature that are designed to address specific areas of disclosure (Popp, 2003; Wu, 2000). Error disclosure is now required by ethicists, professional organizations and increasingly by regulatory bodies.

The goal of this chapter is to combine these accounts, stories and recommendations into a coherent roadmap for guidance in the field of disclosure. To accomplish this goal, we will begin by defining key terms, and will provide evidence that disclosure is a central part of fostering a safety culture. We will examine physician report cards and their relationship to disclosure policies. We will address the significant gap that exists between the principle of error disclosure and actual practice. Although most of the literature on disclosure is based on in-patient adverse event occurrences, most of healthcare occurs in the ambulatory setting. We believe that the principles outlined below apply equally well to the ambulatory setting, but clearly require adapting the actual process of disclosure to accommodate the different time and location of outpatient care. This chapter will then examine the ethical, legal, and regulatory frameworks governing disclosure, and the benefits and drawbacks of disclosure.

Informed Consent and Clinician Accountability: The Ethics of Report Cards on Surgeon Performance. Steve Clarke and Justin Oakley (eds.). Published by Cambridge University Press. © Cambridge University Press 2007.

Definitions

The literature is full of different and conflicting definitions for the same terms, but in this chapter the term 'disclosure' is defined as *any time a member of the clinical team reveals to a patient or the patient's surrogate the occurrence of an adverse event, whether or not this includes an apology and information about causation and responsibility for the event.* An adverse event is defined as 'an event in which preventable harm was caused to the patient' (Jackson Memorial Hospital, 2002). This includes incidents that may or may not be subject to mandatory reporting, such as decubitus ulcers and hospital-acquired infections.

Defining the process of disclosure

Disclosure of adverse events requires a process that will enable clinicians and health care organizations to disclose the occurrence of an adverse event, apologize if warranted, and work to redress the harms suffered by the patient. A detailed discussion of such a process is beyond the scope of this chapter, and there are examples of policies and procedures for disclosure of adverse events in the literature (Devita, 2001; Kraman and Hamm, 1999; Cantor, 2005). However, there are a few key principles that should guide how disclosure is managed.

Criteria should be developed that determine what types of adverse events need to be disclosed, when the disclosure will occur, who will make the disclosure, and how it will be done. Not every adverse event needs to be disclosed: only those that caused significant harm, were not foreseen prior to the care being provided, and require a change in care must be disclosed. One successful approach is a multi-step process similar to that developed at the Lexington, KY, VA Medical Center (Kraman and Hamm, 1999), where a *clinical disclosure* is usually done, firstly, by the clinicians involved in the case, and which only provides basic information about what happened, and advises that an investigation is being launched. The *institutional disclosure* occurs later, and includes the leadership from the healthcare organization, provides an opportunity for an apology if warranted, an explanation of what happened, and advises what will be done to reduce the risk of similar harm to future patients. It is also used to offer compensation to patients for the harm they have suffered. This process also uses a carefully managed approach to create the right environment and to communicate effectively, similar to the approach developed by Buckman (1992) for use in breaking bad news to patients.

Why disclosure?

A major adverse event due to medical errors happens in 3 per cent of all hospitalizations. A 2003 study found that 18 specific human error injuries resulted in 2.4 million extra hospital days and \$9.3 billion in extra costs alone (Penson *et al.*, 2001; Rice, 2002). Disclosure of adverse events is justified because of ethical and legal obligations (see below) and, in addition, it fulfils an important need in the realm of patient safety and medical liability. Disclosure has the potential to significantly promote patient safety and improve error prevention. Much research has focused on the narrative of the event as key to defining and sustaining safety in high risk industries.

Obviously, the optimal solution to safety problems is to prevent all errors. However, safety science research demonstrates that humans make errors even when vigilant. The answer lies in creating safer systems that help to expose errors and to stop them from resulting in adverse events (Reason, 1997). Preventive systems, such as nuclear reactor safety systems, are known as front-end solutions because they are designed to prevent the event from occurring (Apostolakis and Barach, 2003). The danger of another Chernobyl or Three-Mile Island meltdown occurring has stopped all new nuclear power plant construction in the US. Unfortunately, no matter how carefully designed a front-end system is, there is still the possibility that it will fail. This happens because either the system was not comprehensive enough to capture all possibilities or because a 'work-around' (a way of getting around the procedural regulations) was created (Amalberti *et al.*, 2005). While it is true that higher levels of automation tend to reduce errors by decreasing human input into the system, technology can create its own potential cascade of errors, which can be more difficult to identify than human errors.

Ethical rationale for disclosure

There is widespread recognition that disclosing adverse events to patients is the ethically proper response (Cantor *et al*, 2005; Rosner *et al*, 2000; Sweet and Bernat, 1997; Wu *et al.*, 1997). Clinicians, however, face a difficult dilemma when deciding whether and how to disclose a harmful error to a patient. For healthcare professionals, there are three basic ethical rationales for this: utilitarian ethics, which argues that the approach that produces the most good is the proper course to follow (Mill, 1971); deontological, or duty-based ethics, that recognize that professionals have obligations to patients because of their special relationship with patients; and professional standards, that require members of that profession to put the needs and interests of patients ahead of the interests of the individual (Beauchamp and Childress, 2001). Similar reasoning applies to healthcare organizations, with utilitarian ethics supporting disclosure; deontological ethics pointing out that healthcare organizations have duties to patients for whom they provide care; and instead of professional standards, organizational codes of ethics that state organizational values and commit the institution to truth-telling and putting the needs of patients first.

Utilitarian ethics

Utilitarians argue that the process which produces maximum benefit and minimal harm is the proper approach. In the case of disclosing adverse events to patients, it is clear that the benefits of disclosure outweigh the harms. There is even an interest group now pushing for active disclosure of adverse events – a consumer-led group called the *Sorry Works! Coalition* (www.sorryworks.net) has brought together experts in law and medicine with patient representatives, to advocate for changes in organizational policies and state laws that would encourage disclosure of adverse events. Disclosure can result in several benefits to patients, including peace of mind because of the increased knowledge about what happened, better communication and a more trusting relationship with their healthcare providers. For healthcare professionals, disclosure results in relief from the emotional burden of making a mistake; opportunities to learn from errors and improve care in the future; opportunities to improve communication skills and strengthen the clinician–patient relationship; and potential reduction in litigation costs. For institutions, the major benefits are improvement in the quality of care because of greater availability of data on errors; increased transparency and trust from the community served; and a potential reduction in litigation costs.

Benefits for the patient

Patients may gain the most from the disclosure of adverse events. The first benefit for the patient is that disclosure can put the patient's mind at ease, though this may not always be the case. Surveys of patients and anecdotal evidence suggest that they want three things out of a disclosure: an explanation of what happened and why; an apology; and reassurance that something is being done to keep this from happening to the patient and other patients again (Mazor, Simon and Gurwitz, 2004). Research demonstrates that most patients want to be kept informed about the plan of care (Popp, 2003). Providing *consistent* information to the patient about an adverse event can be the sole factor that determines whether or not the patient pursues legal action. One noted physician has published a story recounting an incident where a patient was upset because the physician missed a digit fracture on an X-ray. Initially the patient threatened to sue their physician. The doctor quickly apologized to the patient and admitted the mistake. The patient then returned a few days later to apologize for his reaction and to state that he was not going to sue (Ryan, 1999). This story describes how an incensed patient was 'talked down' by his doctor admitting her mistake and apologizing for it. If we make the reasonable assumption that satisfied patients do not sue, this evidence supports the theory that proper disclosure to patients is reassuring (Hilborne and Kwon, 2000).

procedures are being done unnecessarily to allow opting out of the limited scope of the registry, such as adding a mitral valve plasty when doing a routine coronary bypass surgery (Werner and Asch, 2005).

Several obstacles confront these report cards, including technical measurement challenges, resistance to use these data tools, malpractice litigation concerns, and wariness with the reliability of these tools. The bar for admission of these data into the malpractice litigation appears at present too high and thus seems of limited concern. However, recent efforts in Florida, for example, in which all peer review protection has been pierced by legislation making physician deliberations vulnerable to legal discovery. These examples highlight the risk and challenges of all disclosure data (i.e. near miss as well as adverse event) being used against physicians in addressing patient adverse outcomes (Barach, 2005). This includes non-legal proceedings, such as hospital and state licensing and credentialing boards and other adjudicatory bodies, with more relaxed rules of evidence.

The future of physician performance reports suggests using aggregate patient encounters while focusing on the entire microsystem outcome – that is, the patient journey – and less on individual providers (Barach and Johnson, 2006). By doing this, regulators and insurers will help make these tools truly patient-centered and alleviate the physician concerns. By going down this path, report cards on individual clinicians would be more consistent with, or in the spirit of, adverse event disclosure, given that the latter tends to emphasize systems (in order to encourage greater openness and so promote safety), whereas report cards emphasize individual clinicians. The next few years will need to address this key tension to ensure wider acceptance of physician performance report cards.

Benefits for the healthcare organization

Healthcare organizations may benefit from disclosure, as liability can pass through from the clinician to the hospital or healthcare organization under operation of the common law. Thus, any of the legal benefits that accrue to the clinician will also transfer to the health care organization. This does not take into account the fact that there is a fiduciary duty that exists between the health care organization and the patient (Stewart, 2002; Horton, 1999). Because of this duty, non-disclosure not only prohibits the healthcare organization from gaining the potential legal benefits discussed above, but it might actually *increase* the potential liability of the healthcare organization.

Healthcare organizations should also consider the value of transparency, and growing evidence that disclosure cuts litigation costs. Society is increasingly placing a high value on being honest and forthcoming with information, especially when it is adverse. This generalization is based on the evidence that, while some legal experts have predicted that more disclosure would result in increased liability, the empirical evidence demonstrates that overall liability will likely decrease. The

Lexington, KY, Veterans Administration Medical Center (VAMC), has had a policy of 'extreme honesty' and active disclosure of adverse events since the mid-1980s (Kraman *et al.*, 2002; Lowes, 1997). After introducing the disclosure programme, the Lexington VAMC decreased its total payouts for medical negligence cases. Interestingly, even though the total number of payouts increased, the amount per payout decreased, largely because the medical centre worked with an injured patient or family member to arrive at a sum of money that would provide restitution for additional costs, and avoided punitive damage awards.

More recent evidence has come from medical negligence insurers. COPIC, a major medical malpractice insurance carrier in Colorado, has the '3Rs' programme where physicians participate in a programme to 'Recognize, Respond to and Resolve' adverse events. According to COPIC's 3Rs programme newsletter, in the first 3 years of the programme, there were 435 qualifying incidents, and 153 payouts, with an average cost of $1820 (Copic, 2004). This amount is in contrast to the average cost of all COPIC claims, which was $78 741 per claim, including claims where nothing was paid. The average cost of a typical case where payment was made was in excess of $250 000, in contrast to the 3Rs claims, where the maximum payout was $26 566 and the minimum was $100. Overall, claims have dropped 50% since the programme started, and settlement costs have declined 23% (Kowalczyk, 2005). Similarly, at the University of Michigan Healthcare System, a programme of active disclosure has cut claims in half and reduced attorneys' fees from $3 million a year to $1.25 million per year (Shapiro, 2000).

Society values and will reward a healthcare organization that is transparent and forthcoming with adverse event data. There is evidence that media and regulators are much less hostile to a healthcare organization when a medical error is admitted, and the general public does not have to find out about the error from secondary sources (Pietro *et al.*, 2000). This approach allows the healthcare facility to be proactive and control the narrative, and make it a story about recovery from an adverse event rather than the adverse event itself.

Overall, disclosure of adverse events can lead to increased patient satisfaction, increased trust in the physician, more positive emotional support for patients and professionals, and a decreased chance that the patient will change physicians after the event is disclosed (Mazor *et al.*, 2004). Given that there are multiple benefits to disclosure, why is it still not done universally?

The risks and costs of disclosure

While the potential benefits of a system of disclosure are great, there are also drawbacks. Although disclosure can be beneficial, it appears that most people are so concerned with the potential drawbacks that they fail to act in a way that would capture the benefits of disclosure. Thus, in order to form an effective physician and team are part of the hospital. Additionally, the healthcare organization needs to consider a potential 'conflict of obligations', since it has a duty to help and protect its patients, and a similar responsibility to its staff and clinicians.

The balancing of the healthcare organizations' conflict of obligations is an interesting challenge (Stewart, 2002; Nowicki and Chaku, 1998). The difference between clinicians and the healthcare executives is that the clinician's self-interest affects only the clinician, while the executive's duty affects all employees and patients of the organization. If one accepts the legal arguments that disclosure reduces malpractice payments, it would appear that the healthcare organizations may benefit from full disclosure. However, there are some cases where disclosing the adverse event will harm the organization, whether it is through financial costs, bad publicity, or increased regulatory scrutiny and required corrective actions. Organizational leaders managing such cases face a conflict of obligations – what is best for the patient (disclosure), is harmful to the organization. Upholding both duties is not possible – if disclosure takes place, the organization suffers, if it does not take place, then the patient suffers.

The other drawback that healthcare organizations could face from disclosure is an increase in scrutiny from regulators. Just as clinicians have been reprimanded for being forthcoming about flaws in the system, healthcare organizations can be punished if they fully disclose what is happening within the organization. For example, Duke University Medical Center in the US has recently become a favorite target of regulators after they disclosed an adverse event in which a 17-year-old patient died after receiving a lung transplant from a donor with a different blood type, a known cause of rejection of implanted organs (Campion, 2003). This places healthcare organizations in a difficult position: if they disclose they might be punished, but whether and how they are punished may depend on the severity of the incident. It is also possible that organizations that foster a culture of transparency and disclosure will ultimately be rewarded for this by regulators who recognize the benefits of that approach.

Duty-based ethics

Clinicians and organizations have obligations because of their special relationships with patients that require them to act as fiduciaries and put the needs of the patient ahead of their own. This duty comes from several sources: respect for patient autonomy, and the recognition that patients need complete information in order to make treatment decisions; the need to act as a fiduciary; and because truth-telling enhances and supports patient trust (Cantor *et al.*, 2005). The implication of this duty is that professionals and the organizations they work for are obligated to disclose adverse events, even if it is not beneficial for them to do so, which is in some ways a stronger argument than the utilitarian model, since the duty-based model does not require balancing of harms and benefits (Greely, 1999).

Professional ethics and organizational values

Healthcare professionals are also bound by the values of their profession to tell patients the truth and put the interests of patients ahead of their own. Professional codes of ethics for physicians, nurses and other healthcare professionals uniformly require truth telling, and by extension, disclosure of adverse events. Healthcare organizations are bound by analogous statements of organizational values and mission. For example, the mission of the Veterans Health Administration (2005) is to 'Honor America's veterans by providing exceptional health care that improves their health and well-being.' Embedded within this statement are the core values and beliefs that support provision of high-quality care that helps veterans, and the willingness to disclose and provide for redress when adverse events occur.

Conclusions

Disclosing adverse events is a complex process, but it is increasingly recognized as an important aspect of providing care of patients. Clinicians and organizations have clear ethical obligations to tell the truth about what happened, and to do it in a way that is sensitive, yet informative and clear. A growing body of evidence demonstrates that the benefits of disclosure outweigh the burdens, and that effective disclosure can improve patient safety, quality of care, and reduce costs. Although the ultimate goal is to avoid and eliminate adverse events, it is important to have mechanisms to mitigate the damage caused by these events, and disclosure is an important strategy for mitigation and improvement. Attributing errors to systems failures does not absolve physicians of their duty to care. Disclosure adds to their responsibility to participate in redesign of a safer system.

References

Amalberti, R., Auroy, Y., Berwick, D. and Barach, P. (2005). Five system barriers to achieving ultrasafe health care. *Annals of Internal Medicine*, **142**, 756–64.

Anderson, E. (2001). Learning from my mistakes. *Medical Economics*, **78**, January 8.

Apostolakis, G. and Barach, P. (2003). Lessons learned from nuclear power. In *Patient Safety, International Textbook*, ed. M. Hatlie and K. Tavill. New York: Aspen Publications, pp. 205–25.

Do report cards or performance monitoring reduce complications for patients?

The evidence that feedback of analysed performance data to clinicians can contribute to improved performance is now consistent and widespread. Some of the early work is worth examining to identify factors contributing to the success of the data collection and factors that may be irrelevant.

S. M. Shortell was an early contributor to the healthcare Quality Improvement (QI) literature, and using a QI project in a Los Angeles Urology practice, he and his co-workers demonstrated that timely, appropriate feedback of analysed data improved the outcomes of operative surgery for all practitioners (Shortell *et al.*, 1998; Shortell, 1995). Mark Chassin, as CEO of New York State Department of Health, set up a mandatory data collection in hospitals undertaking cardiac surgery and interventional cardiology. He demonstrated that, by mandating data collection in New York State hospitals undertaking cardiac interventions, there was a demonstrable, consistent reduction in mortality for all interventions (Hannan *et al.*, 1994). The seminal paper describing the success of the data collection with respect to reduced mortality rates for coronary artery surgery observed a reduction in mortality rates of 40% over 3 years for similar patients with identical risk of death prior to surgery (Hannan *et al.*, 1994). Although there were immediate detractors from the New York State scheme, the early theoretical criticisms raised have remained merely hypothetical (Green and Wintfeld, 1995). A separate analysis, to try to clarify some of the theoretical objections to the conclusions produced by Chassin's group that were raised by Green and Wintfeld, was undertaken by Chassin. This analysis provided no evidence to support these criticisms (Chassin, 2002). The outstanding reduction in mortality can now be attributed to improved surgical team and institutional performance.

Another group working in northeast USA soon supported the validity of the early conclusions by Chassin's team. O'Connor and co-workers, in a similar project, undertaken on a voluntary basis by clinicians working in hospitals providing cardiac surgery services, came up with similar findings (O'Connor *et al.*, 1996). The voluntary aspect of the data collection set up by O'Connor and co-workers is important. It indicates that surgical teams can be encouraged to collect the data for the right reasons. Thus the teams are not merely collecting the data because doing so enables them to continue to practice in the field or the hospital, which was the requirement in the New York State study. Surgical teams are collecting the data in order to improve their performance, and this step improvement in their ethical attitude to data collection must be emphasized and acknowledged. Some authors would consider that such surgical teams had moved beyond the 'Four Principles' of medical ethics (Autonomy, Beneficence, Non-maleficence and Justice) enunciated by

Beauchamp and Childress (1973), and had adopted a more 'virtue-based' approach to their professional practice (Bolsin, Faunce and Oakley, 2005). This improvement in ethical behaviour is a point worth emphasizing because ethical behaviour has been shown to deteriorate during training of medical students (Goldie *et al.*, 2003). This deterioration has been attributed to the 'informal' or 'hidden' curriculum of medical training (Hundert *et al.*, 1996; Hafferty and Franks, 1994). In fact, the process is known to begin early in medical training and is well advanced by the time of graduation (Goldie *et al.*, 2003; Goldie, 2004). The cause of the deterioration is difficult to pin point, but the role models provided by junior medical staff have been suggested as a powerful influence towards bad (and sometimes good) ethical behaviour (Paice *et al.*, 2002; Paice *et al.*, 2004). Thus we propose that the collection of surgical outcome data for complex surgical interventions and the feedback to individual surgeons, teams and institutions in a meaningful manner can lead to improved surgical performance. But, we also assert that, if this process occurs as part of a voluntary data collection process, then ethical as well as clinical standards have improved.

These early studies demonstrated the value of feedback to practitioners of risk-adjusted mortality (outcome) data, but are there more valuable data on performance that could be employed? Marc de Leval, working in the field of paediatric cardiac surgery in the UK, used an industrial Quality Assurance methodology, Cumulative summation or Cusum, to identify loss of skill or competence at a particular complex operation, the 'arterial switch' procedure (de Leval *et al.*, 1994). He described re-acquiring competence at that operation through a process of retraining. Kestin and co-workers used the same statistical methodology to identify acquisition of practical skills in anaesthetic trainees (Kestin, 1995). Thus, we have the ability to feed back not only information that will improve the performance of the surgical team at an institution, but we are also in a position to use these data to demonstrate acquisition of competence at individual procedures, and, as a consequence, are able to statistically demonstrate loss of competence (Bolsin, 2000; Bolsin and Colson, 2000; Colson and Bolsin, 2003). This is one of the measures that accreditation, credentialing and professional colleges have attempted to produce for many years. The information is extremely easy to obtain and is of significant value to the clinician, employing organisation, and credentialing agencies (Bolsin, Faunce and Colson, 2005; Bolsin *et al.*, 2005).

At Geelong Hospital we use the same statistical methodology to monitor trainee and specialist performance. However, we include the data collection on a mobile computing platform using a personal digital assistant (PDA) (Bent *et al.*, 2002). The value of PDA technology is that it allows data collection at the time of undertaking the assessed task (Bolsin *et al.*, 2005). The data entry is undertaken initially by the trainee, guided by a supervisor of training, but later becomes a task the trainee is encouraged to complete without supervision.

trusted and acted upon, then they must respect the methods of collection and the source of the analysis (Hannan, 1996; Hannan *et al.*, 1997; Green and Wintfeld 1995). When data collection is suspected as having been dubious, then the analysis that can be undertaken and the value that the analysis contributes can both be reduced (Aylin *et al.*, 2001).

Thirdly, the feedback of the information must be timely and relevant. An example of data feedback that has taken years to achieve is the reports of the Victorian Consultative Council on Morbidity and Mortality (VCCAMM). The 2004 Report contained analysis of data from the years 1996–1999 (Mackay, 2004). The current Chairman of VCCAMM sees this as an unacceptable delay related to the time required to collect and analyse incidents using the original methodology (Personal communication A/Prof Larry McNichol, Chairman VCCAMM). The value added to the data collected by the analysis must be relevant to the clinician and provide extra information that is not immediately available from the raw data. Such timely and appropriate analysis will be valued and sought after by clinicians.

Lastly, the data collection must be relatively easy to undertake, if the clinician is required to complete the task (Kingston *et al.*, 2004). Furthermore, the task of data collection should not be time-consuming but should be designed to take as little time as possible (Bolsin, Faunce and Oakley, 2005; Bent *et al.*, 2002; Kingston *et al.*, 2004; Bolsin, 2005). Data collections using these guidelines are much more likely to be completed by busy clinicians, and to contribute to valuable ongoing database analysis (Bolsin *et al.*, 2005; Chassin, 2002; White, 2004; Runciman 2002). Furthermore, data collections with analysis and feedback showing these features are also much more likely to be valued by clinicians, and the information contained therein is thus more likely to be acted on to change practice (Bolsin *et al.*, 2005; Shortell *et al.*, 1998; Hannan *et al.*, 1994; Chassin, 2002; Spiegelhalter *et al.*, 2003).

What are the barriers to enhanced performance reporting?

The generational factors involved in the introduction of new technology to a complex industry such as healthcare are an obvious barrier to uniform rapid adoption of enhanced performance reporting along the lines we have suggested. This assertion is emphasized by Sir Donald Irvine, who cites the 'Bristol Cardiac Disaster' as pivotal to the change in attitudes that occurred in the medical profession and also the General Medical Council in the 1990s (Irvine 1999; Irvine 2004a, 2006a, 2006b). Coupled with the revelations in the UK about the GP Dr Harold Shipman and the 'rogue' gynaecologist Anthony Ledward, the public pressure for the profession to change their ethical stance was irresistible (Irvine 2004a, 2006a, 2006b; Klein, 1998). Similar changes are being urged in Australia in response to parallel disclosures and inquiries revealing sub-standard care in many different states including the problems associated with the rogue surgeon at Bundaberg hospital (Faunce and Bolsin, 2004). Sir Donald Irvine picked up this similarity in a requirement for ethical change during a trip to Australia in 2004 (Irvine, 2004b). We would suggest that, in fact, the old ethical standards were inadequate and always suspect, relying as they did on clinical autonomy and a professional collegial stance that did not serve patients' best interests. One important component of this analysis is to identify the characteristics of the senior and middle management represented in the Federal, State, professional and organizational structures providing the leadership to healthcare policy makers, healthcare providers and healthcare professionals across Australia.

One of the conclusions from this analysis is that the medical profession has not always been ethically sound in its dealing with patients and the general public. This conclusion is partly supported by the publications of Sir Donald Irvine, who is the past President of the General Medical Council in the UK (Irvine, 2006a, 2006b; Smith, 1998). In 1997 Sir Donald identified that the implementation of a coherent strategy of quality-assured professional self-regulation would require 'a clear ethical framework' (Irvine, 1997). In 2004 Sir Donald stated, 'There was the widening gap between the profession's laid-back approach to accountability and transparency, and the public's increasingly explicit requirements. Hence, the growing public criticism of the profession's secretive attitude to risk and to the disclosure of information that would shed light on doctors' personal conduct and performance' (Irvine, 2004a). Sir Donald identified the need for a cultural change in the profession and set about producing 'a New Professionalism' for doctors the United Kingdom (Irvine, 1999, 2004a, 2004b). Commenting on a publication from the Royal College of Physicians of London, Sir Donald proposes that the basis for a new 'moral contract' be a commitment to integrity, compassion, altruism, continuous improvement, excellence and partnership in healthcare care teams (Irvine, 2006b).

At the conclusion of the GMC Disciplinary Committee hearing into the professional behaviour of the paediatric cardiac surgeons and CEO in Bristol, Richard Smith, in his now famous editorial entitled 'All changed, changed utterly', stated 'The Bristol case has already accelerated the move to provide patients with data on the performance of doctors and hospitals, and this has to be a good outcome' (Smith, 1998). This move was seen as linked to improved professional and ethical standards, and implies that the pre-existing ethical standard was inadequate or less satisfactory. Summarizing the history of the GMC in 2006, Sir Donald Irvine concluded that 'The stark reality is that, from the beginning in 1858 right up to the early 1990s, statutory self-regulation as operated by the GMC failed the public and conscientious doctors' (Irvine, 2006a). In the same article he also states 'But in the case of the British medical profession the underlying cause is surely professional culture. In too many ways the culture today still reflects medical practice as it was in the latter half of the 19th and first half of the 20th centuries' (Irvine, 2006a). This was an outmoded culture of paternalism, self-protection and introspection. While not criticizing all medical practice as unethical, we would assert that in the area of informed consent, performance monitoring and healthcare errors, the profession has tended to behave unethically for many years, and this breach must be urgently addressed.

What evidence exists to help us decide which possibility is the most likely to explain the attitudes of the management of our healthcare structures? The evidence we have accumulated suggests that the medical profession has certainly subverted the ethical standards of its trainees in the medical curriculum, with many authors describing 'hidden' or 'informal' ethics curricula at work in medical school training as recently as 2004 (Bolsin, 2003; Goldie *et al.*, 2003; Hundert *et al.*, 1996; Hafferty and Franks, 1994). Other evidence comes from the attitudes to implementation of the type of performance monitoring programme described in this chapter. Funding for these monitoring projects from professional bodies has been obtained only from the Australian and New Zealand College of Anaesthetists (ANZCA). However United Medical Protection, the Victorian Managed Insurance Authority, the Medical Defence Association of Victoria and the Federal Department of Trade and Industry (DTI) have committed other contributions. The affiliations of the sponsors indicate that, while insurers and medical indemnity organizations consider programmes for collecting performance data to be a considerable advance on current clinical governance arrangements, there is little support from the profession, healthcare managers and credentialing organizations, for whom there would be considerable benefit. Furthermore, the allocation of AU$500 000 from the DTI, to develop the other specialty versions of the programme indicates a belief at Federal level that the thinking underlying the model will lead to commercial and healthcare benefits in the future.

The striking absence from the list of sponsors or funding organizations apart from the ANZCA is any senior healthcare safety or quality organization. Our concern is that many patients, providers and payers of healthcare cannot afford to wait passively for that change. Too many patients will die unnecessarily, and too many unnecessary costs to healthcare funding bodies will have been incurred, for inaction to be a reasonable option for these groups.

Conclusions

Although the interest in report cards to date has centred on complex surgical interventions, there is no reason to consider that other specialties should not be subject to similar assessments (Bolsin, 2000; Bolsin and Colson, 2000; Bolsin and Day, 1998; Colson and Bolsin, 2003; Spiegelhalter *et al.*, 2003; Bolsin and

Colson, 2003). In a retrospective analysis of mortality data from UK General practices, Speigelhalter and co-workers demonstrated that such an analysis of routinely collected data (if it had been current at the time) would have detected the abnormally high mortality rate of patients in Dr Harold Shipman's practice, and could have triggered an inquiry after as few as 40 deaths had occurred (Spiegelhalter *et al.*, 2003). Thus, the analysis of routinely collected outcome data in General Practice in the UK NHS could lead to the early detection of both adverse and favourable trends in that practice. This could identify and eradicate potential bad practice, and could identify and encourage the spread of practices associated with improved patient outcomes (Bolsin, 2000). Thus, it is possible to conclude that no specialty is too complex or non-procedural to make it immune or insulated from the voluntary collection of outcome data (Bolsin, 2000; Bolsin and Day, 1998). The potential benefit of a 40% reduction in risk-adjusted mortality over 3 years suggested in the studies by both Hannan and co-workers and O'Connor and co-workers, is too large an improvement to ignore (Hannan *et al.*, 1994; O'Connor *et al.*, 1996).

Conversely, we would consider that the number of deaths and iatrogenic injuries that would result from failing to implement such data collections is an unjustified risk to future patient safety. Medicine has been aware of its contribution to patient mortality and morbidity for hundreds of years. More recently, detailed studies of the developed healthcare systems of the Western world have confirmed that 'medical error' and 'systems failings' still contribute to adverse outcomes for patients. However, at the same time, the medical literature contains many studies demonstrating the improvements in performance that result from the feedback of outcome data to practising clinicians (Shortell, 1998; Hannan *et al.*, 1994; O'Connor *et al.*, 1996). Thus, report cards improve practice and save lives, and we can count the lives saved. Furthermore, it has been demonstrated that analysis and feedback of routinely collected data in paediatric cardiac surgery and UK General Practice would have led to the early identification of poor outcomes at the Bristol Royal Infirmary and in Harold Shipman's general practice (Spiegelhalter *et al.*, 2003). An estimated minimum number of 200 lives were lost as a result of not having this routine analysis.

Early mandatory data collections were necessary to ensure uniform collection of data of the required quality for trusted analysis and feedback of information that was valued by the participating clinicians (Hannan *et al.*, 1994). Subsequent voluntary data collections have demonstrated similar quality improvements as well as an improved ethical standard (Bolsin, Faunce and Oakley, 2005; Bolsin, 2000; O'Connor *et al.*, 1996; Bent *et al.*, 2002; Clarke and Oakley, 2004). The next step in improving that ethical standard will be to make the data available to the patient and public as part of the consent to treatment process (Clarke and Oakley, 2004). When these stages have been followed through, it will be possible for those members of the medical and healthcare professions participating in such voluntary, open data collections to demonstrate that not only are they actively contributing data to optimise outcomes for their patients, but they are also demonstrating an improved standard of ethical behaviour over those data collections which were mandatory and secret to the profession.

References

Aylin, P., Alves, B., Best, N. *et al.* (2001). Comparison of UK paediatric cardiac surgical performance by analysis of routinely collected data 1984–96: was Bristol an outlier? *The Lancet*, **358**, 181–7.

Beauchamp, T. L. and Childress, J. F. (1973). *Principles of Biomedical Ethics*. 1st edn., New York: Oxford University Press.

Becher, E. C. and Chassin, M. R. (2001). Improving the quality of health care: who will lead? *Health Affairs*, **20**, 164–79.

Benson, K. and Hartz, A. J. (2000). A comparison of observational studies and randomised controlled trials. *New England Journal of Medicine*, **342**, 1878–86.

Bent, P., Creati, B., Bolsin, S. N., Colson, M. and Patrick, A. (2002). Professional monitoring and critical incident reporting using personal digital assistants. *Medical Journal of Australia*, **177**, 496–9.

Bion, J. F. and Heffner, J. E. (2004). Challenges in the care of the acutely ill. *The Lancet*, **363**, 970–7.

Black, N. (1997). Developing high quality clinical databases. *British Medical Journal*, **315**, 381–2.

Black, N. (1999a). High-quality clinical databases: breaking down barriers. *The Lancet*, **353**, 1205–6.

Black, N. (1999b). What observational studies can offer decision makers. *Hormone Research*, **51** (Suppl. 1), 44–9.

Black, N. and Payne, M. (2003). Directory of clinical databases: improving and promoting their use. *Quality and Safety in Health Care*, **12**, 348–52.

Bolsin, S. N. (2000). Routes to Quality Assurance: Risk adjusted outcomes and personal professional monitoring. *International Journal for Quality in Health Care*, **12**, 367–9.

Bolsin, S. N. (2003). Whistle blowing. *Medical Education*, **37**, 294–6.

Bolsin, S. N. (2005). Personal digital assistants (PDAs) – improving patients' safety. *British Medical Journal*, **331**, 57–8.

Bolsin, S. N. and Day, C. J. (1998). Risk evaluation, quality of practice and audit. In *A Short Practice of Anaesthesia*, ed. G. Hall and M. Morgan. London: Chapman Hall, pp. 111–22.

Bolsin, S. N. and Colson, M. (2000). Methodology Matters; CUSUM. *International Journal for Quality in Health Care*, **12**, 433–8.

Bolsin, S. N. and Colson, M. (2003). The use of statistical process control methods in monitoring clinical performance. *International Journal for Quality in Health Care*, **15**, 445.

Bolsin, S. N., Patrick, A., Creati, B., Colson, M. and Freestone, L. (2004). Electronic incident reporting and professional monitoring transforms culture. *British Medical Journal*, **329**, 51–2.

Bolsin, S. N., Faunce, T. and Colson, M. (2005). Using portable digital technology for clinical care and critical incidents: a new model. *Australian Health Review*, **29**, 297–305.

Bolsin, S. N., Faunce, T. and Oakley, J. (2005). Practical virtue ethics: healthcare whistleblowing and portable digital technology. *Journal of Medical Ethics*, **31**, 612–18.

Bolsin, S. N., Patrick, A., Colson, M. and Creati, B. (2005). New technology to enable personal monitoring and incident reporting can transform professional culture: the potential to favourably impact the future of health care. *Journal of Evaluation in Clinical Practice*, **11**, 499–506.

Bourn, J. A. (2005). *A Safer Place for Patients: Learning to Improve Patient Safety*. London: National Audit Office.

Brook, R. H. (1994). Health care reform is on the way: do we want to compete on quality? *Annals of Internal Medicine*, **120**, 84–6.

Charlton, B. G., Taylor, P. R. and Proctor, S. J. (1997). The PACE (population-adjusted clinical epidemiology) strategy: a new approach to multi-centred clinical research. *Quartely Journal of Medicine*, **90**, 147–51.

Chassin, M. R. (2002). Achieving and sustaining improved quality: lessons from New York State and cardiac surgery. *Health Affairs*, **21**, 40–51.

Chassin, M. R., Park, R. E., Lohr, K. N., Keesey, J. and Brook, R. H. (1989). Differences among hospitals in Medicare patient mortality. *Health Services Research*, **24**, 1–31.

Chassot, P-G., Delabays, A. and Spahn, D. R. (2002). Preoperative evaluation of patients with, or at risk of, coronary artery disease undergoing non-cardiac surgery. *British Journal of Anaesthesia*, **89**, 747–59.

Clarke, S. and Oakley, J. (2004). Informed consent and surgeon's performance. *Journal of Medicine and Philosophy*, **29**, 11–35.

Codman, E. A. (1914). The product of a hospital. *Surgery, Gynecology and Obstetrics*, **18**, 491–6.

Concato, J., Shah, N. and Horwitz, R. I. (2000). Randomised, controlled trials, observational studies, and the hierarchy of research design. *New England Journal of Medicine*, **342**, 1887–92.

Colson, M. and Bolsin, S. N. (2003). The use of statistical process control methods in monitoring clinical performance. *International Journal for Quality in Health Care*, **15**, 445.

De Leval, M. R., Francois, K., Bull, C., Brawn, W. and Spiegelhalter, D. (1994). Analysis of a cluster of surgical failures: application to a series of neonatal arterial switch operations. *Journal of Thoracic and Cardiovascular Surgery*, **107**, 914–23.

Duff, E. (1998). Florence Nightingale: basing care on evidence. *Royal College of Midwifery Midwives Journal*, **1**, 192–3.

Faunce, T. and Bolsin, S. N. (2004). Three Australian whistleblowing sagas: Lessons for internal and external regulation. *Medical Journal of Australia*, **181**, 44–7.

Freestone, L., Bolsin, S. N., Colson, M., Patrick, A. and Creati, B. (2006). Voluntary incident reporting by anaesthetic trainees in an Australian hospital. *International Journal for Quality in Health Care*, **18**, 452–7.

Goldie, J. G. S. (2004). The detrimental ethical shift towards cynicism: can medical educators help prevent it? *Medical Education*, **38**, 232–4.

Goldie, J. G. S., Schwartz, L. and McConnachie, A. (2003). Students' attitudes and potential behaviour with regard to whistle blowing as they pass through a modern medical curriculum. *Medical Education*, **37**, 368–75.

Green, J. and Wintfeld, N. (1995). Report cards on surgeons. Assessing New York State's approach. *New England Journal of Medicine*, **332**, 1229–32.

Hafferty, F. W. and Franks, R. (1994). The hidden curriculum, ethics teaching and the structure of medical education. *Academic Medicine*, **69**, 861–71.

Hannan, E. L. (1989). The relation between volume and outcome in health care. *New England Journal of Medicine*, **340**, 1677–9.

Hannan, E. L. (1996). Report cards: are they passing or failing? One New Yorker thinks they're passing. *Clinical Performance and Quality Health Care*, **4**, 218–19.

Hannan, E. L., O'Donnell, J. F., Kilburn, H. Jr., Bernard, H. R. and Yazici, A. (1989). Investigation of the relationship between volume and mortality for surgical procedures performed in New York State hospitals. *Journal of the American Medical Association*, **262**, 503–10.

Hannan, E. L., Kilburn, H. Jr., O'Donnell, J. F. *et al.* (1992). A longitudinal analysis of the relationship between in-hospital mortality in New York State and the volume of abdominal aortic aneurysm surgeries performed. *Health Services Research*, **27**, 517–42.

Hannan, E. L., Kilburn, H., Racz, M., Shields, E. and Chassin, M. R. (1994). Improving the outcomes of coronary artery bypass surgery in New York State. *Journal of the American Medical Association*, **271**, 761–6.

Hannan, E. L., Siu, A. L., Kumar, D., Racz, M., Pryor, D. B. and Chassin, M. R. (1997). Assessment of coronary artery bypass graft surgery performance in New York: is there a bias against taking high-risk patients? *Medical Care*, **35**, 49–56.

Hlatky, M. A., Califf, R. M., Harrell, F. E. Jr., Lee, K. L., Mark, D. B. and Pryor, D. B. (1988). Comparison of predictions based on observational data with the results of randomized controlled clinical trials of coronary artery bypass surgery. *Journal of the American College of Cardiology*, **11**, 237–45.

Hundert, E. M., Douglas-Steele, D. and Bickel, J. (1996). Context in medical education: the informal ethics curriculum. *Medical Education*, **30**, 353–64.

Irvine, D. (1997). The performance of doctors. II: Maintaining good practice, protecting patients from poor performance. *British Medical Journal*, **314**, 1613–15.

Irvine, D. (1999). The performance of doctors: the new professionalism. *The Lancet*, **353**, 117.

Irvine, D. (2004a). Health service reforms in the United Kingdom after Bristol. *Medical Journal of Australia*, **181**, 27–8.

Irvine, D. H. (2004b). Time for hard decisions on patient-centred professionalism. *Medical Journal of Australia*, **181**, 271–4.

Irvine, D. (2006a). A short history of the General Medical Council. *Medical Education*, **40**, 202–11.

Irvine, D. (2006b). New ideas about medical professionalism. *Medical Journal of Australia*, **184**, 204–5.

Kestin, I. G. (1995). A statistical approach to measuring the competence of anaesthetic trainees at practical procedures. *British Journal of Anaesthesia*, **75**, 805–9.

Kingston, M. J., Evans, S. M., Smith, B. J. and Berry, J. G. (2004). Attitudes of doctors and nurses towards incident reporting: a qualitative analysis. *Medical Journal of Australia*, **181**, 36–9.

Klein, R. (1998). Competence, self-regulation and the public interest. *British Medical Journal*, **301**, 1740.

Kohn, C. T., Corrigan, J. M. and Donaldson, M. S. (1999). *To Err is Human: Building a Safer Health System*. Washington: Institute of Medicine.

Mackay, P. (2004). *Eighth Report of the Victorian Consultative Council on Anaesthetic Mortality and Morbidity*. Melbourne: DHS Victoria.

Michel, P., Quenon, J. L., de Sarasqueta, A. M. and Scemama, O. (2004). Comparison of three methods for estimating rates of adverse events and rates of preventable adverse events in acute care hospitals. *British Medical Journal*, **328**, 199–204.

Monteiro, L.A. (1985). Florence Nightingale on public health nursing. *American Journal of Public Health*, **75**, 181–6.

O'Connor, G. T., Plume, S. K., Olmstead, E. M. *et al.* (1996). A regional intervention to improve hospital mortality associated with coronary artery bypass graft surgery. *Journal of the American Medical Association*, **275**, 841–6.

Paice, E., Heard, S. and Moss, F. (2002). How important are role models in making good doctors? *British Medical Journal*, **325**, 707–10.

Paice, E., Aitken, M., Houghton, A. and Firth-Cozens, J. (2004). Bullying among doctors in training: cross sectional questionnaire survey. *British Medical Journal*, **329**, 658–9.

Rubin, G. L. and Leeder, S. R. (2005). Health care safety: what needs to be done? *Medical Journal of Australia*, **183**, 529–31.

Runciman, W. B. (2002). Lessons from the Australian Patient Safety Foundation: setting up a national patient safety surveillance system – is this the right model? *Quality and Safety in Health Care*, **11**, 246–51.

Shortell, S. M. (1995). Physician involvement in quality improvement: issues, challenges, and recommendations. In *Improving Clinical Practice*, ed. D. Blumenthal and A. Scheck. San Francisco: Jossey-Bass, pp. 205–28.

Shortell, S. M., Bennet, C. L., Byck, C. R. (1998). Assessing the impact of continuous quality improvement on clinical practice: what it will take to accelerate progress. *The Milbank Quarterly*, **76**, 593–624.

Smith, R. (1998). All changed, changed utterly. British medicine will be transformed by the Bristol case. *British Medical Journal*, **316**, 917–18.

Spiegelhalter, D., Grigg, O., Kinsman, R. and Treasure, T. (2003). Risk-adjusted sequential probability ratio tests: applications to Bristol, Shipman and adult cardiac surgery. *International Journal for Quality in Health Care*, **15**, 7–13.

Vincent, C., Neale, G. and Woloshynowych, M. (2001). Adverse events in British hospitals: preliminary retrospective record review. *British Medical Journal*, **322**, 517–19.

White, C. (2004). Doctors mistrust systems for reporting medical mistakes. *British Medical Journal*, **329**, 12.

Wilson, R. M., Runciman, W. B., Gibberd, R. W., Harrison, B. T., Newby, L. and Hamilton, J. D. (1995) The quality in Australian healthcare study. *Medical Journal of Australia*, **163**, 458–71.

Wilson, R. M. and Van Der Weyden, M. B. (2005). The safety of Australian healthcare: 10 years after QAHCS. *Medical Journal of Australia*, **182**, 260–1.

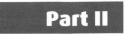

Part II

Informed consent

Part introduction

Informed consent

One of the main lines of argument for publishing surgeon performance information appeals directly to the doctrine of informed consent. It is a commonplace in medical ethics that a significant medical procedure cannot ordinarily be conducted on a patient without that patient's consent. It is also widely accepted that consent cannot be effectively provided unless it is grounded on a proper basis of relevant information. Hence the phrase 'informed consent'. It has become standard in medical practice, and indeed in medical law, to hold that medical professionals have a responsibility to ensure that patients have given their effective informed consent, before a significant medical procedure can be conducted.

The first chapter in this section, by Steve Clarke and Justin Oakley, argues that standard treatments of the doctrine of informed consent, such as that due to Faden and Beauchamp (1986), have implicitly been committed to the provision of surgeons' performance information to prospective patients before a surgical operation can take place. Standard treatments of the doctrine of informed consent concur on the requirement that all significant risks involved in undergoing an operation must be disclosed to a patient before that operation can take place. The significant risks of an operation will vary, *inter alia*, according to the performance abilities of the surgeon undertaking the operation. Clarke and Oakley argue that, because standard treatments of the doctrine of informed consent require that the actual risks of an operation be disclosed, this doctrine implicitly requires that the performance abilities of prospective surgeons who may be conducting the operation in question be disclosed.

Merle Spriggs is supportive of the argument from the doctrine of informed consent to the requirement that surgeon performance information be provided to patients. In her paper she attends to recent criticisms by Carl Schneider (1998) and Onora O'Neill (2003) of the doctrine of informed consent, which is claimed to establish an impossible goal, or involves consent procedures that may become empty rituals. Spriggs argues that these criticisms can be effectively addressed and that we are left with a robust enough version of the doctrine of informed consent to require the provision of surgeons' performance information to patients. The following chapter is a response to Clarke and Oakley from David Neil. Neil argues that the requirement of providing risk information for the purposes of informed consent does not extend to a requirement to provide patients with *comparative* performance information. He argues that considerations of autonomy and informed consent are not, by themselves, sufficient to justify devoting the substantial public resources necessary for the collection, publication, and disclosure to patients of fine-grained surgeon-specific performance data, over competing demands for such resources.

The next chapter in the section, by David Macintosh, is concerned with the impact that surgeon report cards may have on patients' trust of their surgeons. Macintosh argues that the provision of surgeon's performance information has the potential to increase the level of trust between surgeons and patients and thereby enable better decisions about consent to surgery to be made. The chapter that follows Macintosh's chapter is concerned with the practicalities of presenting performance information to patients for the purposes of enabling effective informed consent. The author, Steve Clarke is concerned with the ways in which patients' understanding of comparative surgeon performance information may be subject to well-known psychological biases. He offers suggestions as to how the effects of these can be minimized when performance information is provided to patients. In the final chapter of this section, Adrian Walsh is concerned to properly contextualize the notion of informed consent. He relates the doctrine of informed consent to the idea of consumer sovereignty in economics and considers the moral implications of making surgeons' performance information available commercially.

References

Faden, R. R. and Beauchamp, T. L. (1986). *A History and Theory of Informed Consent.* New York: Oxford University Press.

O'Neill, O. (2003). Some limits of informed consent. *Journal of Medical Ethics*, **29**, 4–7.

Schneider, C. E. (1998). *The Practice of Autonomy: Patients, Doctors, and Medical Decisions.* New York: Oxford University Press.

Informed consent and surgeons' performance

Steve Clarke

Centre for Applied Philosophy and Public Ethics, Charles Sturt University
and Program on the Ethics of the New Biosciences, James Martin
21st Century School, University of Oxford, UK

Justin Oakley

Monash University, Centre for Human Bioethics, Australia

Risk and disclosure

In order to qualify as an instance of informed consent, a patient's decision to consent to an operation needs to be grounded on an adequate basis of relevant information. Without such a basis of relevant information, a patient's decision to consent to an operation is not an effective informed consent, and is not, therefore, sufficient to authorize that operation. Because many of the categories of information that inform effective decisions by patients to consent to an operation are categories of specialist medical information, patients must rely on the disclosure of such information by medical professionals. A patient must receive an adequate disclosure of a variety of categories of information that are relevant to their decision to undergo an operation, as a precondition to the provision of effective informed consent.

Exactly which categories of information should be disclosed, for the purposes of providing informed consent, is in dispute.[1] What is not disputed by any commentators who accept a doctrine of informed consent is that a necessary component of disclosure, for the purposes of informed consent, is disclosure of the reasonably foreseeable risks of an operation. In this chapter, we argue that disclosures made for the purposes of obtaining patients' informed consent to an operation ought to include material information about a subcategory of risk information: that is, information about the ability of available surgeons to perform the operation in question. Disclosures that do not include at least some relevant, material information about the performance ability of available surgeons are an inadequate basis for the provision of effective informed consent. Our argument is for the disclosure of a class of information that has not hitherto been recognized in standard treatments of disclosure in informed consent.[2]

Informed Consent and Clinician Accountability: The Ethics of Report Cards on Surgeon Performance.
Steve Clarke and Justin Oakley (eds.). Published by Cambridge University Press. © Cambridge
University Press 2007.

However, we do not understand ourselves to be opposed to standard treatments of disclosure in informed consent, such as those provided by Faden and Beauchamp (1986), Appelbaum, Lidz, and Meisel (1987), and Wear (1998). The disclosure requirement that we argue for is a hitherto unrecognized consequence implied by these treatments of disclosure, which can be made explicit when we think carefully about risk, one of the 'elements of disclosure'.

Our main point is simple and, we think, very hard to deny. The risks that should be disclosed to patients are the risks that we can reasonably expect that patients will face when undergoing an operation. These risks will vary, *inter alia*, according to the level of ability of the surgeons who are available to perform that operation. So, information about the performance ability of surgeons is a necessary component of the disclosure of the reasonably foreseeable risks of a surgical intervention. And, as the disclosure of the reasonably foreseeable risks of a surgical intervention is a necessary requirement for the provision of effective informed consent, the disclosure of information about the performance ability of available surgeons is a necessary requirement for the provision of effective informed consent to a surgical intervention.

Before we go on, we should stress that we fully accept the 'received view', that the overriding purpose of the doctrine of informed consent in medical ethics is to ensure that patient autonomy is respected in medical decision making. Faden and Beauchamp state that an '... analysis of the nature of autonomy provides the essential foundation for our analysis of the nature of informed consent' (1986, p. 235). According to Appelbaum, Lidz and Meisel, informed consent is 'an ethical value rooted in our society's cherished value of autonomy' (1987, p. 3). We share these sentiments. It is because we ought to uphold the value of patient autonomy that material information about a surgeon's ability should be disclosed to patients as a part of the informed consent process.[3] We best uphold a patient's autonomy by enabling that patient to properly understand the risks that they are exposing themselves to when choosing to be operated on by a particular surgeon.

Appelbaum *et al.* (1987, p. 51) provide a useful analysis of the disclosure of risks, identifying the following four components: (1) the nature of the risk; (2) the magnitude or seriousness, of the risk; (3) the probability that the risk might materialise; and (4) the imminence of the risk. The following example is a simple application of their analysis. Recently, Clarke was diagnosed with a cartilage tear in his right knee. He was advised that arthroscopic surgery could be conducted on his knee to alleviate the condition, and that this would involve the risk of severing a nerve in the knee area causing permanent numbness in that region, immediately. The likelihood of this happening was reported, by Clarke's surgeon, as 1 in 1000. The nature of the risk (1) was severing a nerve. The magnitude or seriousness (2), is determined by understanding the consequences of the risk occurring and depends, *inter alia*, on how much Clarke values feeling in his right knee.[4] The probability of the risk materializing (3) was reported to be 1 in 1000, and the consequences of the operation going wrong (4) would be experienced immediately.

What does it mean to say that the probability of this risk materializing was 1 in 1000? The surgeon advising Clarke appeared to be asserting that if he (call him Bloggs) were to operate on Clarke, the probability of severing a nerve would be 1 in 1000. But why would Bloggs have thought this? Presumably, because he was in possession of information about the success rates of actual instances of arthroscopic surgery performed by a suitably large class of surgeons, of which he is a member (let us suppose this class is the class of Australian surgeons), on a suitably large class of patients, of which Clarke is a member (let us suppose that this is the class of Australians). Furthermore, Bloggs presumably believed that the probability of severing a nerve, if he were to perform arthroscopic surgery on Clarke, would be no different, *ceteris paribus*, from the probability of severing a nerve when any given Australian surgeon performs this form of surgery on any given Australian.

Measures of the probability that a risk might materialize as a result of an operation are typically presented as if it were unproblematically the case that the probability of a risk materializing in a particular operation simply was the average probability for operations performed by all surgeons within a suitably large reference class, on all patients within the same suitably large reference class. However, this will not always be the case. It might be, for example, that Clarke is a member of a subclass of the population, which has a different probability of the risk materialising from the risk for the population as a whole. Suppose that Clarke is a Torres Strait Islander, and that for Torres Strait Islanders it has been demonstrated that there is a significantly higher probability of this risk materializing – say 1 in 100, rather than 1 in 1000. As an Australian, Clarke has a 1 in 1000 chance of ending up with a severed nerve in his knee, but as a Torres Strait Islander, Clarke has a 1 in 100 rate of ending up with a severed nerve in his knee if he goes ahead with the operation. Which rate should Bloggs quote when disclosing the risks of the operation to Clarke? If Bloggs is aware of the substantially higher risk rate for Torres Strait Islanders, then Bloggs should cite this information. Bloggs should provide Clarke with the information available that most closely reflects his actual circumstances. All things being equal, the information that will more closely approximate the actual rate at which a risk to Clarke can be expected to materialize will be information about the most specific reference class to which Clarke belongs and, clearly, information about Torres Strait Islanders is information about a more specific reference class than is information about Australians generally.[5]

Just as specific information about Clarke may be relevant to the rate at which a risk materializes, so too information about Bloggs can be relevant. In particular, information about Bloggs' ability to perform the operation will surely affect the rate at which injuries can be expected to occur. Suppose, for the sake of argument, that Bloggs has performed arthroscopic surgical operations of the type being contemplated 10 000 times, and 100 of these operations have resulted in severed nerves – i.e. 1 in every 100 times. If Clarke is to be operated on by Bloggs, then is the expected risk of a severed nerve for Clarke closer to 1 in 1000 or closer to 1 in 100? Surely, all things being equal, 1 in 100 is the more accurate figure, because it represents the probability of the occurrence of an event that is closer in description to the event that is actually being contemplated. It is more fine-grained information, and as we have already argued, all things being equal, we ought to provide more fine-grained information where it is available, because it more closely approximates to the actual probability of the relevant possible event.

The actual probability of a severed nerve, when Bloggs operates on Clarke, will depend on many factors, such as the quality of the lighting in the operating theatre, peculiarities about Clarke's right knee, the occurrence of unforeseen events that interrupt the operation and even whether or not Bloggs slept properly the night before the operation.[6] To provide precise information about the actual probability of a risk materializing, for a particular operation, we would have to anticipate the probability of all such relevant effects and make appropriate adjustments to our assessment of the probability of a risk. As a complete list of factors that can potentially affect the probability that a risk may materialize would be extremely long, if not infinite, this would be impractical, if not impossible. Furthermore, even for those factors that we can anticipate, we will be unable to provide reliable information about some of them. Suppose that Clarke is a member of a distinct population group with, say, less than 100 members. Even if we have reason to suspect that members of this group may be susceptible to the risk in question at a rate which is different to that for the overall population, we may simply be unable to obtain enough reliable information about such a small group to confirm this suspicion.

It is not reasonable for a patient to expect medical professionals to anticipate all factors relevant to a given risk. And nor is it reasonable for patients to expect that medical professionals will be able to provide reliable information about all such factors, even if they are made aware of the materiality of such factors to the decision making of a particular patient. However, it surely is reasonable to expect medical professionals to make the effort to anticipate some of the factors that will be most important for the decision-making of the majority of patients. And, it surely is reasonable to expect medical professionals to collect such information about those important factors and to provide it to patients for the purpose of enabling effective informed consent. With many operations, a surgeon's level of performance will be one of the most important factors causing risks to patients; and so it is plausible to believe that many patients will appreciate having such information available (see Marshall, Shekelle, Leatherman, Brook, and Owen, 2000, pp. 60–2). So it is reasonable to require that relevant information about surgeons' performance abilities be made available to patients for the purpose of enabling effective informed consent. Commonly, surgeons already maintain records of their performances in operations, so it would not be an onerous administrative imposition to require that material information derived from such records be made available so that it may be provided to patients for the purposes of enabling informed consent.

Recent institutional and legal developments

We are unaware of other philosophers who have explicitly advocated the provision of material information about the performance of surgeons for the purpose of disclosure in informed consent in medicine, but we are not the first advocates of the provision of information about the performance of surgeons. In some American hospitals information about the performance of surgeons is already collected and made publicly available on the internet. The best known and longest established such internet site is one maintained by the New York State Department of Health, which issues annual reports, known as 'report cards', comparing the mortality rates of individual surgeons who have conducted coronary artery bypass graft operations.[7] This is a commonly recommended form of surgery for people with severe atherosclerotic coronary artery disease. There are also sites available providing data about the performance of heart surgeons in Pennsylvania, and of the results of patient satisfaction surveys of practitioners of general medicine, obstetrics, surgery and intensive care in Cleveland.[8]

There are moves under way to introduce report cards into the public health-care systems in both the United Kingdom and in Australia. In 1998, the UK Department of Health released a comprehensive set of performance indicators against which to measure hospital data for the purposes of developing report cards on hospitals, and general practitioners have access to data that enable them to give their patients detailed information about the success rates for a given procedure in a particular hospital, and how that compares with the national average (Department of Health, 1998). The case for public reporting in Britain has gained considerable impetus as a result of the Bristol Royal Infirmary scandal. In response to a recommendation of the subsequent public inquiry into the events at Bristol, *inter alia*, the UK Department of Health decided that data on the mortality rates for individual cardiac surgeons would be made available to the public in 2004.[9] (They were eventually made available to the public (on the UK Healthcare Commission's website) in April 2006.)

In Australia the use of report cards on hospitals has been strongly advocated in the State of Victoria. The Health Services Performance Review, carried out in 1999 under the leadership of Professor Stephen Duckett, produced a discussion paper recommending that a set of comprehensive consumer-orientated performance indicators be developed and that the Victorian Department of

Human Services publish annual data on the comparative performance of individual hospitals and day centres for specific procedures.[10] These data on the comparative performance of hospitals have now been made available to the public in Victoria. Although the information contained in report cards on hospitals is not as fine-grained as information contained in report cards on individual surgeons, provision of such information is a step in the right direction. Information about the likelihood of a risk materializing, if an operation is performed at a particular hospital, is more fine-grained information than information about the likelihood of such a risk materializing if the reference class in question is all surgeons performing that operation in an entire nation.

Consider the recent scandal at the Bristol Royal Infirmary. In that case the anaesthetist 'whistleblower', Dr Stephen Bolsin, collected figures which showed that two surgeons had mortality rates for two particular operations that were well above the British national average for those operations. The data collected by Dr. Bolsin throw into sharp relief the importance of providing to patients (and hospital administrators) sufficiently fine-grained information about surgeons' performance. For paediatric cardiac operations in 1990–1992, the mortality rate at the Bristol Royal Infirmary was three to four times higher than the national average. For one of the surgeons at the centre of the scandal, Mr Wisheart, the mortality rate for paediatric cardiac operations in that period was reported as being five to six times the national average.[11] Clearly, parents who were informed about the mortality rate of paediatric cardiac surgery, for operations conducted by Mr Wisheart, would be in a better position to give effective informed consent to a paediatric cardiac operation conducted by Mr Wisheart than would parents who had been told only about the mortality rate for all surgeons conducting paediatric cardiac operations at the Bristol Royal Infirmary. And parents in the latter group would, in turn, be in a better position to give effective informed consent than those parents who were only told about the national average mortality rate for all surgeons operating in the United Kingdom.

Our view is also broadly in line with the ruling in a recent Australian legal case, *Chappel v Hart* (1998) whose details are as follows. Mrs Hart consulted an ear, nose and throat specialist, Dr Chappel, following a sore throat that she had had for a period of nine months. It turned out that Mrs Hart had a pharyngeal pouch and this had caused a narrowing of her oesophagus. Dr Chappel recommended surgery, but failed to warn Mrs Hart that surgery would involve a slight risk of vocal damage, despite the fact that Mrs Hart had indicated to him that she considered such a risk material to her, informing him that she 'didn't want to end up with a voice like Neville Wran' (the ex-premier of New South Wales, who had a famously croaky voice). Surgery was performed by Dr Chappel, and while he was deemed by the court not to have performed the surgery negligently, Mrs Hart's oesophagus was inadvertently perforated during the operation, an accident that indirectly caused the permanent impairment of her voice. Mrs Hart's concern about the state of her voice was particularly well motivated because her position as an Education Officer required that she be able to speak clearly. Following the operation, she was assessed as medically unfit to continue her work and had no option but to retire.

Mrs Hart was awarded a sum of AUS$172 500 in damages by the NSW Supreme Court, a decision which was subsequently upheld by the High Court of Australia. Mrs Hart did not contend that she would not have undergone the operation had she known about the risk to her voice. Instead, she contended that she would have gone ahead with the operation, but with a more experienced surgeon – the most experienced surgeon in the field available, whom, Mrs Hart believed, would be the best performing surgeon.[12]

It seems clear from the context of the court's decision that, had Dr Chappel advised Mrs Hart merely of the average risk of such a complication for any Australian patient being operated on by any Australian surgeon, he would not have done enough to escape liability. Because the court's decision turned on accepting Mrs Hart's claim that, had she known of the risk to her voice, she would have sought the most experienced surgeon in the field available, it seems the court believed that Dr Chappel had an additional obligation to inform Mrs Hart that his experience was limited. One of the presiding judges, Justice Gaudron, argued that, if the risk to Mrs Hart is understood as a loss of an opportunity to undergo surgery at the hands of a more experienced surgeon, then Dr Chappel should be understood to have had a duty to inform Mrs Hart that there were more experienced surgeons practising in the field.

Both the High Court of Australia's judgement and Mrs Hart's reasoning appear to be premised on the assumption that greater experience straightforwardly equates to better performance. Here we must demur.[13] While, all things being equal, performance and experience are positively correlated, the relationship between the two is far from straightforward, exceptionless and linear. Some very experienced surgeons may be 'past their prime', and in such cases marginal increases in experience will negatively correlate with performance. In some cases performance ability may 'plateau' and further experience may make little or no difference to it. In his sceptical study of professional psychology and psychotherapy, Robyn Dawes cites evidence, due to Howard Garb (1989), of such plateauing. In professional psychology, once the rudiments of technique are mastered, experience does not produce any measurable increase in diagnostic performance (Dawes, 1996, pp. 106–7).

The overall relationship between experience and performance is extremely complicated and can be expected to vary across different areas of human endeavour. According to Dawes, one generalization that is reliable is that experience enhances performance when practitioners are given regular and explicit feedback about performance and are thus prompted to alter their practices in light of failure (Dawes, 1996, pp. 118–21). Potentially, report cards could have a role in improving overall performance and in making experience correlate more positively with performance. In any case, report cards can be used to indicate performance levels without recourse to indications of experience. Had Dr Chappel had ready access to reliable statistical information about surgeons' performance, he would have been able to provide Mrs Hart with very accurate information about his ability to perform the operation that she underwent, as well as accurate information about the relative ability of other surgeons in his field.

It should be noted here, however, that the fact that particular details about an individual surgeon would be material to a given patient's decision about whether or not to consent to that surgeon operating upon them does not by itself suffice to show that those details ought to be provided to the patient. Patients may regard all manner of details about an individual surgeon as material to their decisions about whether or not to consent to that surgeon operating upon them, but the surgeon's privacy is another important factor to be considered in determining what sorts of disclosures are justifiable. Some facts about surgeons are justifiably kept private, even when those facts might be considered material to a particular patient's decision about whether to be operated upon by a given surgeon. For instance, a homosexual surgeon, who preferred that his sexual orientation be kept from his patients, would surely be justified in keeping such information private, even where a patient would regard this information as being material to her decision about whether to be operated upon by this surgeon. The promotion of patient autonomy is justifiably limited by the value of respect for a surgeon's privacy here.

The value of privacy clearly licenses the withholding of certain sorts of information about individual surgeons, even where this information would be material to a given patient's decision. However, it is hard to see how this sort of rationale could plausibly be applied to mount an argument for the withholding of information about a surgeon's performance. Even if some surgeons actually do regard details about their surgical performance as equally personal and private as information about, say, their sexual orientation, the moral foundations of professional obligations provide good reason for thinking that, while the public may not have a claim on the latter information, they do have a strong claim on the former. It seems very plausible to hold that, in exchange for the community entrusting professionals with a monopoly of expertise on the provision of certain key goods, professionals owe the community the means to ascertain and monitor whether the requisite expertise is indeed being provided. And surely the provision of information about professional performance is a key way of meeting this demand.[14]

Two objections

Although we see our argument as based on drawing out a logical implication of the doctrine of informed consent, a doctrine that enjoys widespread support, the argument's consequences ensure that it will be controversial. So, it is important that we examine some objections to our position. Two objections seem to us especially worthy of consideration.

The threshold objection

It might be argued that surgeons can meet their professional obligations by providing performance data regarding their ability, up to a particular threshold, and that it is supererogatory for surgeons to provide further performance data beyond that threshold, even where a surgeon is aware that this further information is material to a particular patient. If this is right, then surgeons need merely to demonstrate that they have met this threshold. If this is to be a low threshold, then a mere demonstration that they are entitled to be called competent might be all that is sufficient, or so our objector may tell us. This objection is plausibly motivated by a general view about professional obligations. According to this view, those of us in need of the services of a professional have a right to know only that the skills of the particular professional in question pass a certain standard of competence and we are not entitled to be given any further details about the individual characteristics of different practitioners.[15] This sort of view is sometimes claimed to be well suited to contemporary professional practice, given that doctor–patient relationships tend to be more impersonal than they have been previously, and given that what those seeking the help of a professional need to know, above all, is that the professional will adhere to a certain charter of norms and values, no matter what their personal characteristics may be (see Dare, 1998a; Veatch, 1985).

To evaluate this sort of objection properly, we would need to be told more about the point at which it is said to become supererogatory for surgeons to provide data on their performance that was material to a particular patient. If this threshold for surgeons was set quite high, then we might not find this suggestion particularly problematic. Nevertheless, we do find rather implausible the general suggestion that our rights to know details about the performance of individual professionals extend only as far as the information necessary to establish that they meet some threshold of basic competence. Sometimes, the services that we are engaging a professional to provide are of a relatively high level of significance to us. In fact, this is typically the case when we are choosing a surgeon. In such situations, the suggestion that a surgeon who has demonstrated their basic competence has no obligation to provide any further performance information that would be material to our decision seems particularly implausible. Indeed, in some professions it has been thought appropriate to make information available to the public about individual members that goes beyond their meeting a baseline of competence. For example, in Anglophone countries a barrister's advanced level of skill is indicated by their being accepted as a Senior Counsel or a Queen's Counsel. At the very

data was ethically unjustified, all things considered. Different ethical theories might well provide different answers here. If the publication of surgeons' report cards is shown to result in a reduction in medical utility overall, utilitarians would regard this as a strong reason to reject the use of report cards, while some Kantians might (depending, perhaps, on the extent of this reduction) view this as a price worth paying in order to uphold respect for patient autonomy. In any case, our argument has not been directed at giving an overall ethical assessment of surgeons' report cards. Rather, we aim to show that standard requirements of informed consent and respect for patient autonomy entail that the information contained in these report cards ought to be provided to potential patients, for whom it would be material when they make decisions about surgery. To settle conclusively whether surgeons' report cards should be made publicly available for all would require further argument, which is beyond the scope of this paper.

Practical considerations

Let us now consider some practical difficulties that have been raised about the implementation of surgeons' report cards, and suggest some ways in which these might be dealt with. A fairly common objection to the implementation of report cards is that it is likely that patients will misinterpret such data, because they will fail to appreciate the difficulties and complexities involved in assessing surgeons' performance.[18] Indeed, it is sometimes suggested that patients should *not* be provided with performance data about individual surgeons, since these data are likely to be so misleading that patients will make *mis*informed decisions about which surgeon to engage. For example, patients might infer, from the fact that a particular surgeon has a relatively high mortality rate for a given procedure, that this surgeon is poorly skilled at this procedure. But such an inference would be mistaken, as different surgeons' mortality rates for a given procedure are affected not only by their levels of surgical skill, but also, *inter alia*, by variations in the health conditions of the patients they operate on, the degree of surgical support available at the institution where they practise, and the sort of post-operative care provided to each patient. A high mortality rate need not indicate a lack of surgical skill. In fact, some very skilful surgeons may actually have quite high mortality rates, since they may be more likely than other surgeons to be called on to perform high-risk operations.

A related problem is that the presentation of performance data can be deliberately manipulated in order to create the impression that a surgeon is considerably more skilled than he or she actually is. Surgeons with objectively poor outcomes may be able to find ways of framing their performance data, in an attempt to mislead patients into believing that they are more successful surgeons than they in fact are. Attempts to counter such distortions by providing additional information threaten to compound the difficulties facing patients. If patients are already confused by the data they are presented with, then they may be further confused by being given more information.

We think these problems can be alleviated, to a large extent, by the use of processed rather than raw data, which is intended to take into account the particular difficulties faced by doctors in particular circumstances. In addition to publishing raw mortality rates, the New York State Department of Health also publishes 'risk-adjusted' mortality rates, which indicate what a particular surgeon's mortality rate would have been had he or she had a mix of patients identical to the state average. An analogy that can be made here is to the difference between a raw batting or bowling average in the game of cricket, and the 'processed' rating that the LG International Cricket Council (ICC) rankings provide.[19] The raw batting average fails to take into account various factors such as the difficulty of batting conditions on particular grounds that a particular batsman may be more likely to encounter, and the quality of bowling attack that he may happen to face. The LG ICC ratings account for these factors by statistically adjusting raw data to take into account the ways in which the overall conditions that a batsman faces deviate from the norm.[20]

It is unlikely that risk-adjusted statistics could be so well adjusted as to fully represent the complete range of variables that a surgeon encounters. However, it is surely absurd to insist that anything less than perfectly accurate information about surgeons' performance should be withheld from patients. From a patient's point of view, information that is reasonably accurate and fairly representative can be of significant value, despite its imperfections, and is usually better than having no performance data at all.

From the point of view of surgeons and health policy makers, it may appear justifiable to withhold certain sorts of imperfect performance information from patients, if the provision of such information is likely to have highly deleterious effects on the availability and practice of surgical care generally. But the question of the extent – if at all – to which imperfect performance data can be justifiably withheld from an individual patient to whom it would be material, in order to maintain or promote better overall medical practice, will depend importantly on how one balances such factors as patients' rights to medical information, rights to treatment, surgeons' duties as professionals to make their services broadly available, and the promotion of medical utility overall. And the bearing such factors will have on one's answer here will depend importantly on whether one relies on, for example, a Kantian or a Utilitarian ethical theory. Thus, Kantians may argue here that the public has a right to know about surgeons' performance data, imperfect or not, particularly if such data can enhance the autonomy of patients' decisions about surgery. Utilitarians, on the other hand, might argue that imperfect performance information should not be released to patients, where the provision of such information is likely to lead patients to make decisions that are contrary to their best interests, or is likely to result in a lowering of the quality of surgical care offered to the community overall.

In any case, the worry that patients may misuse or fail to comprehend performance information contained in report cards can be addressed by considering the nature of the informed consent process itself. In standard models of the informed consent process, such as the account given by Wear (1998, Chap. 6), the doctor provides relevant information to the patient and then takes reasonable measures to ensure that the patient comprehends that information. Comprehension typically involves placing the significance of the information provided in an appropriate context for the patient to interpret. Consistent with this approach, cardiologists in New York State are encouraged by the Department of Health to discuss and contextualize the different risk-adjusted mortality rates of various cardiac surgeons, as part of the development of an appropriate treatment plan. Report cards made publicly available may well be improperly interpreted by the public at large. However the relevant issue, for the purposes of providing for informed consent, is not whether to make such information available to the public generally, but whether to provide such information to patients who are contemplating the surgical procedure in question.

It might seem unrealistic to expect surgeons with poor report cards and a lack of plausible explanations for those poor results, to own up and say that they are poor surgeons. Some might suggest it is more likely that such surgeons will provide implausible explanations, but dress them up in such a way as to make them appear plausible to patients. This problem prompts thinking about ways in which the informed consent process might be adjusted to minimize the potential for surgeons to mislead patients as to their ability. One idea is to involve third parties in the informed consent process. Although it may be unrealistic to expect a surgeon to divulge that he or she is of poor ability when it comes to performing a particular operation, there is no reason why a third party might not be able to indicate that the surgeon's reports are poor and that his or her explanations for these poor results are inadequate. To an extent, third parties are already involved in the informed consent process in situations where patients seek a 'second opinion'. Further, in the UK, Patient Care Advisers are now employed by the National Health Service to assist cardiac patients with making various decisions about surgery. The role of these advisers currently includes assisting cardiac patients who have been awaiting surgery for over six months to decide whether to be transferred to another cardiac unit (elsewhere in the UK), which can provide surgery sooner than the unit that the patient is currently listed with. In assisting patients with their decisions, these advisers help patients to consider a range of information, including performance data on individual cardiac units. All indications are that these advisers will also be asked to assist patients with considering performance information on individual cardiac surgeons, once that information becomes publicly available in

2004.[21] Another consideration is that surgeons with merely average performance data might be able to make their services more attractive to patients, offering their services at cheaper rates than those of surgeons with better results, and might be prepared to acknowledge their average results to patients, as a way of explaining their lower fees. In public hospital situations where doctors' fees are not at issue, surgeons with merely average performance results may be able to offer patients reduced waiting times for non-emergency operations.[22]

Another practical issue to consider is the impact of report cards on the training of new surgeons.[23] It takes a long time to become a fully qualified surgeon. Practitioners will typically spend many years as surgical residents, performing operations under close supervision, before they are permitted to play a leading role in a surgical procedure.[24] It seems to follow from our argument that a surgeon's status as a trainee, or as a newly qualified practitioner, should be disclosed to those patients who would regard this as material to their decisions about whether or not to be operated upon by a given practitioner.[25] Likewise, where significant data are collected on a trainee's performance in order to monitor the trainee's progress, our argument seems to imply that these data should be made available to those patients who would regard these as material information. However, there may not be sufficient data on an individual practitioner, during their training and immediately after qualifying as a surgeon, to enable a satisfactory report card on their performance to be created. Typically, a satisfactory report card will need to be based on data collected over several years. Attempts to construct a report card on fledgling surgeons, who have conducted only a small number of surgical procedures, can be expected to yield data that are very unreliable.

The problem of adequately informing patients about the performance of trainees and newly qualified surgeons, in a way that minimizes the chance of such information being misinterpreted, is a difficult one to resolve. Much research is currently being done on ways of improving and possibly standardizing measures of trainee surgeons' progress along the learning curve, but the problem of how to adequately inform patients about trainee surgeons' performance is widely acknowledged, and the medical profession itself has not so far been able to come up with a solution to this problem.[26] Close supervision of trainees is clearly important, as are the proliferation of skills laboratories where trainees can practise under simulated conditions. However, there will still be occasions where the trainee must perform a procedure themselves for the first time, and outcomes for patients in such cases are commonly worse than if the procedure was carried out by a fully qualified surgeon (Gawande, 2002, pp. 21–30). Nevertheless, the difficulties of adequately informing patients about trainees may not be entirely intractable. Perhaps there are better ways of helping patients to understand a trainee surgeon's performance than by attempting to develop statistically valid report cards on trainees. After all, records are kept to enable a trainee's progress to be monitored by their superiors, and if suitably contextualized, these records could be provided to patients who see this information as material to their decision about surgery. Because performance information on trainees and newly qualified surgeons is particularly likely to mislead those unfamiliar with the circumstances and procedures surrounding surgical training,[27] it is especially important to assist patients who are provided with such information to properly contextualize that information.

However, disclosing information to patients about a trainee surgeon's status and their level of performance, raises a further concern. That is, such disclosures may lead patients to avoid the trainee in favour of more experienced practitioners, and this will potentially impede the trainee's development of those surgical skills that can be effectively learnt only by operating on actual patients. Given these implications, we need to address the question of whether there are any reasons that would suffice to justify withholding such information about trainee surgeons from patients who would regard this as material to their decision about surgery.

An argument that some might advance for withholding such information appeals to the notion of justice as reciprocity. According to this argument, because each of us has been, or is likely to be, the beneficiary of a practitioner's surgical skills at some stage in our lives, there is a reciprocal (*prima facie*) moral obligation upon each of us to accept a trainee surgeon, on some occasion, when we need surgery. Analogous reciprocity-based arguments are sometimes put in the context of medical experimentation, and in regard to blood donation (see for instance, Caplan, 1988). To accept the benefits of medical experimentation or donated blood, without being prepared to make comparable sacrifices, is to act as a 'free rider'.

Such arguments, while intuitively appealing, are controversial, because they assume that free riding must be wrong in all contexts, and this assumption has been strongly challenged.[28] However, even if we agreed that free riding is always immoral, and so accepted that these reciprocity-based arguments create obligations in the case of medical experimentation or blood donation, this would not justify withholding information about a trainee surgeon's status or their performance from patients who would regard such information as material to their decision about surgery.

The provision to patients of materially relevant information about trainees follows from standard informed consent requirements, and none of the reciprocity-based arguments about medical experimentation or blood donation holds that our obligations here require us to sacrifice our right to be informed about the risks of a particular experiment or of donating blood. In any case, accepting the services of a surgeon might not create any reciprocal obligation on the patient's part, since, as we have argued earlier, surgical services can be seen as something that practitioners are obligated to make broadly available to society, in exchange for society granting surgeons a monopoly of expertise on the provision of these services. Perhaps there are other arguments for creating exceptions to standard informed consent requirements in the case of trainee surgeons. But in the absence of such arguments, we hold that such exceptions would be unjustified.

A consequence of disclosing trainee surgeons' status and performance information to those patients who see this as material information, may be that it begins to take longer to train surgeons. This would be a significant public policy issue, which each community would have to confront for themselves, with reference to the particular healthcare system in place there. There are many issues raised here. Several measures might be considered, to help mitigate this effect. The community might decide that greater resources ought to be invested in the training of surgeons, to ensure that their progress is not unduly delayed by a possible reduction in the number of patients willing to have surgery performed by a trainee.[29] Thus, closer supervision of trainees by highly proficient surgeons could be made a mandatory part of surgical training regimes, and this could be clearly explained to patients. Also, the distinction between experience and performance could be emphasized, so that patients do not automatically assume (before seeing a trainee's performance data) that an inexperienced trainee surgeon will have poor performance data, and so that patients may be attracted to the services of trainees with good performance data. Another possibility would be to offer certain incentives to patients who are prepared to have surgery by trainees, such as shorter pre-operative waiting periods.[30] Communities with fee-for-service health systems might also consider requiring lower fees to be charged for surgery carried out by trainees, though patients would need to be assured that they would not have to bear any added costs that might eventuate, should extra follow-up procedures prove to be necessary.[31]

Conclusion

We have argued that a proper understanding of the doctrine of informed consent, in conjunction with a proper understanding of the concept of risk, implies that we should support the provision of performance information about surgeons as part of the informed consent process. We have considered some commonly voiced objections to this chain of implication and found them to be lacking in substance. We have not shown how our proposal could be turned into sound policy – that would be a major undertaking – but we have addressed some common practical objections to its implementation.[32]

Notes

1. Those who adopt a maximal approach include Faden and Beauchamp (1986), Appelbaum, Lidz, and Meisel (1987), Wear (1998), and the state of Georgia

15. This view has been put to us in conversation by Michael Davis, among others.

16. A conclusive answer to these sorts of resource allocation questions would require details about the costs of collecting performance data, and some principle of healthcare resource allocation that would enable us to judge whether preventative health measures ought to receive funding priority over measures to promote informed decision-making by patients in acute care. Examining these issues would take us too far afield here.

17. See *Coronary Artery Bypass Surgery in New York State 1997–1999*, New York State Department of Health, September 2002, p. 1.

18. This concern was expressed by the Australian Medical Association, and the Royal Australasian College of Surgeons, in their submissions to the Victorian Department of Human Services Health Services Policy Review. See Duckett, Casemix Consulting and Hunter (1999, 114–117).

19. See: http://cricketratings.com/.

20. LG ICC use purely mechanical processing procedures to take account of abnormal conditions, when producing weighted batting and bowling averages. This is not the only way to weight raw data. It may be that additional non-mechanical processing is appropriate in some cases, including the development of risk-adjusted surgeons' report cards.

21. The NHS booklet, *Extending Choice for Patients – Heart Surgery: Your Guide to Your Choices* (2003), explains that the Patient Care Adviser's '. . . job is to work for you. Although they work closely with the cardiac team in your local hospital they do not answer to them. Your Adviser is managed by the local Patient Advocacy and Liaison Service to ensure that he or she is an independent voice acting on your behalf'.

22. Of course, the implementation of such strategies is complicated, considerably, by the involvement of the insurance industry in the financing of medical procedures.

23. Thanks to an anonymous referee for raising this concern.

24. See Gawande (2002) for a lively personal account of the difficulties commonly encountered in learning to perform surgery.

25. Note that, as explained earlier, there is no simple and direct correlation between experience and performance. Some very experienced practitioners may have declining levels of surgical performance, and some inexperienced trainees may have relatively high levels of surgical performance. Also, obtaining statistically valid figures on risks for individual surgeons would seem to require that they have performed a minimum number of operations.

26. It is not only novice surgeons whose performance follows a learning curve. Even well-qualified surgeons face a learning curve when mastering new surgical techniques into surgical practice. So, the question of how to adequately inform patients about where a surgeon's level of performance is in relation to that surgeon's learning curve is more pervasive than might initially be apparent.

27. This point is clearly made by Tony Eyers (2003) in a paper describing a first-hand account of surgical training.

28. This assumption is challenged, *inter alia*, by Cullity (1995), and Dare (1998b).

29. Indeed, given that the increased surgical risks posed by trainees are commonly borne disproportionately by lower socioeconomic groups in society, there is a strong distributive justice argument for greater societal investment in surgical training, to

enable these increased risks to be spread more evenly across different socioeconomic groups in the community. (See for instance, Eyers, 2003, on this point.)

30. There is some evidence from the UK that cardiac patients are prepared to make certain sorts of trade-offs – such as travelling significant distances to have surgery at a different cardiac unit – in order to shorten their wait for surgery. See *Extending Choice for Patients – Heart Surgery: Your Guide to Your Choices* (2003).

31. The implications of such incentives for private health insurance would also need to be considered. Further, careful attention would need to be given to each suggested incentive, on a case-by-case basis, to minimise the possibility that such incentives would impair a patient's judgement about the surgery.

32. Informed consent and surgeons' performance, by Steve Clarke and Justin Oakley, *The Journal of Medicine and Philosophy*, vol. 29, no. 1 (2004), pp. 11–35. Copyright © *The Journal of Medicine and Philosophy*, Inc. Reprinted by permission. We would like to thank the journal's anonymous referees for their helpful comments on a previous draft of this paper. For useful feedback on earlier drafts, we also wish to thank Joe Ibrahim, Hugh Martin, David Neil, Tim Van Gelder, the Melbourne-Monash bioethics journal club and audiences at the Children's Hospital, Westmead NSW, the Australian Association for Professional and Applied Ethics annual conference 2001 and CAPPE Melbourne and Wagga Wagga. Research that led to this paper was supported in part by National Health and Medical Research Council Project Grant 236877.

References

Appelbaum, P. S., Lidz, C. W. and Meisel, A. (1987). *Informed Consent: Legal Theory and Clinical Practice*. New York: Oxford University Press.

Bolsin, S. N. (1998). Professional misconduct: the Bristol case. *Medical Journal of Australia*, **169**, 369–72.

Caplan, A. L. (1988). Is there an obligation to participate in biomedical research? In *The Use of Human Beings in Research, with Special Reference to Clinical Trials*, ed. S. F. Spicker, I. Alon, A. de Vries and H. T. Engelhardt, Jr. Dordrecht: Kluwer.

Chappel v Hart, High Court of Australia HCA 55, 2 September 1998, 195 CLR 232.

Chassin, M. R., Hannan, E. L. and DeBuono, B. A. (1996). Benefits and hazards of reporting medical outcomes publicly. *New England Journal of Medicine*, **334**, 394–8.

Clarke, S. (2001). Informed consent in medicine in comparison with consent in other areas of human activity. *The Southern Journal of Philosophy*, **39**, 169–87.

Coronary Artery Bypass Surgery in New York State 1997–1999 (2002). New York State Department of Health.

Cullity, G. (1995). Moral free riding. *Philosophy and Public Affairs*, **24**, 3–34.

Dare, T. (1998a). The secret courts of men's hearts: legal ethics and Harper Lee's *To Kill a Mockingbird*. In *Ethical Challenges to Legal Education and Conduct*, ed. K. Economides. Oxford: Hart Publishing.

Dare, T. (1998b). Mass immunisation programmes: some philosophical issues. *Bioethics*, **12**, 125–49.

Dawes, R. M. (1996). *House of Cards: Psychology and Psychotherapy built on Myth*. New York: The Free Press.

Department of Health (1998). The new NHS performance tables 1997/98. Available: http://www.performance.doh.gov.uk/tables98/index.htm.

Duckett, S., Casemix Consulting and Hunter, L. (1999). Health Services Policy Review: Final Report, Victorian Government Department of Human Services. Available: http://www.dhs.vic.gov.au/ahs/archive/servrev/.

Dworkin, G. (1988). *The Theory and Practice of Autonomy*. Cambridge: Cambridge University Press.

Erickson, L. C., Torchiana, D. F., Schneider, E. C., Newburger, J. W. and Hannan, E. L. (2000). The relationship between managed care insurance and use of lower-mortality hospitals for CABG surgery. *Journal of the American Medical Association*, **283**, 1976–82.

Eyers, T. (2003). Teaching trainee surgeons how to operate. Master of Bioethics research paper, Monash University Centre for Human Bioethics.

Faden, R. R. and Beauchamp, T. L. (1986). *A History and Theory of Informed Consent*. New York: Oxford University Press.

Freckelton, I. (1999). Materiality of risk and proficiency assessment: the onset of report cards? *Journal of Law and Medicine*, **6**, 313–18.

Garb, H. N. (1989). Clinical judgement, clinical training and professional experience. *Psychological Bulletin*, **105**, 387–92.

Gawande, A. (2002). *Complications: A Surgeon's Notes on an Imperfect Science*. London: Profile Books.

Green, J. and Wintfeld, N. (1995). Report cards on cardiac surgeons – assessing New York State's approach. *New England Journal of Medicine*, **332**, 1229–32.

Hannan, E. L., Stone, C. C., Biddle, T. L. and DeBuono, B. A. (1997). Public release of cardiac surgery outcomes data in New York: 'What do New York State cardiologists think of it?' *American Heart Journal*, **136**, 1120–8.

Heinemann, R. A. (1997). Pushing the limits of informed consent: Johnson v Kokemoor and physician-specific disclosure. *Wisconsin Law Review*, **1079**, 1083.

Lambert, B. (2002). Infected doctor told to get patients' consent. *The New York Times*, April 19th.

Marshall, M. N., Shekelle, P., Leatherman, S., Brook, R. and Owen, J. W. (2000). *Dying to Know: Public Release of Information about Quality of Health Care*. Los Angeles: RAND Corporation/Nuffield Trust.

New York State Department of Health (2002). Coronary artery bypass surgery in New York State 1997–1999. Available: http://www.health.state.ny.us/nysdoh/heart/1997–99cabg.pdf.

New York State Department of Health (2003). Percutaneous coronary interventions (PCI) in New York State 1998–2000. Available: http://newyorkhealth.gov/nysdoh/reports/pci_1998-2000.pdf#search=%22Percutaneous%20coronary%20interventions%20(PCI)%20in%20New%20York%20State%201998%E2%80%932000%22.

NHS (2003). Extending choice for patients – heart surgery: your guide to your choices. Available: http://www.dh.gov.uk/assetRoot/04/07/36/17/04073617.pdf.

Oakley, J. and Cocking, D. (2001). *Virtue Ethics and Professional Roles*. Cambridge: Cambridge University Press.

Pennsylvania Health Care Cost Containment Council (2000). Pennsylvania's Guide to Coronary Artery Bypass Graft (CABG) Surgery 2000. Available: http://www.phc4.org/reports/cabg/00/.

Peterson, E. D., De Long, E. R. and Jollis, J. G. (1998). The effects of New York's bypass surgery provider profiling on access to care and patient outcomes in the elderly. *Journal of the American College of Cardiology*, **32**, 993–9.

Quality Information Management Corporation, The Greater Cleveland Consumer Report of Hospital Performance, Cleveland, Ohio (1998). Discussed at http://www.insightsandoutcomes.com/cgi-bin/article.cgi?article_id=55.

Schuck, P. H. (1994). Rethinking informed consent. *The Yale Law Journal*, **103**, 899–959.

Taffinder, N. J., McManus, I. C., Gul, Y., Russell, R. C. G. and Darzi, A. (1988). Effect of sleep deprivation on surgeon's dexterity on laparoscopy simulator. *The Lancet*, **352**, 1191.

The Bristol Royal Infirmary Inquiry. Available: http://www.bristol-inquiry.org.uk/index.htm.

Veatch, R. M. (1985). The physician as stranger: the ethics of the anonymous patient–physician relationship. In *The Clinical Encounter*, ed. E. Shelp. Dordrecht: Reidel.

Wear, S. (1998). *Informed Consent: Patient Autonomy and Physician Beneficence within Healthcare*, 2nd edn. Dordrecht: Kluwer.

8

The value and practical limits of informed consent

Merle Spriggs

Murdoch Childrens Research Institute, Parkville, Australia

Introduction

Obtaining informed consent from patients and research subjects is often seen as an impossible goal. Practical difficulties abound in the disclosure of information, the processing of information and with patient understanding of information. Some people view these practical difficulties as limitations of informed consent. These difficulties and perceived limitations are some of the objections appealed to when it is suggested that patients offered surgery should have access to information about individual clinicians' performance (Clarke, this volume; Clarke and Oakley, 2004). In this chapter I outline the requirements for informed consent and comment on the moral authority of informed consent. I then outline recent influential criticisms of informed consent by Onora O'Neill and Carl Schneider and assess the main practical limitations these authors identify. Based on this assessment, I argue that the practical difficulties can be dealt with – they do not rule out the possibility of informed consent. Instead of practical difficulties, major impediments to achieving informed consent are the result of a failure to adequately value patient autonomy (the value underlying informed consent) and relying on an impoverished or underdeveloped view of autonomy. I argue that a proper understanding of informed consent and patient autonomy clarifies the ethical obligations of health care professionals. A proper understanding of informed consent and patient autonomy also shows us that there is an ethical obligation to provide information about individual clinicians' ability to perform an intervention. I conclude by considering the effect on the doctor–patient relationship of providing information about clinician performance.

Requirements for informed consent and information about persons offering or performing interventions

In the endeavour to obtain informed consent, great emphasis is placed on things patients need to know about and understand, such as 'diagnoses, prognoses, the

Informed Consent and Clinician Accountability: The Ethics of Report Cards on Surgeon Performance.
Steve Clarke and Justin Oakley (eds.). Published by Cambridge University Press. © Cambridge University Press 2007.

nature and purpose of the intervention, risks and benefits and recommendations' (Beauchamp and Childress, 2001, p. 89). While these things are typically considered essential for patients to make informed decisions, there seems to be no requirement to provide information about those offering or performing the intervention. There are only a few philosophers or commentators on informed consent who explicitly advocate the provision of information about persons performing interventions (Clarke and Oakley, 2004, p. 6; Wilkinson, 2001; Kluge, 1999).

Informed decisions and information about risk

It is well recognized that, in order for patients to make meaningful decisions, i.e. decisions with moral weight, reflecting their preferences and values, patients need not only information about procedures, but they also need to understand how the intervention is likely to impact on their life and the things that they value. In other words, patients need 'material' information, i.e. information on which a patient is likely to place significance. Information is 'material' if a patient views it as 'material' information (Faden and Beauchamp, 1986, p. 304). It includes information about benefits and risks on which a person is likely to place significance. Patients are likely to place significance on information that is uncertain, missing or not available. In order to make a properly informed decision, patients also need to understand the information they are given. Information must be *presented* in a way that patients can understand it (NHMRC, 2004a, b).

Risk associated with a procedure can be statistically quantified to some extent, but risk is also an individual thing that must be tailored to individual patients. Risk varies from patient to patient depending on things like health, age, gender, and the presence of co-morbid factors (Lloyd *et al.*, 2001, p. 147). Risk also varies from doctor to doctor and the risk associated with some doctors is greater. Reports such as the following appear regularly in the media: doctors with limited surgical experience operating on patients (Nader, 2005, p. 7); a Sydney neurosurgeon charged with cocaine possession while attending a brain surgeons' conference (Maher, 2005, p. 11); abuse of alcohol and drugs among doctors is about two to three times that of the general population (Cresswell, 2005, p. 5).

These may be extreme examples, but given the risk these behaviours pose for patients, it is reasonable for patients to want to know something about those who are offering and performing interventions, especially when patients are constantly hearing about high rates of medical errors (Braithwaite, Healy and Dwan, 2005, p. vi; Carvel, 2005; Hobgood *et al.*, 2005, p. 1276). The existence of medical errors adds weight to the view that consent that is informed and meaningful in the sense that it reflects a patient's preferences and values requires individualized information about clinicians, specifically their performance – for the same reason that patients need information about their own individual level of risk. Performance data on individual clinicians will reflect things that may be concealed from the public and which have a bearing on the risk that patients face. Patients need this information to be properly informed.

The level of risk a person is prepared to take on is also an individual thing. Only I know what level of risk I am willing to accept, and while competent, it is not up to any other person to decide on my behalf what level of risk is acceptable to me. Therefore, in order to make an informed and meaningful decision, 'material' information includes information about: (a) how an intervention is likely to affect my life or the things that I value; (b) information about my individual risk factors; (c) information on the level of risk associated with the clinician performing the intervention, i.e. individual performance data. I then deliberate on this information in light of my particular values and preferences.

The moral authority of informed consent

In health, law and ethics, moral authority is given to the informed consent of competent adults about their own healthcare. A competent adult's decision to undergo (or forego) treatment is justification to proceed (or desist) despite risks – as long as relevant information has been provided (including risks, uncertainties and alternative options); the individual understands the information; and makes a voluntary decision (is not coerced or deceived), based on their own values and preferences. The moral authority of an individual's consent is therefore grounded in the degree of autonomy of the decision. And the ethical significance we give to autonomy will depend on the underlying ethical theory we hold. Autonomy can be regarded as good because it has instrumental value, because it has intrinsic value, or it can be viewed as a side-constraint that we ought not to violate, apart from exceptional circumstances (Spriggs, 2005, p. 247).

Criticisms of informed consent

I begin by outlining the influential critiques of Onora O'Neill and Carl Schneider whose arguments represent the major and most prevalent criticisms of informed consent. I then assess in detail the main practical limitations that these authors identify.

Onora O'Neill claims that she takes informed consent 'sufficiently seriously to identify some of its limitations' and that her intention is not to deny the importance of informed consent or recommend a return to medical paternalism. The 'ethical importance' of informed consent she claims, is not that 'it secures some form of individual autonomy, but that it provides assurance that patients and others are not deceived or coerced' (O'Neill, 2003, pp. 4–5). O'Neill's arguments deal with medical treatment, research and the use of human tissue, although she focuses mostly on the latter two. Carl Schneider focuses on informed consent in clinical practice. He is sceptical about the possibility of obtaining informed consent and sceptical about its value.

In *The Practice of Autonomy*, Schneider presents a case for the conclusion that patient decisions are often made on other than rational grounds (Schneider, 1998, p. 99). He presents a caricature of the idea of autonomy (the underlying value of informed consent) which he refers to as 'mandatory' autonomy and then proceeds to criticize that (Schneider, 1998, pp. 17–32, 137–79). He equates this conception of autonomy with independence and self-sufficiency (Schneider, 1998, pp. 153–4), and implies that autonomy involves patients taking full decisional control, having full information and achieving full understanding even in the technical sense (Schneider, 1998, pp. 52–6, 107). Based on this conception of autonomy, he argues that autonomy is an 'unattainable and unwise standard' (Schneider, 1998, p. 174). He also claims that many patients are reluctant to make their own medical decisions (Schneider, 1998, p. 46). In a more recent article he continues in this vein to argue that the goals of informed consent are not achieved because more disclosure does not lead to better decisions (Schneider, 2005, p. 13).

Practical limitations: an assessment

The requirements for informed consent are an impossible goal

According to Schneider, full disclosure is required for informed consent and patients need (on the extreme view that he presents) to understand all information, even technical medical information (Schneider, 1998, pp. 52–3, 128–30). Schneider rightly predicts that satisfying such a standard would lead to information overload and that would interfere with understanding (Schneider, 1998, p. 60). Schneider also worries that patients are basing their decisions on missing or unreliable information because the data on which diagnosis and prognosis are made are fraught with uncertainty and doubt (Schneider, 1998, p. 52). The existence of uncertainty, together with less than full information contributes to Schneider's view that informed consent is not achievable (Schneider, 1998, pp. 52–5). For Schneider, informed consent seems to be an impossible goal because full information is problematic and less than full information is also problematic.

I would argue that the requirements for informed consent are not an impossible goal. Of course, *full* autonomy requiring *full* information and knowledge of outcomes is indeed an unrealistic ideal. While achieving this ideal is often not possible, it is also not necessary. *Substantial* rather than *full* autonomy is a more appropriate standard, i.e. having 'material' information on which the individual places importance. On this standard, individuals need enough information to feel that their choice is a responsible choice relative to the available evidence – irrespective of what the outcome may be. In other areas of life, significant choices involving intentional action, substantial understanding and freedom from constraint are justifiably respected and not interfered with – even when we do not know how things will turn out, e.g. making financial investments, hiring employees and buying a house (Beauchamp and Childress, 2001, pp. 59–60). Some patients might want access to technical information, but full technical information is not necessary for someone to gain an appreciation of how an intervention may affect the things they value.

Contrary to Schneider, it is possible to make medical decisions that are autonomous even though they include information that is uncertain. We can give meaningful consent to complicated surgery even though we are uncertain about what the outcome might be – even though the outcome may turn out not to our liking. The things that matter are the relevance and quality of the information that is disclosed, the voluntariness of the decision and the quality of our deliberation. Uncertainty can be perceived and evaluated and factored into a decision, e.g. there is uncertainty about the best treatment for breast and prostate cancer but certainties and uncertainties can be identified. Doctors and patients can talk about what is known, unknown and that which is conjecture (Katz, 1984, pp. 167–9). By taking uncertainty into account rather than disregarding uncertainty, patients can make an informed decision and choose the option they prefer – knowing that there is an element of uncertainty. Likewise, research participants can give informed consent to enter a trial with the knowledge that they will not know and will not be told which treatment arm they are assigned to.

Lack of understanding

Lack of understanding is a practical limitation to achieving informed consent. Patients cannot give informed consent if they cannot understand the thing for which their consent is sought. Lack of understanding due to information processing problems has received much attention (Clarke, 2007; Gilovich, Griffin and Kahneman, 2002; Beauchamp and Childress, 2001; Faden and Beauchamp, 1986). O'Neill provides a different take on this limitation with the claim that consent is a 'propositional attitude'. According to O'Neill, propositional attitudes are opaque. Consent is directed at a proposition that 'describes an intended intervention' but there may be 'other true descriptions of the same intervention, or its more obvious effects' (O'Neill, 2005, p. 4). O'Neill cites the example of parents who consented to the removal of tissue from their dead children but did not understand that that entailed removal of entire organs (O'Neill, 2003, p. 6). According to O'Neill, in trying to get 'explicit' and 'specific' consent (O'Neill, 2005, p. 5), we end up performing a 'ritual' rather than achieving what she calls 'genuine' consent. When the focus is on documents, signatures and avoiding litigation, there is a danger of overwhelming patients with 'excessive or technical detail' and obtaining consent becomes a 'matter of ticking boxes' (O'Neill, 2003, pp. 5–6).

O'Neill exaggerates the difficulty with understanding when she claims that 'the descriptions to which consent is given are always incomplete' (O'Neill, 2005, p. 6) and that 'the quest for perfect specificity is doomed to fail since descriptions can be expanded endlessly, and there is no limit to a process of seeking more specific consent' (O'Neill, 2003, p. 6). There are ways to help people understand those things that are entailed or caused by medical interventions. O'Neill seems to be suggesting that providing more and more information is the typical response and that this is problematic because it will lead to longer, more complex consent forms with the result that informed consent will be undermined (O'Neill, 2003, pp. 5–6).

In the example cited by O'Neill, adding the words 'this may include entire organs' would surely aid understanding. This is not an onerous task and is not likely to overtax or create information overload – especially as it is likely to be 'material' information. A further case illustrates this point. A man, who did not intend to consent to being sterilized, was sterilized when he consented to prostate surgery. Sterilization was an inevitable outcome of the specific procedure he consented to but he was not aware of that (Beauchamp and Childress, 2001, p. 88). This should not be interpreted as a problem with the 'quest for perfect specificity'. It should be viewed as withholding or failing to disclose information necessary for informed consent and as a failure on the part of the consent seeker. When something significant like sterilization or the removal of entire organs from dead children is entailed in a procedure, it is surely an obligation of health professionals to make sure that those things are spelled out. It is the responsibility of clinicians or researchers seeking consent to make sure what is entailed in a procedure is understood.

Clinicians need effective communication skills to facilitate patient understanding. There are strategies and technologies to help communicate unfamiliar, novel, and specialized information to laypersons, e.g. pictures, drawing analogies and the use of computer-based patient education (Jimson and Sher, 2000, pp. 335–61; Faden and Beauchamp, 1986, pp. 318–19). The facilitation of patient understanding may benefit from the use of a professional health educator who is skilled in these approaches, especially in situations where doctor and patient do not have a shared world view or knowledge base. The use of an educator may also help overcome certain obstacles to patient understanding, e.g. patient's fear of 'appearing to waste the physician's time' and their reticence to articulate informational needs and acknowledge their ignorance (Faden and Beauchamp,

1986, pp. 314–15). On the other hand, patient understanding and the doctor–patient relationship may be enhanced when both parties to an intervention participate in the informational exchange – doctors also achieve understanding, e.g. understanding of patients concerns, false beliefs and confusions. Ideally, the acquisition of effective communication skills and taking time to converse with patients will be viewed as part of good patient care. However, time and 'time costs' involved in talking with patients are sometimes invoked as constraints that impose a burden on doctors (Katz, 1984, p. xi).

Excessive emphasis on informed consent procedures

The main target of O'Neill's criticism about incomplete descriptions and lack of understanding is the emphasis on procedure – the 'ritual' of informed consent (O'Neill, 2003, p. 5). This is a legitimate concern. Informed consent procedures are important but when the idea of informed consent is reduced to a procedure or 'ritual' it can make consent meaningless. When satisfying the procedure and getting a signature on the consent form become the focus, this can displace concern about the quality of deliberation or the quality of understanding required to give informed consent. When the focus is on the procedure, the guiding value may have nothing to do with patient's interests or level of understanding. The guiding value may be fear of legal liability and the interests of institutions, and be altogether unrelated to the patient and to medical considerations (Spriggs, 2005, pp. 125–6). An emphasis on the procedure may regulate the behaviour of the person seeking consent but it has nothing to say about the quality of patients' decisions.

The difficulty in knowing what information is 'material'

The difficulty in knowing what information is 'material' to an individual patient can be viewed as a limitation. O'Neill compares this to trying to achieve 'specific and generic' consent and with trying to answer the question 'how long is a piece of string?' (O'Neill, 2005, pp. 6–7). O'Neill, however, overstates the problem and makes light of the importance of the issue. Helping patients obtain information about what is 'material' to them does not entail having to provide 'full' information in order for patients to pick out what is personally relevant.

The simple act of talking with patients is effective and efficient. The crucial role of conversation in informing patients, as promoted by Jay Katz, illustrates its importance. Katz says that John Stuart Mill, whose argument for liberty is often mistakenly interpreted as an argument for non-intervention, anticipates his views on the need for conversation:

[Mill] most insistently asserted instead that 'Considerations to aid his judgment, exhortations to strengthen his will, may be offered to him, even obtruded on him, by others.' Only after such an enforced conversation must individual men and women be allowed to be 'the final judge' since 'they have means of knowledge [about their feelings and circumstances] immeasurably surpassing those that can be possessed by anyone else'. (Katz, 1984, p. 123)

Conversation incorporates the obligation of healthcare professionals to provide information and helps clarify misconceptions and misunderstandings. It involves patients asking or being prompted to ask questions, and physicians providing answers. In this way, it delivers the awareness of relevant information required by patients for making informed meaningful decisions (Katz, 1984, p. 124, p. 155).

Informed consent does not lead to better choices or good or palatable outcomes

Some people expect that the requirements for informed consent should bring about good or palatable outcomes. O'Neill complains that informed consent procedures protect choices that are not worthy of being protected. They protect choices that are 'timid, conventional, and lacking in individual autonomy' as much as they protect choices that are 'bursting with individual autonomy (variously conceived)' (O'Neill, 2003, p. 5). For Schneider, 'the goal of disclosure requirements' in the doctrine of informed consent 'is to improve the decisions recipients make' and 'success means improving decisions enough to justify the costs of the disclosure requirement' to disclosers and recipients. The 'baseline for evaluation' he claims, is 'the quality of the decisions people would make were there no disclosure laws' (Schneider, 2005, pp. 12–13).

To some extent, the above concerns can be attributed to a flawed view of informed consent and autonomy. Informed consent does not necessarily lead to 'good' or palatable choices, e.g. making an informed decision from a restricted range of options can result in outcomes that are not ideal or not to our liking. Indeed, people sometimes have to make tragic choices but there is still value in choosing in accordance with their values and preferences. Having to make a tragic choice does not take away a person's need or desire for information. Nor does it cancel the obligation of healthcare professionals to provide patients with information.

O'Neill's worry that informed consent procedures protect choices that are not worth protecting is a legitimate concern when the emphasis is on procedures. But, as discussed above, informed consent involves more than disclosure and a signature. It involves disclosure of 'material' information, understanding on the part of patients and conversation has an important role. Conversation between patient and doctor (or educator) can help identify what is material – and can help ensure that decisions are worthy of respect. O'Neill's concern may be more applicable in the research context where a patient's best interests are not the primary concern and informed consent does not rule out the possibility of exploitation. Properly informed, some people may consent to an offer which is to their advantage but nevertheless exploitative. Exploitation is consistent with freedom to choose – it may be 'mutually advantageous and consensual' (Carling, 1998, p. 220; Wertheimer, 1996, p. ix).

Schneider is also concerned with problems of disclosure and understanding but he has an additional concern. Schneider thinks that the effort expended in addressing these problems needs to be justified – and that the effort is not justified. According to Schneider, 'people's decisions do not always change, much less improve, with more information' (Schneider, 2005, pp. 12–13).

First of all, the idea that costs to the discloser should figure in the justification seems contrary to the standard interpretation of the doctrine of informed consent. Furthermore, studies tell us, and Schneider acknowledges, that patients value disclosure and want information about their medical circumstances (Schneider, 1998, pp. 35–41), so, if some decisions do not change with more information it is reasonable to conclude that the value is not to be found by justifying costs or by looking for 'improved' decisions.

Expecting informed consent to produce 'happy' or 'improved' outcomes means that we overlook the value of disclosure. Disclosure of relevant information demonstrates respect for patients and their autonomy and the act of respect is not conditional upon outcomes. Disclosure that is an act of respect has nothing to say about how the information should be used.

Information about individual clinician's performance

Assessment of the practical limitations and the value of informed consent provide some lessons for the inclusion of information about clinician's performance.

Information about a clinician's ability to perform an intervention is necessary for meaningful consent

When competent adults make decisions about their own healthcare, such as when they are offered a surgical intervention, informed consent is important and valuable. In the clinical setting, the best interests of the patient are the primary concern. There are no competing aims impacting on the disclosure of information as may happen in the research setting. There should be no opposition to the provision of 'material' information. As mentioned previously, patients need information about risks, what the surgery entails and how it could impact on the things they value. Not all patients will want to know about risks associated with the procedure but for those that do, information about clinician performance, to the extent that it is an element of the risk a patient faces, is 'material' and therefore necessary for making an informed decision.

Information about clinician performance might not be available but it is not impossible to provide. It is not unknowable. This is an important distinction and in terms of meaningful consent, there is a significant difference between making a decision that would take into account information that is unknowable, e.g. unforeseeable effects of an intervention – and making a decision without specific information – information that has not been collected and centrally collated but could be collected and collated to provide comparative performance information. Information not available in the sense that it has not been collected and collated is more akin to information that is withheld. Not collecting the information is not sufficient justification for not providing this information to patients.

Surgeons' performance data may be hard to interpret but this difficulty can be addressed. Consider the complex nature of genetic information. When individuals are offered interventions such as genetic testing and pre-natal diagnosis, patient autonomy is the guiding principle. Great emphasis is placed on giving patients and prospective parents as much information as possible about risks and probabilities despite the number of variables, complexity of the information and the possibility of false positives. Genetic counselors are trained and utilized to help patients understand these things. A standard of information considered necessary for significant decisions, should apply for all significant decisions. Counseling or education (guided by the desire to respect patient autonomy) to help individuals understand complex information, should be provided for patients undergoing other significant interventions as well, e.g. surgery.

Disclosing clinician performance information to patients may strengthen the doctor–patient relationship

Clinicians may feel threatened by being required to provide information about their performance. From the clinician's perspective the doctor–patient relationship may be adversely affected. From the patient's perspective however, disclosure and consent do not put an end to trust. Jay Katz argues convincingly that disclosure and consent 'make mutual trust possible for the first time' because they 'banish unilateral blind trust' (Katz, 1984, p. xvi).

Clinicians may feel threatened by a requirement to provide information about their performance but being accountable to patients in this way is not incompatible with trust. It may increase trust. This has been demonstrated in one study in which medical students informed patients of their inexperience (Santen et al., 2005). Experience and performance ability are different but they are comparable in the sense that they both influence the level of risk patients are exposed to. The aim of the study was to determine whether patients would consent to a procedure performed by inexperienced medical students in a hospital emergency department when informed by the medical student of their inexperience. It was found that acceptance of medical students in clinical situations may be higher than has been predicted in hypothetical studies. Patients seemed to welcome the involvement of students in their care as long as they felt assured that medical care would not be compromised. Although most patients wanted to be informed if it was the first time a student performed the procedure, the majority of patients (90%) consented to the student performing the procedure. An obvious limitation of the study is that the procedures were of a minor nature such as sutures, putting in an intravenous line or splinting. Studies are needed to see if the results differ for more invasive and complicated procedures such as surgery. The lesson in this, and the relevance to providing surgeon's performance data, lies in the researchers' speculation that the increased consent rate (compared to theoretical survey studies) was due not only to the lack of complexity of the procedure, but was also a result of talking with the patient and the 'increased comfort' for the patient from 'having established a rapport with the medical student' (Santen et al., 2005. p. 368). This suggests that, rather than eroding trust, talking with patients (even talking about risk) may strengthen the doctor–patient relationship and increase trust. Having a role in helping patients interpret and understand the data should allay fears about the fairness of the ranking system.

Atul Gawande's book *Complications: A Surgeon's Notes on an Imperfect Science*, attests to the rapport that is possible despite the risk and uncertainty associated with medicine and surgery. Gawande concedes the fallibility of individual doctors, and he does not shirk from acknowledging the uncertainty of medicine: 'It's not science that you call upon but a doctor. A doctor with good days and bad days ... A doctor with three other patients to see and, inevitably, gaps in what he knows and skills he's still trying to learn' (Gawande, 2002, p. 5). This book nevertheless generates confidence, empathy and trust through its candour and by way of an obvious respect for patients.

A distrust of doctors is more likely to occur with a policy of not providing information about the performance ability of individual surgeons. Important information that is withheld and that has relevance to patients (such as a high mortality rate) is likely to be known by some people informally. Distrust is likely to follow if it becomes known that information has been withheld (Williamson, 2005, p. 1079). Distrust will be further exacerbated when information withheld from the public is used by the connected and the knowledgeable. Those with inside knowledge are unlikely to ignore information that indicates a significant risk.

Providing performance data may or may not bring about happy outcomes. Nevertheless, the primary justification for providing information about clinician's performance is that it will help make consent informed and meaningful and it demonstrates respect for patients.

Conclusions

Gaining informed consent is not a practical impossibility. As we have seen, there are challenges and difficulties but major obstacles to achieving informed consent are not valuing autonomy and relying on an impoverished or under-developed view of autonomy.

Contrary to O'Neill (2003, pp. 4–5), the ethical importance of informed consent is that it secures some form of individual autonomy – and the account of autonomy we rely on is important. Well-developed accounts of autonomy do exist (Spriggs, 2005; Mele, 1995; Christman, 1991; Meyers, 1989; Dworkin, 1988; Young, 1986). On these accounts, autonomy has a deeper sense than mere freedom from coercion or deception. These accounts all have something to say about the quality of patient's deliberation and understanding.

Finally, an understanding of what gives moral weight to informed consent, together with a well-developed account of autonomy emphasizing deliberation and understanding, will help us recognize the ethical obligation of health care professionals to respect and promote patient autonomy. And, because clinician performance data is an element of risk information, it is clear that the obligation of healthcare professionals includes making that information available and helping patients understand that information.

References

Beauchamp, T. and Childress, J. (2001). *Principles of Biomedical Ethics*, 5th edn. New York: Oxford University Press.

Braithwaite, J., Healy, J. and Dwan, K. (2005). *The Governance of Health Safety and Quality*, Commonwealth of Australia. Available at http://www.safetyandquality.org/governance0705.pdf (Accessed 4 November 2005).

Carling, A. (1998). Exploitation. In *Encyclopedia of Applied Ethics*, Volume 2, ed. Chadwick, R. Academic Press, pp. 219–32.

Carvel, J. (2005). More than 1 m patients fall victim to mistakes in NHS hospitals. *The Guardian*, 3 November. Available at http://www.guardian.co.uk/uk_news/story/0,3604,1607108,00.html (Accessed 4 November 2005).

Christman, J. (1991). Autonomy and personal history. *Canadian Journal of Philosophy*, **21**, 1–24.

Clarke, S. and Oakley, J. (2004). Informed consent and surgeons' performance. *Journal of Medicine and Philosophy*, **29**, 11–35.

Cresswell, C. (2005). Drugged up doctors. *The Weekend Australian*, 1–2 October, p. 5.

Dworkin, G. (1988). *The Theory and Practice of Autonomy*. Cambridge: Cambridge University Press.

Faden, R. R. and Beauchamp, T. L. (1986). *A History and Theory of Informed Consent*. New York: Oxford University Press.

Gawande, A. (2002). *Complications: A Surgeon's Notes on an Imperfect Science.* New York: Picador.

Gilovich, T., Griffin, D. and Kahneman, D. (2002). *Heuristics and Biases: The Psychology of Intuitive Judgment.* Cambridge: Cambridge University Press.

Hobgood, C., Tamayo-Sarver, J., Elms, A. and Weiner, B. (2005). Parental preferences for error disclosure, reporting, and legal action after medical error in the care of their children. *Pediatrics*, **116**, 1276–86.

Jimison, H. and Sher, P. (2000). Advances in presenting health information to patients. In *Decision Making in Health Care: Theory, Psychology and Applications*, ed. G. Chapman and F. Sonnenberg. Cambridge: Cambridge University Press, pp. 335–61.

Katz, J. (1984). *The Silent World of Doctor and Patient.* London: Collier, Macmillan Publishers.

Kluge, E. (1999). Informed consent in a different key: physicians' practice profiles and the patient's right to know. *Canadian Medical Association Journal*, **160**, 1321–2.

Lloyd, A., Hayes, P., Bell, P. R. F. and Naylor, A. R. (2001). The role of risk and benefit perception in informed consent for surgery. *Medical Decision Making*, **21**, 141–9.

Maher, S. (2005). Surgeon does drug rehab program away from spotlight. *The Weekend Australian.* 1–2 October, p. 11.

Mele, A. (1995). *Autonomous Agents: From Self-Control to Autonomy.* Oxford: Oxford University Press.

Meyers, D. T. (1989). *Self, Society and Personal Choice.* New York: Columbia University Press.

Nader, C. (2005). Doctors 'operate without skill checks'. *The Age*, 29 September, p. 7.

NHMRC (2004a). *Communicating With Patients: Advice for Medical Practitioners.* Commonwealth of Australia. Available at: http://www7.health.gov.au/nhmrc/publications/_files/e58.pdf (Accessed 4 October 2005).

NHMRC (2004b). *General Guidelines for Medical Practitioners on Providing Information to Patients.* Commonwealth of Australia. Available at: http://www7.health.gov.au/nhmrc/publications/synopses/e57syn.htm (Accessed 4 October 2005).

O'Neill, O. (2003). Some limits of informed consent. *Journal of Medical Ethics*, **29**, 4–7.

O'Neill, O. (2005). Informed consent and public health. SARS conference, Royal Society.

Santen, S., Hemphill, R., Spanier, C. and Fletcher, N. (2005). 'Sorry, it's my first time!' Will patients consent to medical students learning procedures? *Medical Education*, **39**, 365–9.

Schneider, C. E. (1998). *The Practice of Autonomy: Patients, Doctors, and Medical Decisions.* New York: Oxford University Press.

Schneider, C. E. (2005). Reaching disclosure. *Hastings Center Report*, **35**, 12–13.

Spriggs, M. (2005). *Autonomy and Patients' Decisions.* Maryland: Lexington Books.

Wertheimer, A. (1996). *Exploitation.* New Jersey: Princeton University Press.

Wilkinson, T. M. (2001). Research, informed consent, and the limits of disclosure. *Bioethics*, **15**, 341–63.

Williamson, C. (2005). Withholding policies from patients restricts their autonomy. *British Medical Journal*, **331**, 1078–80.

Young, R. (1986). *Personal Autonomy: Beyond Negative and Positive Liberty.* London: Croom Helm.

9

Against the informed consent argument for surgeon report cards

David Neil

University of Wollongong, Australia

The publication of outcomes information, or 'report cards', for individual surgeons can be argued for on three distinct grounds. One kind of argument appeals to healthcare quality, and focuses on the value of individual perform-ance auditing for patient safety and for an evidence-based approach to best practice. A second kind of argument constructs the patient as a healthcare 'consumer' and appeals to a notion of consumer rights, such that patients have a right to comparative information about the healthcare products and services that they consume. Some proponents of this kind of argument believe that enabling patients to be more informed consumers will introduce productive market incentives into the healthcare system. A third kind of argument appeals to respect for patient autonomy and the requirement of informed consent to any medical intervention. I will refer to these arguments, respectively, as 'the argu-ment from quality', 'the argument from consumer sovereignty' and 'the argu-ment from informed consent'. In advocating the publication of surgeon-specific outcomes data, it matters which argument we take to be fundamental, because the basic rationale for having surgeon-specific report cards has implications for the form, content and funding of such a system.

With respect to the argument from quality, the literature examining the effect of public reporting of comparative performance information on health-care quality presents an increasingly compelling argument that such reporting is necessary for sustainable quality improvement (Chassin, 2002; Marshall *et al.*, 2002). From this perspective, the value of surgeon-specific performance data is that it assists with a sophisticated analysis of the factors contributing to medical errors. As Mark Chassin (1996) puts it:

Some of the new tools of quality improvement permit us to understand much better how errors creep into clinical practice. This kind of analysis, adapted from industrial models, involves studying in detail all the steps involved in providing a particular kind

Informed Consent and Clinician Accountability: The Ethics of Report Cards on Surgeon Performance. Steve Clarke and Justin Oakley (eds.). Published by Cambridge University Press. © Cambridge University Press 2007.

of care. It does not seek to identify errors in order to assign blame, but instead assumes that faulty systems of care are very often responsible for errors. Fixing systems by reducing unwarranted variations in the provision of care can be much more effective in reducing errors than punishing people.

The argument from quality and the argument from consumer sovereignty are not necessarily incompatible. The quality approach focuses on the technical analysis of the sources of error in complex medical systems. The argument from consumer sovereignty sees the value of surgeons' report cards, not in terms of the analytical value of the data, but as a means of introducing incentives that reward doctors and institutions for good outcomes. Whether the market effects of report cards for medical service providers advances or hinders the goal of quality is a substantive empirical question, and the available evidence is mixed.

UK government reforms requiring patients to be given a choice of hospitals provide a case in point. The University College London Hospitals Trust announced, in December 2005, that it would advertise for patients by claiming that it has the lowest death rates in the National Health Service (Templeton, 2005). The claim is based on the findings of the independent health research group Dr Foster. This kind of initiative aims to force hospitals to compete on the grounds of safety and quality. However, it may turn out that link-ing surgeons' 'market value' to their mortality rates may introduce counter-productive disincentives into the system. For instance, there is some evidence from New York that cardiac surgeons are turning away some high-risk patients who might benefit from surgery, in order to protect their published mortality rates (Kolker, 2005). Similarly, Sir Bruce Keogh, president-elect of the Society of Cardiothoracic Surgeons, has said that:

There is absolutely no doubt in my mind that the publication of mortality data in England has had a negative effect on surgeons taking on high-risk cases . . . There will, inevitably, be some people who don't get an operation now, who might have got one in the past. (Fracassini and Nutt, 2005)

I am sceptical about the idea that consumer preference, informed by access to report cards, could be an effective mechanism for driving improvements in surgical safety. However, the question of whether market mechanisms can promote healthcare quality is not the subject of this paper. Rather, this paper examines the argument from informed consent.

The argument from informed consent is important because it is independ-ent of the argument from quality. The argument from informed consent attempts to sidestep questions about the actual effects that report cards will have on the healthcare system, by arguing that access to surgeon-specific performance information falls within the ambit of an existing right. This is not an argument that rests on empirical claims about the costs and benefits of performance reporting, but instead appeals directly to a general principle of medical ethics – the principle of respect for patient autonomy.

I will argue that the informed consent argument for surgeon report cards is actually fairly weak; too weak in fact to provide a sufficient justification for developing a surgeon-specific outcomes reporting system. The right to such information cannot be derived from the general requirement to respect patient autonomy. Consequently, calls for a report card system need to be justified in terms of their value for realizing improvements in quality and safety standards.

The idea that, as patients, we have a right to know about our surgeon's experience and success rates has an immediate appeal. It is the kind of demand that follows naturally in the wake of revelations of clinical incompetence, and indeed it did follow in the wake of the Bristol Royal Infirmary scandal. The UK national paper, *The Express*, offered one of the more shrill responses to the findings of the Bristol Royal Infirmary Inquiry (Parker, 2001):

Not until we have eradicated a culture in which doctors can be more interested in furthering their ambitions than in telling the truth about their success rate or a patient's chances, will we prevent another scandal like that at Bristol Royal Infirmary happening again.

It is important, however, not to conflate our right, as patients, to be protected from medical negligence and incompetence, with a proposed right to have fine-grained comparative performance information about all surgeons.

The argument from informed consent has been developed primarily by Steve Clarke and Justin Oakley in their paper 'Informed consent and surgeons' performance' (2004). My critique of the argument from informed consent will focus on Clarke and Oakley's paper. Their basic strategy is very straightforward. It is uncontroversial, under the doctrine of informed consent, that the reasonably foreseeable risks of an operation must be disclosed to patients in the consent process. Clarke and Oakley contend that relevant risk information includes 'information about the ability of available surgeons to perform the operation in question' (2004, p. 12):

Our main point is simple and, we think, very hard to deny. The risks that should be disclosed to patients are the risks that we can reasonably expect that patients will face when undergoing an operation. These risks will vary, *inter alia*, according to the level of ability of the surgeons who are available to perform that operation. So, information about the performance ability of surgeons is a necessary component of the disclosure of the reasonably foreseeable risks of a surgical intervention. And, as the disclosure of the reasonably foreseeable risks of a surgical intervention is a necessary requirement for the provision of effective informed consent, the disclosure of information about the performance ability of available surgeons is a necessary requirement for the provision of effective informed consent to a surgical intervention. (2004, p. 12)

Clarke and Oakley stress that they accept the 'received view' that the moral principle which grounds the doctrine of informed consent is respect for patient autonomy. They insist that the availability of surgeon report cards will give patients more autonomy with respect to decisions about surgery:

We best uphold a patient's autonomy by enabling that patient to properly understand the risks that they are exposing themselves to when choosing to be operated on by a particular surgeon. (2004, p. 13)

There are two problems with this argument. The first concerns Clarke and Oakley's use of the notion of 'disclosure'. A medical practitioner's obligation to disclose information applies to information that she knows or should know – crucially, information that is *available*. Standard obligations of disclosure cannot be extended to generate an obligation to *discover* information that is not presently known. Clarke and Oakley expand the obligation of disclosure in a way that has counter-intuitive consequences. The second problem with their argument is that it fails to respect a formal constraint on any argument from autonomy – namely, that any substantive right derived from the principle of respect for autonomy must be universalisable. I will consider these problems in turn.

   Clarke and Oakley point out that, where it is available, stratified risk information is more relevant than very general risk information. For instance, a risk algorithm such as the European System for Cardiac Operative Risk Evaluation Score (EuroSCORE) takes into account a range of factors in determining percentage predicted mortality for cardiac surgery. These risk factors include age, gender, history of pulmonary disease, previous cardiac surgery, unstable angina as well as 14 other criteria. If you were considering consenting to a coronary artery bypass graft, you should be told your mortality risk as predicted by an algorithm such as EuroSCORE, rather than merely being told less 'personalized' information, such as the average mortality rate for all cardiac patients. Clarke and Oakley tell us that 'we ought to provide more fine-grained information where it is available, because it more closely approximates the actual probability of the relevant possible event' (2004, p. 14).

   The phrase 'where it is available' is misleading in this context. Clarke and Oakley recognize that 'a complete list of factors that can potentially affect the probability that a risk may materialize would be extremely long, if not infinite' and that this would be 'impractical if not impossible' (2004, p. 15). Having noted, on pain of absurdity, that some restrictions must apply to the scope of the disclosure obligation, Clarke and Oakley do not give any sustained consideration to the difficult question of how the appropriate boundary between obligatory and supererogatory disclosure should be drawn. Instead, they assert that a surgeon's level of performance is a factor that many patients would consider important. They further claim that:

Commonly, surgeons already maintain records of their performances in operations, so it would not be an onerous administrative imposition to require that material information derived from such records be made available so that it may be provided to patients for the purposes of enabling informed consent. (2004, p. 15)

Many surgeons may indeed keep detailed case notes. However, no individual surgeon's records can contain the kind of information that advocates of report cards are calling for; that is, *comparative* risk information. It is important to understand what is involved in meaningful comparative surgical audit. Comparison of surgeons' performance, with adequate risk adjustment to account for case-mix, requires all units to collect and report data against a uniform set of data standards, sufficient to apply a well-verified algorithm for assessing pre-operative risk.

To gain a sense of the kind of research necessary to provide risk-adjusted mortality comparisons for individual surgeons, consider the experience of the Society of Cardiothoracic Surgeons (SCTS) Britain. Anticipating the results of the Bristol Royal Infirmary Inquiry, the SCTS instituted the collection of data on surgeon specific activity and in-hospital mortality for several index procedures (Keogh *et al.*, 2004). The Society established a national database in 1994 which collects data on all adults undergoing cardiac surgery, beginning with 12 hospitals and now taking data from all NHS cardiac surgery units (SCTS, 2003). The main aim of the database was to develop reliable, UK-orientated risk stratification models. In the UK the process of developing an agreed minimum required dataset and standards for data reporting, and of bringing all units into a centralized data collection system was a major project, requiring national cooperation and considerable research and innovation. A study designed to assess the quality and completeness of the SCTS database was conducted by the SCTS in co-operation with the Nuffield Trust in Britain and the RAND Health Program in the United States. Sampling of the database 'revealed it to be both incomplete and unreliable in its ability to yield accurate, risk adjusted outcomes data' (Fine *et al.*, 2003, p. 28). Thus, when the SCTS published surgeon specific results, in 2004, it did so on the basis of raw, unadjusted mortality figures because it was not yet in a position to provide validated risk-adjusted mortality rates (Keogh *et al.*, 2004). Along with New York State, the SCTS in the United Kingdom has been at the forefront of surgical outcomes data collection in the world, and yet a decade of groundbreaking work is only now bringing individualised outcomes reporting within reach. The impressive work done by the SCTS in this area shows what is really involved in providing meaningful, validated, risk-adjusted, comparative outcomes data for individual surgeons. The suggestion that this kind of information could be harvested from existing records without 'onerous imposition' is rather too sanguine about the scale and analytical complexity of the task.

Once we acknowledge that determining risk-adjusted mortality rates for individual surgeons requires the kind of nationally co-ordinated database development that the SCTS has been engaged in since the early 1990s, it is immediately evident that it is misleading to talk about the 'disclosure' of such information. The obligation to disclose risk information to a patient is relative to the current state of medical knowledge. For almost any medical intervention we could name, it is likely that future research will yield information that is not currently available, but would be material to patients' treatment decisions if it were available. There may be obligations to undertake certain kinds of research, but if research obligations exist they are not derived from disclosure obligations. Standard obligations of disclosure do not generate any obligation to produce new information that will require substantial work to discover.

Outside of those places where report cards systems are under development, the information which Clarke and Oakley want to see published would require a considerable research and infrastructure investment to produce. Resources are scarce and there is any number of potential research and infrastructure projects that could improve the understanding and treatment of disease (and by extension the quality of informed consent to such treatment). The provision of surgeon specific performance information may ultimately make an important contribution to quality and safety in surgical practice, and so it may be worthwhile to invest resources in the development of report cards. However, a demand that surgeon report cards be made publicly available is a demand that substantial resources be allocated to that end. To justify such a project, we need to show that the benefits outweigh the costs.

I am not disputing the claim that comparative information about surgeons' performance would be valuable, both for the profession and for some patients. But no individual surgeon themselves can discover that information. Inter-surgeon comparison requires comparison of their respective case-mix in terms of a valid, standardized measure of patients' pre-operative risk. The resource expenditure required to produce comparative tables is not mandated by the requirements of informed consent. Rather, a compelling argument for surgeon report cards needs to justify the significant opportunity costs of developing such a system.

The publication of risk adjusted mortality rates may promote transparency in healthcare, but is of quite limited value in terms of patient safety. Because a surgeon's reputation and practice can be damaged, publicly reported outcomes data must be thoroughly validated and reliable. In New York the validation process typically means that data is 3 years old when it is published. Dated information is of limited use for informed consent. The way to deal with substandard surgeons is not to publish their poor results and hope that patients will choose to avoid them. What is needed is a system of continuous audit that identifies early signs of poor performance and calls surgeons and units to account well before the evidence of excessive mortality has reached the confidence level required for public reporting. In the UK the SCTS has adopted that role. It should not be via adverse publicity that a problem surgeon first comes to the attention of his or her hospital.

Clarke and Oakley briefly consider concerns that the publication of surgeon report cards will lead to defensive medicine and cite evidence suggesting that this has not happened in the case of New York. They then make the striking claim that, even if turns out that the publication of surgeon report cards does have 'certain deleterious effects' on the practice of medicine, their publication might still be ethically justified. They note that different ethical theories give different answers here, and while utilitarians will need to see a cost/benefit balance sheet to make up their minds, 'some Kantians might . . . view this as a price worth paying in order to uphold respect for patient autonomy' (2005, p. 23).

I claimed above that Clarke and Oakley's argument violates a formal requirement on arguments based on the principle of respect for autonomy. We now turn to this second problem with the argument from informed consent. Their view that patient autonomy is enhanced by knowing the comparative, risk-adjusted mortality of available surgeons is mistaken – particularly on a Kantian conception of autonomy.

It is common to conflate autonomy with a broader and more consumerist conception of individual choice, and a version of this confusion infects Clarke and Oakley's argument. According to Clarke and Oakley, the fact that a piece of information is material to a patient's decision about whether or not to consent to an operation is not a sufficient condition for the patient having a right to that information. A homophobic patient might consider the surgeon's sexual orientation material, but such information is protected by privacy rights. However they suggest that 'it is hard to see how this sort of rationale could plausibly be applied to mount an argument for the withholding of information about a surgeon's performance' (2005, p. 19).

The notion of a piece of information being 'material' to a patient's decision is essentially a legal concept. In the important Australian case of *Rogers* v *Whitaker* the High Court found that a doctor has a duty of care to disclose 'material' risks, and stated that a risk is material if:

In the circumstances of the particular case, a reasonable person in the patient's position, if warned of the risk, would be likely to attach significance to it or if the medical practitioner is, or should reasonably be aware that the particular patient, if warned of the risk, would be likely to attach significance to it. (Skene and Smallwood, 2002)

Clarke and Oakley cite, with approval, the judgment in the case of *Chappel v Hart*, to make the point that they endorse a subjective conception of materiality; that is, information is material if the patient herself considers it material.

However, it is a mistake to hold that the principle of respect for autonomy always weighs in favour of giving patients information they regard as material. There are types of information that may be material to a patient's decision, that are not protected by privacy or other rights, and yet the patient has no autonomy-based right to that information.

The principle of autonomy is complex, but on any viable version of the principle it involves a commitment to the moral equality of individuals. The demand that others respect my autonomy implies a duty on my part to reciprocate that respect towards others. For a Kantian, an agent acts autonomously only where she intends that her actions comply with the Categorical Imperative, which means that it must be possible for all others, similarly situated, to act in the same way. For the purpose of this argument, the relevant constraint on autonomous decisions is roughly this: respect for a person's autonomy does not confer on her a right to arrogate to herself resources or limited opportunities, where by so doing those resources or opportunities are thereby denied to others. An example may help to illustrate the point.

Ms Scalpel is a surgeon whose overall performance is exceptionally good. Suppose that the majority of her work consists of one procedure, normally taking 3 hours, which she typically performs twice a day. She has kept meticulous records and has discovered that her risk-adjusted mortality rate is slightly better for the first operation of the day, in the morning, than for patients who are operated on in the afternoon. Perhaps her concentration and dexterity are diminished after several hours at the operating table. Her overall long-run mortality rate is considerably better than average, and the difference between the first and second operations of the day is slight. Suppose that, other factors being equal, her afternoon patients have a 1% higher probability of in-hospital mortality than her morning patients. Ms Scalpel knows this fact about her performance. Does she have an obligation to disclose to her patients the increased risk associated with her afternoon operations, compared with her morning operations?

No she does not. At least there is no obligation to disclose this information deriving from considerations of patient autonomy and informed consent. Any patient who knew this fact, and had the option of choosing morning or afternoon surgery, would rationally opt to be the first patient of the day. Yet the option of a morning operation cannot be given to *all* of Ms Scalpel's patients, and no patient can claim that, *on grounds of respect for autonomy*, she is entitled to a resource or an opportunity which cannot be made available to other similarly situated patients. For this reason, a patient cannot, in the name of informed consent, demand comparative performance information in order to seek out an above average surgeon or unit. The purpose of informed consent is not to help patients compete for undeserved advantage over other patients.

A patient may well want the best surgeon in the country, but a patient whose demand for the best surgeon is not met cannot thereby claim her autonomy has been violated. In general, the principle of autonomy does not require us to furnish patients with information to facilitate choices that are not universalisable. Importantly, a threshold model of publication of surgeon performance information is compatible with a Kantian view of autonomy. Threshold reporting simply shows that a surgeon meets or fails to meet a specified performance standard. A patient can reasonably demand evidence her surgeon is safe and competent, and threshold reporting would fulfil that demand without compromising other patients.

It might be objected that providing information and providing an option are not the same thing, and that a patient may want comparative performance information for reasons other than selecting the best surgeon. A patient may simply want to know, for instance, and in such a case would not providing such information enhance autonomy? Even if we accept a subjective test for the materiality of information, such that information is material just if a patient regards it as material, it does not follow that respect for autonomy requires the development of surgeon-specific performance tables. This conception of informed consent only entitles patients to information that is both unprotected and available. Where information is unavailable and costly to produce, the mere fact that a patient would like to have that information does not generate a claim on the public dollar.

Sir Bruce Keogh, co-ordinator of the National Adult Cardiac Surgery Database in the UK (and former president of the SCTS) has noted that, if the purpose of publishing individual surgeon performance information is for patient choice, then the information must be presented in a comparative fashion as detailed, risk-adjusted tables. However, publishing to indicate whether a surgeon is safe or not 'requires agreeing a threshold of unacceptable mortality and then showing where each individual surgeon's results lie relative to that threshold' (Keogh *et al.*, 2004, p. 451). I have argued that considerations of informed consent, at best, support a threshold model of surgeon performance reporting. Against Clarke and Oakley, I have argued that the doctrine of informed consent in medical ethics does not require the publication of comparative performance information on surgeons of a kind that constitutes a league table.

References

Chassin, M. (2002). Achieving and sustaining improved quality: lessons from New York State and cardiac surgery. *Health Affairs*, **21**, 40–51.

Chassin, M. (1996). Health care quality of service. *New England Journal of Medicine*, **335**, 1060–4.

Clarke, S. and Oakley, J. (2004). Informed consent and surgeons' performance. *Journal of Medicine and Philosophy*, **29**, 11–35.

Fine, L. G., Keogh, B. E., Cretin, S., Orlando, M. and Gould, M. M. (2003). How to evaluate and improve the quality and credibility of an outcomes database: validation and feedback study on the UK Cardiac Surgery experience. *British Medical Journal*, **326**, 25–8.

Fracassini, C. and Nutt, K. (2005). Secrecy sliced open; a 10 month battle has forced the NHS to reveal its death rates. *The Sunday Times* – Scotland, Dec 11.

Keogh, B., Spiegelhalter, D., Baily, A., Roxburgh, J., Magee, P. and Hilton, C. (2004). The legacy of Bristol: public disclosure of individual surgeons' results. *British Medical Journal*, **329**, 450–4.

Kolker, R. (2005). Heartless: To manipulate their crucial personal-fatality ratings, New York heart surgeons are turning away needy patients. http://newyorkmetro.com/nymetro/health/features/14788/index1.html (accessed Dec. 2005).

Marshall, M. N. and Brook, R. H. (2002). Public reporting of comparative information about quality of healthcare. *Medical Journal of Australia*, **176**, 205–6.

Parker, S. (2001). What the papers say: extracts from the leader columns of the national press on the findings of the Bristol Royal Infirmary inquiry. *The Guardian*, July 19.

Skene, L. and Smallwood, R. (2002). Informed consent: lessons from Australia. *British Medical Journal*, **324**, 39–41.

Society of Cardiothoracic Surgeons of Great Britain and Ireland (2003). National adult cardiac surgical database [Online]. http://www.scts.org/sections/audit/cardiac/index.html (Accessed March 2007).

Templeton, S. K. (2005). Hospital to woo patients with death rate boast. *The Sunday Times*, Dec. 4.

10

Trust and the limits of knowledge

David Macintosh

James Cook University, Cairns, Australia

I would be true, for there are those who trust me.   *Howard Arnold Walter*, 1906

The old song by Walter implies that, if we are trusted, we will feel the need to take up some personal obligation to those who trust us. This is interesting, as it suggests that trust is not merely a device for cementing some certainty and commitment in relationships, but imposes an obligation on the trustee that goes to the core of his character. If surgeons are to be trusted to look after the interests of their patients, does this mean that they can also be expected to develop a corresponding sense of duty that is an integral part of the way they see themselves? It would be good if this were so. This chapter examines the effect that trust, or lack of it, may have on surgeons and how it can influence the way they behave. The use of report cards may increase the knowledge we have about particular surgeons, but how does the revelation and application of that knowledge affect surgeons and their relationship with patients?

Difficulties interpreting information

In many situations in life we have to make decisions where we would like to have more or a deeper understanding of the information that is available. We may not be able to access what we need to know or this is couched in terms we do not understand. At worst, we suspect that we are being deliberately kept in the dark and at best we feel disadvantaged and impotent. For instance, workers in Australia were recently offered a choice in which funds their superannuation could be invested. Alan Wood (2004, p. 40) argues that a pre-condition for the choice of a fund is an informed investor supplied with information that is easily understood. Wood claims that some in the superannuation industry are not keen to disclose 'how much money juicy fees and kickbacks can cost you'. The Australian Consumers Association and others want investors to know how much fees will reduce an employee's final super payout. The industry and the

Informed Consent and Clinician Accountability: The Ethics of Report Cards on Surgeon Performance. Steve Clarke and Justin Oakley (eds.). Published by Cambridge University Press. © Cambridge University Press 2007.

government both claim that it is too difficult to supply this information. Whilst the government has announced it will warn people to be wary of costs and will offer access to detailed fee disclosure models, Wood claims 'you might even understand it if you happen to be an actuary, but it won't help most people'. If we cannot obtain or understand the information we need, we can only make sensible decisions if we can trust someone to find and interpret it for us.

Some aspects of trust

Francis Fukuyama (1995, p. 26) defines trust as 'the expectation that arises within a community of regular, honest and cooperative behaviour, based on commonly shared norms, on the part of other members of that community'. Bernard Barber (1983, p. 9) also describes trust as an expectation that people will act within a persistent moral order and in a sense sees trust as social capital based on common values. Broad social expectations are necessary in everyday life and without some trust of this nature, the world would be so disorganized that we would feel unable to get out of bed in the morning (Luhmann, 1979, p. 22). Institutions have the power to make decisions about individual members of the community without those individuals being aware of either the process of decision-making or the attitudes of those people within the institutions. But what if we see the superannuation industry as acting outside our own community of interest with very different values to us? There is a danger, if we are to blindly rely on the internal mechanisms of institutions, that they will operate more in their own interests than ours.

Trust, however, is not simply a matter of calculation or an assessment of a 'spectrum of behaviour dealing with risk' (Mitchell, 2001, pp. 591–607). We are more inclined to trust people whom we feel have some understanding of our needs and who have motivation to protect us. It is possible to legislate for a degree of good behaviour, to forbid certain practices, to set up rules of conduct and to encourage best practice in an industry, but important information may have to be interpreted for a layperson by an expert with some understanding of the needs of the client. It is hard to legislate for good, honest judgement. Perhaps the best we can do with legislation in this situation is to demand some fiduciary duty from those who advise and act for us.

Self-interest, trust and professionalism

Fiduciary duty requires a person who has specific knowledge or expertise to use this in a way consistent with the proper role of his profession or organization and in the interest of his client. That requires him to have a commitment to this role and an understanding of the client's abilities and needs. As Mitchell claims (Mitchell, 2001, p. 598), he must act as a trustee for his client. 'One could not understand fiduciary duty without understanding trust, and for that to be effective, fiduciary duty must rely on the willingness of business actors to trust and be trusted'.

What can we do to make our advisers trustworthy? Russell Hardin (1991, p. 26) believes that we can rationally trust people only while it is in their interest to be trustworthy, and that a person becomes untrustworthy when that incentive goes. Thus, according to Hardin, we should think of trust as 'essentially rational expectations about the mostly self-interested behaviour of the trusted'. Hardin also claims it is not rational to trust anyone without having sufficient knowledge of that person's beliefs, needs and desires which might influence his attitude towards us. This appears to preclude that we can rationally trust strangers. Yet we seem to trust strangers all the time. Not only do we trust surgeons we have never met before, we sometimes trust strangers in the street and used car salesmen, even when we suspect we should not (Baier, 1986, p. 235). Baier looks at trust from the point of view of her particular expectations about people, which is, that others will treat her well and generally be trustworthy, because they recognize her as being important in her own right. The idea that a stranger might not show her ill will suggests to her that her identity as an individual is important. Baier thinks of trust as not merely a broad social expectation, but something that individuals take into account as affecting them personally. Yet it does seem true that the more we know about the trustee the surer any decision to trust will be.

A rational expectation about the self-interest of those we trust is probably an essential part of the trusting relationship, but it is insufficient to fully explain the relationship. We often get very upset if a trusting relationship fails. If trust is purely a matter of rational expectation, then what reason is there for us to be upset if this expectation does not come to fruition? If we have rationally assessed the situation and come to conclusions on the facts available to us, we should expect to feel nothing but some sense of inadequacy in our poor judgement if the trust fails to achieve the results we expected. For instance, if I were to allow my young son to go with his friend's family for a holiday and during that holiday he became ill, and he was neglected by the family and suffered badly from this, how would I react? If I was thinking purely rationally, I might conclude that I had made a bad decision in trusting my son to this family and think no more about it. However, it is unlikely that I would think this way, as I would be very angry with that family and believe that they had not behaved in the way that they should. I would not say that that is all one could expect, as it is human nature to forget things or to sometimes neglect the children of others. On the contrary, unlike Hardin, I would strongly believe that the family had some obligation to look after someone that I valued that did not just depend on their self-interest.

A trustee needs to have the characteristics of a trustworthy person, which we implicitly assume means having certain personal characteristics and an inclination to use them well. Hegel argued that 'I can trust a person if I believe he has sufficient insight to treat my cause as if it were his own and to deal with it in the light of his own best knowledge and conscience.' (Hegel, 1998, p. 392). To have insight into another person's cause requires knowledge, empathy and understanding and to deal with it requires commitment and integrity. The trustee's judgement may turn out to be different from that of the truster, particularly if considered in retrospect, but as long as the trustee has acted in good faith with the truster's interest at heart, then the 'trust' has not been violated. In such a case the truster may have an obligation, due to the nature of the trusting relationship, to forgive the trustee if things go wrong.

When dealing with superannuation funds, it may be sufficient for us to obtain reliable and understandable information about fees and profits. In other situations, however, we can get understandable, comparable and reasonably objective information about quality of performance and yet feel we need to know more about the character of the people we are dealing with. When I used to take my children into their classrooms, it was not just the quality of the work produced that impressed me, but all of the teacher's skills that made the classroom a good place to be. The good teachers were warm, kind, encouraging and caring. These qualities are much harder to measure than literacy and numeracy.

Schools are relatively safe places, but there are always risks, and despite the disclaimers and waivers presented to be signed by administrators and teachers I usually trusted the teachers to look after the children as well as they could. I made personal judgements about the attributes of individual teachers, but I also trusted them because they were professional teachers whose role it was to care for children. A good teacher has certain values and ideals that are particular to her role as a teacher. The compassion and care that the good teacher gives to her student may be additional to, and in a way, distinct from, the sort of compassion or concern that she might have for people outside the teaching relationship. This is a role morality that is personal, although Blum and Kohl (Blum, 1990, pp. 179–85; Kohl, 1984) argue that it is also impersonal, as it is independent of, and in addition to, the teacher's personal characteristics, as it is an obligation of the role itself.

At its best, the profession of medicine shares with teaching the idea that its members can have ideals and values that go beyond the specifications and duties expected of other professions. If I need to have a heart operation and have managed to organize my superannuation so that I can afford to choose my own surgeon, I will assess him in a number of ways, not the least of which will be his technical competence and the reputation of the hospital in which he works. Yet I will look for more. I feel that my surgeon should have some particular care for me, as a human individual, apart from his technical ability and clinical judgement. I would like my surgeon to have some sense of vocation.

> The notion of a vocation implies that the ideals it embodies are ones that speak specifically to the individual in question. There is a personal identification with the vocation, that is, its values and ideals, and a sense of personal engagement that helps to sustain the individual in her carrying out the activities of the vocation. (Blum, 1990, p. 179)

I expect my surgeon to have personally embraced the values and ideals of a good surgeon and for him to use those values to both guide and sustain him. If my operation goes wrong and my life is in danger I would like to know that, whatever the outcome, my surgeon will care for me to the limits of his personal as well as his surgical abilities. I would expect him to go home that evening tired and emotionally drained. As much as he can, I wish to trust him to deal with my needs as if they were his own and to deal with them in the light of his own best knowledge and conscience.

Trust and surgeons

How a surgeon should relate to his patient is not necessarily overtly stated, as there is assumed some sense of obligation of one person to another. Certain rules of behaviour may start simply as matters of convention or convenience but over time can 'take on the characteristics of a moral obligation' (Thibaut and Kelley, 1959, p. 128) as these rules are internalized. The community assumes that surgeons will follow rules particular to their occupation, whether stated or not, and it is to be expected that they have incorporated these rules into a commitment that has become part of their own sense of vocation.

The good surgeon, in an Aristotelian sense (Aristotle, 1991), practises all the appropriate skills until he has mastered them, but he may not become trustworthy in a professional sense until he has reached a degree of practical wisdom or clinical judgement and internalized certain moral obligations. This requires him to have the ability, firstly to make independent decisions in particular situations, based on his own experience and judgement, and secondly, to apply them in a trustworthy manner. Aristotle suggests that the only person who could fully appreciate whether he is good at the first would be another surgeon. We cannot, as a community, however, accept only the judgement of a surgeon's peers, as we know that professional groups have a tendency to look after their own interests. Whether a surgeon is trustworthy or not is difficult to assess and, in part, will depend on the personal experience of the patient as well as the measurement of outcomes.

In the process of obtaining consent, it is appropriate that the patient has any questions answered that are worrying her. But is there a limit to how far she can go? Imagine the situation if a patient starts to ask more probing questions of the surgeon. 'If your mortality rate is 5 per cent why did they die? If one of these bled to death what measures did you take to stop it? What was the cause of the bleeding and what is the evidence that you used best practice to assess and control the anti-coagulant effect of surgery and anaesthesia? What suture material do you use? Are you sleeping with the scrub nurse and does that affect your concentration?' These are all legitimate questions, but sooner or later the surgeon is likely to respond that the patient is going too far, as she does not trust his professional autonomy and he may wish to withdraw from the relationship and not operate on her. She may have crossed a line that offends his sense of his own personal integrity and professionalism. Yet the patient could argue that she was simply seeking information relevant to her. Penetrating questions such as these ought to be asked on behalf of all patients as part of peer review.

Managing risk

A community that demands information may publish report cards and do it as part of 'a right to know', but it risks changing the attitude of surgeons from one of obligation and caring, which most would like it to be, to a self-serving preservation of professional power associated with strategies designed to avoid risk. The modern consent form, with its pages of disclaimers, is a good example of a technique, clothed in nobility and produced ostensibly to protect the patient, which is really designed to protect the doctor and hospital from being sued. Demands for accountability, reasonable in themselves, may risk reducing a surgeon's trustworthiness in areas where trust really matters. Sometimes we need to trust surgeons to make decisions in our interest in situations where we have no control and no real choice, say in an emergency situation or if something unexpected happens during an operation.

Whenever we trust someone with something that matters to us, we take a risk that the trustee will not care enough for us or is not able or sufficiently dedicated to look after our interests properly. If surgeons, as a collegiate group, wish to be trusted, then they have to convince us that they have the attributes of a trustworthy group. Any institution, such as a college of surgeons or a hospital, can appear trustworthy by regulating the behaviour of its members, but these measures must have real substance. Machiavelli (1961, p. 101) considered that, in order to be seen as trustworthy, one did not have to be really so, as it was only necessary that a person 'should appear a man of compassion, a man of good faith, a man of integrity, a kind and religious man'. Machiavelli reasoned that 'Men in general judge by their eyes rather than by their hands; because everyone is in a position to watch, few are in a position to come in close touch with you. Everyone sees what you appear to be, few experience what you really are.' Thus, on this view, it is sufficient to maintain only an illusion of trustworthiness in order for an institution to successfully maintain its own independence and control. But decisions in surgery have to be made that depend on the knowledge and integrity of the individual surgeon involved and in difficult circumstances his judgement needs to be trusted. How he performs will depend on his own character and training.

Any illusion of trustworthiness will soon be seen to be false if the surgeon does not himself have those virtues that are necessary for him to act fully in the interests of his patients. Hegel argued that a person in an institution has to be more than a mere follower of rules, he has to be able to make good decisions for others, and 'a doctrine of virtues is not a mere doctrine of duties' (Hegel, 1967, p. 108). An institution cannot for long sustain the appearance of trustworthiness unless its members are genuinely trustworthy. Even Machiavelli (1950, p. 247) realised this and warned that a state (or a hospital for that matter) might not be able to function if 'by ill chance the populace has no confidence in anyone at all, as sometimes happens owing to its having been deceived in the past'.

The perspective of the trustee

Whilst it is clear that the truster usually has a significant emotional involvement in a trusting relationship, less has been said about the feelings of the trustee. It may be instructive to look at the surgeon–patient relationship from the point of view of the surgeon. Why might surgeons wish to be trustworthy? Trustees of any sort are vulnerable to loss of friendship and abuse from others and even to having legal action taken against them if things go wrong. It is necessary for a trustee to understand, take care of and sometimes to make decisions on behalf of the truster. It might be a lot easier, if it were possible, to have some type of formal contract so that trust is not required.

When we are trusted, we have a burden placed upon us. The truster takes a risk in trusting, but at the same time she places a responsibility upon the trustee, as now he is expected to care and act well towards her, simply because of the very idea that she does trust him. In being trusted, the trustee is expected and must try to be trustworthy.

To understand trust from the perspective of the trusted is to understand that trust is more than a device for reducing transaction costs or worldly complexities, for smoothing the way of business, for building successful economies or even coherent societies. To understand the importance of being trusted is to understand the way in which the responsibility for trust reposed can affect character. (Mitchell, 2001, p. 599)

One of the interesting things about trust is how being trusted can affect the trustee. Karen Jones (1996) looks at trust as an attitude of optimism, concerned, amongst other things, with the good will of the one being trusted and the idea that the trustee will be 'favourably moved' by the thought that we are counting on him. Jones believes that such confidence is an affective attitude rather than a judgement of the facts she knows or believes about her trustee as a trustworthy person. The optimism is based on the trustee being favourably moved by the thought that someone is in some way including her in a personal relationship. The truster is thus expecting the trustee to form some kind of affective attitude towards her. Philip Pettit (1995) argues that any affectivity a trustee may feel may also include the enjoyment of the goodwill of the truster, particularly if he values her good opinion, and this may actually increase his trustworthiness as he desires to please. The opposite also applies, as if the trustee does not care for the opinion of the truster then he is likely to be less trustworthy, unless he has another reason to be trustworthy, for instance if he identifies himself with an institution that depends on trust or wishes to have a good opinion of himself as a trustworthy person.

Trust and moral character

Being a trustee may impose a major burden of time, effort and emotion; yet the realisation that he is being trusted can make a person want to be trustworthy. Mitchell (2001) uses the example of some characters in a Steinbeck novel (*Tortilla Flat*, 1953), who are moved to act honestly, against their original intentions, by the simple trust of an acquaintance. The fact that he trusts them changes their attitude to him and forces them to examine their own consciences and they begin to sympathize with him. Their characters are changed as they respond to the emotional challenge of recognizing the needs of a fellow human; indeed, eventually it seems to them that they have no choice but to be trustworthy and so they are. We have all had similar experiences, although, alas, we do not always respond so well. If we recognize our failure, we often feel guilty and resolve to do better in the future. Over time, we may notice an improvement in our character. Mitchell argues that the moral psychology of being trusted, in that it helps to create trustworthiness in people, makes personal trust a rational process. A sense of vocation, with its inbuilt moral structure, can reinforce this character building and lead a teacher or a surgeon to see being trustworthy as an end in itself. Looking at this argument another way, it may be that report cards could lead surgeons to be less caring about their patients if patient trust is transformed into, or becomes subsidiary to, no more than mere reliance on published data.

On the other hand, those who trust too easily, or refuse to take any responsibility for their own actions, diminish the relationship. If patients were never to question surgeons and trusted all implicitly, it would probably not take long for the surgeons to lose the sense of obligation derived from the relationship, as no one likes to be taken for granted. Indeed, many surgeons are wary of patients who appear to trust too easily, as they feel a patient needs to take some responsibility for his own decisions and should accept that there are risks involved that have to be shared and they are not just the responsibility of the surgeon. There are other reasons to continually question surgeons, as being trusted too readily can lead to carelessness and indifference. The process of consent, if it involves questioning and answering and is done sincerely, may well develop the relationship and the commitment between surgeon and patient. When a patient is able to talk through her fears and hopes, it reveals her humanity and a responsive surgeon may empathize with her and, in so doing, develop genuine personal trust in addition to any that may have been there because of his professional role.

The danger in distrust

There is a reverse process: not being trusted can lead to untrustworthiness. We find it difficult to live or work with someone who does not trust us. If our actions and motives are constantly being checked, we eventually lose confidence in the relationship and become unable to make appropriate decisions. At the same time, we may lose confidence in ourselves, as we see the other person does not honour our integrity and we begin to doubt our own self-worth. One of the rewards of being a surgeon is the sense of being trusted and the self-confidence and the sense of self-worth that this brings. If we feel we are not trusted, we often respond with anger, at least partly due to a sense of loss and the feeling we are not appreciated, but eventually this anger cools and is replaced with indifference. Once we become indifferent and cease to care about the other, we lose the impetus to act well towards them and we may become untrustworthy. Failure to trust may eventually lead to loss of trustworthiness on the part of the trustee. Untrustworthy behaviour leads to further lack of trust and a lamentable situation exists with a vicious downward spiral that is hard to break. It would be unfortunate if surgeons reacted to a perceived loss of trust by becoming indifferent and less trustworthy.

Conclusions

It is appropriate for us to expect the highest standard of technical skill from cardiac surgeons and to monitor their performance. The use of report cards is one way of doing this. We should expect professional behaviour, including peer review and good personal skills, from surgeons. In order to foster trustworthiness in surgeons, the community must first trust the surgeons and show them they are trusted, as without being trusted in the first place an individual cannot develop and practice the specific skills of a trustworthy surgeon. At the same time, surgeons have to continually demonstrate that they are worthy of being trusted. The surgeons must have a commitment to their vocation and what that implies. Appropriate and well-judged trust encourages good behaviour and, whilst patients should not trust too easily, the relationship between surgeon and patient does not usually work well if the patient does not trust him and the surgeon does not feel he is trusted. This means that, if report cards are to be used, they should be presented and used in such a way as to foster trust, rather than appear to be a controlling or censoring device. This requires sensitivity on behalf of legislators and co-operative understanding amongst surgeons.

References

Aristotle (1991). *The Nicomachean Ethics.* Tr. D. Ross, Oxford University Press: Oxford.

Baier, A. (1986). Trust and antitrust. *Ethics,* **96**, 231–60.

Barber, B. (1983). *The Logic and Limits of Trust,* New Jersey: Rutgers University Press.

Blum, L. A. (1990). Vocation, friendship, and community; limitations of the personal-impersonal framework. In *Essays in Moral Psychology,* ed. O. Flannigan and A. O. Rorty. Cambridge MA: Massachusetts Institute of Technology Press, pp. 179–85.

Fukuyama, F. (1995). *Trust, the Social Virtues and the Creation of Prosperity,* London: Penguin Books.

Hardin, R. (1990). Trusting persons, trusting institutions. In *The Strategy of Choice,* ed. R. J. Zeckhauser. Cambridge MA: Massachusetts Institute of Technology Press.

Hegel, G. (1967). *Hegel's Philosophy of Right.* Tr. T. M. Knox, Oxford: Oxford University Press.

Hegel, G. (1998). Ethical life, the philosophy of right. In *The Hegel Reader,* ed. S. Hulgate, Oxford: Blackwell.

Jones, K. (1996). Trust as an affective attitude. *Ethics,* **107**, 4–25.

Kohl, H. (1984). *Growing Minds: On Becoming a Teacher,* New York: Harper and Row.

Luhmann, N. (1979). *Trust and Power,* New York: John Wiley and Sons.

Machiavelli, N. (1961). *The Prince,* London: Penguin Classics.

Machiavelli, N. (1950). *The Prince and the Discourses,* New York: The Modern Library.

Mitchell, L. E. (2001). The importance of being trusted. *Boston University Law Review,* **81**, 591–617.

Pettit, P. (1995). The cunning of trust. *Philosophy and Public Affairs,* **24**, 203–25.

Thibaut, J. W. and Kelley, H. H. (1959). *The Secret Psychology of Groups,* New York: Wiley.

Walter, H. A. (1906). I would be true. *Folksongs,* http://ingeb.org/songs/iwouldbe.html, accessed 14/11/05.

Wood, A. (2004). *The Weekend Australian Newspaper.* Nationwide News Pty. Ltd., Melbourne, June 19–20, p. 40.

11

Surgeons' report cards, heuristics, biases and informed consent

Steve Clarke

Centre for Applied Philosophy and Public Ethics, Charles Sturt University
and Program on the Ethics of the New Biosciences, James Martin
21st Century School, University of Oxford, UK

Informed consent and surgeons' performance information

An important reason for providing patients with performance data on individual surgeons is to enable patients to make better decisions about surgery, as a part of the informed consent process. Surgeons' performance data can be utilized to enable a variety of types of decision that a patient may face. A patient can utilize performance data on individual surgeons to enable a choice between available surgeons. A patient can utilize surgeons' performance data when deciding between surgery involving an available surgeon and a non-surgical alternative form of treatment. Also, a patient can utilize surgeons' performance data to help decide whether or not to wait for a high-performing surgeon, who is not currently available, to become available.

Traditionally, performance data on individual surgeons have not been disclosed to patients, and such data have not usually been thought necessary to disclose for the purposes of providing effective informed consent. Canonical treatments of the doctrine of informed consent, such as Faden and Beauchamp (1986), do not consider the possibility of making such information available to patients. However, it has recently been argued that the doctrine of informed consent implicitly requires that surgeons' performance data be made available to patients (Clarke and Oakley, 2004). The gist of this argument is easy enough to grasp: it is uncontroversial that the significant and material risks associated with an operation should be disclosed to a patient who is contemplating that operation. If an operation is known to involve a 10 per cent risk of mortality, and there is a failure to disclose that it involves a 10 per cent risk of mortality, before the operation takes place, then effective informed consent has not been provided. However, the actual risks of an operation will vary, according *inter alia* to the performance ability of the surgeon conducting the operation. An operation that has a 10% risk of mortality, on average, may only have a 5% risk of mortality when conducted by one surgeon and a 15% risk of mortality when conducted by

Informed Consent and Clinician Accountability: The Ethics of Report Cards on Surgeon Performance.
Steve Clarke and Justin Oakley (eds.). Published by Cambridge University Press. © Cambridge
University Press 2007.

another surgeon. So, a disclosure of the actual risks of an operation, for the purposes of enabling effective informed consent, needs to include information about the performance abilities of available surgeons.

In the United States and in the United Kingdom, the two countries in which cardiac surgeons' performance data have been made publicly available, considerations other than a concern to enable effective informed consent have led to the publicising of individual surgeons' performance data. The motive for making cardiac surgeons' performance data publicly available in the United Kingdom has been a desire to change the closed culture of medicine that led to the Bristol Royal Infirmary Scandal, and to ensure that high standards of professional accountability are now met (Neil *et al.*, 2004, p. 266). In the United States, an explicit aim of public release, which has taken place in New York, Pennsylvania and New Jersey, has been to improve clinical quality. This is to be done by providing information that can improve the quality of patients' decisions and then allowing market mechanisms to influence the behaviour of surgeons (Neil *et al.*, 2004, p. 267; Marshall *et al.*, 2000).

In New York State, tables of surgeons' comparative performance information (known colloquially as 'report cards') for coronary artery bypass graft (CABG) operations, the most common form of cardiac surgery, have been made publicly available for over 15 years. If we look at the most recent report card on CABG (2001–2003) in New York State, we find information such as the following:

St Francis Hospital

Name	Cases	No. of Deaths	OMR	EMR	RAMR	95% CI for RAMR
Berkow N	697	27	3.87	2.35	3.36	(2.21, 4.89)
Colangelo R	751	17	2.26	2.33	1.97	(1.15, 3.16)
Damus P	501	5	1.00	1.73	1.17	(0.38, 2.74)

Source: (New York State Department of Health, 2005, p. 23).

OMR: The observed mortality rate is the number of observed deaths within 12 months, of isolated CABG surgery, divided by the number of patients.
EMR: The expected mortality rate is the sum of the predicted probabilities of death for each patient, divided by the total number of patients.
RAMR: The risk-adjusted mortality rate is the best estimate of what the provider's mortality rate would have been, if the provider had a mix of patients identical to the state-wide mix.
95% CI for RAMR: The 95% Confidence Interval (CI) for RAMR is indicative of the degree of confidence that we are warranted in attaching to RAMR figures for individual surgeons. N. Berkow has a RAMR of 3.36 with a 95% CI (2.21, 4.89). This means that we can be 95% confident that his actual RAMR falls between 2.21 and 4.89.

Doctors operate at different hospitals, which receive different mixes of patients. And not all surgeons at a particular hospital will treat a similar mix of patients. More experienced surgeons, and surgeons whose ability is regarded as superior by their peers, may be asked to conduct more of the difficult, higher-risk operations that need to be conducted. To achieve a fair reflection of a surgeon's performance, given his or her OMR, we need to adjust for the EMR of his or her particular mix of patients, producing the surgeon's RAMR. Risk adjustments are made by considering a variety of factors that affect outcomes, such as age, gender, ventricular function and the presence of significant 'comorbidities'.

In the United Kingdom, risk-adjusted performance information for individual cardiac surgeons is also collated and made available to the public. These data were released in a very coarse-grained form, from 2004 to 2006, with British cardiac surgeons being rated with the use of a three-point scale (Neil *et al.*, 2004). However, Britain has now moved to a system of providing percentile risk-adjusted survival rates (RASR) for individual cardiac surgeons conducting CABG operations and aortic valve replacement operations.[1] These data are not currently complete, with surgeons from only 17 of the 33 heart units in England and Wales now providing RASR for their operations. Figures will be updated annually and, although participation is voluntary, it is expected that these data will soon become much more comprehensive (Healthcare Commission, 2006).

Here, I consider evidence from the field of behavioural decision-making, which suggests that ordinary decision-making is affected by a variety of systematic biases, and I investigate some ways in which this research bears on issues concerning the presentation of comparative surgeons' performance data for the purposes of enabling informed consent.[2,3] These are biases that are particularly relevant to the interpretation of statistical information and which can be extremely serious. Consider a recent study by Yamagishi (1997). Most participants in this study of lay estimates of risk rated a cancer as riskier, when it was described as one that 'kills 1286 out of 10 000 people', than when it was described as one that 'kills 24.14 out of 100 people'. But, in actual fact, a risk of 1286 in 10 000 is approximately half as severe as a risk of 24.14 in 100. This result is an instance of the bias of base-rate neglect (Tversky and Kahneman, 1974). 1286 is a large number relative to 24.14 and it appears that participants in this study directly compared these two numerators, while losing sight of the fact that they are intended to be understood in relation to different denominators.

Along with Faden and Beauchamp (1986, p. 235) and most other contributors to the literature, I hold that the overriding goal of the informed consent process is to uphold the value of patient autonomy. While the autonomous choices of patients need not be based solely on rational factors, a patient is not able to make a fully autonomous choice to provide consent, unless it is possible for that patient to rationally deliberate about the alternative courses of action available to her.[4] But, if psychological biases seriously erode a patient's deliberative capacities, then that patient is not able to deliberate rationally and is hence not fully able to act autonomously; and the key value that the doctrine of informed consent is designed to uphold cannot be upheld. So it is crucial, if we are to enable effective informed consent, that we are sensitive to the ways in which surgeons' performance information is processed by patients and the ways in which that processing may become distorted.

Heuristics, biases and dual-processing

The phenomenon of base-rate neglect can be explained by appeal to the activation of the 'representativeness' heuristic (Tversky and Kahneman, 1974). Rather than adjusting the two fractions to be compared to a common denominator, and then making a comparison, most of Yamagishi's (1997) subjects looked for an implicit cue indicative of the relative size of the two fractions. We can often make comparisons of the relative size of numbers intuitively, just by looking at the number of digits contained in those numbers. In one case, we have a numerator with four digits, while, in the second case, we have a numerator with only two digits (ignoring the digits after the decimal point). Generally, numbers with more digits are larger numbers and we may be inclined to apply this intuitive cue and judge the fraction containing the larger of the two numerators to be the larger of the two fractions, instead of performing the laborious calculations that would lead us to be able to directly compare the two. Unfortunately, in some circumstances, the application of such quick and easy heuristics produces the wrong result.

Another systematic bias that can be explained by the activation of the representativeness heuristic is the 'conjunction fallacy', memorably described in Tversky and Kahneman's (1983) 'Linda' example. In their (1983) study subjects were given the following information:

Linda is 31 years old, single, outspoken and very bright. She majored in philosophy. As a student, she was deeply concerned with issues of discrimination and social justice, and also participated in anti-nuclear demonstrations. (Tversky and Kahnemann, 1983, p. 297)

Having read the above statement, subjects were asked to rank the probability of a set of eight descriptions, which included the following (along with six 'fillers'):

6. Linda is a bank teller.
8. Linda is a bank teller and is active in the feminist movement.

An application of elementary logic would lead to the conclusion that description 8 cannot be more probable than description 6. Description 8 is a conjunction, description 6 is one of its conjuncts, and a conjunction can never be more probable than one of its conjuncts. Nevertheless, 85% of the research subjects concluded that description 8 was more probable than description 6. Rather than reasoning logically, it appears that they approached the problem

intuitively, applying implicit stereotypes. Linda represents the common stereo-
type of a 'feminist' much more closely than she represents the common stereo-
type of a 'bank teller', and so the representativeness heuristic was activated in
85% of the research subjects, who intuited that description 8 was more probable
than description 6.

As well as various biases that have been explained by appeal to the representativeness heuristic, there are many other cognitive biases that psychologists have
assembled evidence for and have been explained by appeal to the operation of
other heuristics. These include biases explained by appeal to the 'availability
heuristic' (Tversky and Kahneman, 1974), in which the easy availability of
certain sorts of information leads to people giving disproportionate weighting
to that information, at the expense of less available information. There are also
biases that have been explained by appeal to the 'affect heuristic', in which
intuitive judgements of goodness or badness influence assessments of likelihood
and influence a variety of other assessments (Slovic *et al.*, 2002).

The conjunction fallacy is often committed by people who are capable of
reasoning logically about conjunction, but who nevertheless apply heuristics,
such as the representativeness heuristic. Why do we employ heuristics in our
thinking, when these can lead us astray and when we could often avoid being
led astray by applying systematic logical reasoning? The best answer to this
question, that I am aware of, starts with the plausible assumption that our
minds are 'dual processors'. We employ two very different sorts of cognitive
processes, a controlled effortful reasoning process and an automatic effortless
intuitive process (Kahneman and Frederick, 2002). Dual-processing theorists
Stanovich and West (2002) refer to automatic intuitive processes as instances
of the application of 'System 1' and effortful reasoning processes as instances of
the application of 'System 2'. It is probably not feasible to use System 2
processing much more than we do, in the view of most dual-processing
theorists, because conscious attention, required for System 2 processing, but
not for System 1 processing, is a precious resource, which we need to deploy
sparingly (Moskowitz *et al.*, 1999, pp. 26–30).

The operation of particular instances of System 1 and System 2 processing
occur independently of one another. However, System 1 is an adaptive system,
and complex cognitive operations that form a part of System 2 may influence
the development of System 1 over the course of time. For example, a dedicated
chess player can, over time, acquire an ability to intuitively 'read' a position,
using intuitions that have been 'trained up' by the repeated application of
System 2 to the game of chess. Switching between System 1 and System 2
processing generally takes place automatically and often goes unrecognized.
Even when we do recognize that we have been applying System 1 processing, in
circumstances where it may be more appropriate to employ System 2 processing, and we then go on to apply System 2 processing, it may be hard to prevent
ourselves from automatically reverting to System 1 processing. Steven Jay

Gould's account of the Linda case study as one in which '. . . a little homunculus in my head continues to jump up and down, shouting at me – but she can't just be a bank teller; read the description' (1991, p. 469), appears to be an example of such automatic reversion taking place.

It is sometimes assumed that Tversky and Kahneman (1974, 1983) have demonstrated that human judgements are frequently in error. But, although it is easy enough to demonstrate that some System 1 judgments are liable to systematic bias, there is a long way to go if we want to establish that the use of System 1 processing leads us to commit frequent errors of judgement in natural settings. Gerd Gigerenzer and his colleagues have mounted a spirited defence of reasoning based on System 1 processing, against the charge of frequent error (Gigerenzer and Todd, 1999). They argue, roughly, that heuristics are adaptive tools that enable us to employ effective System 1 processing in situations that require rapid decision-making, and in which it would be impractical to employ System 2 processing to make decisions in a time-effective manner.[5] They also hold that the dramatic demonstrations of failures of natural decision-making, in the sorts of experiments that Tversky and Kahneman (1974, 1983) have made famous, are largely confined to the artificial experimental settings that they are conducted in.[6]

The presentation of comparative surgeons' performance information is one setting that appears to approximate closely to the artificial experimental settings that Tversky and Kahneman (1974, 1983) and others have examined. Comparative surgeons' performance information is typically presented in an abstract mathematical format, as exemplified by the earlier extract from the New York State Department of Health (2005). So it seems very doubtful that Gigerenzer and Todd's (1999) defence of the use of System 1 processing in natural settings – even if it were judged to be successful for typical natural settings – would be sufficient to erase our concerns about the use of System 1 reasoning in an unusual natural setting that approximates closely to the artificial experimental settings that Tversky and Kahneman's experiments have mostly been conducted in. It is, of course, possible that in the future Gigerenzer and his colleagues, or some other researchers, will produce evidence that will be sufficient to enable us to set aside concerns about biased System 1 processing in the interpretation of comparative surgeons' performance information. However, in the absence of such evidence, it seems prudent to err on the side of caution and assume that the lay interpretation of comparative surgeons' performance information will be subject to systematic bias.

Responding to bias

A number of different policy responses to the problem of cognitive bias in patient's interpretation of surgeons' performance information in the informed consent process have been suggested to me. One response is to seek to avoid bias by encouraging patients to employ System 2 processing when incorporating surgeons' performance information into their decision-making processes for the purposes of informed consent. A second suggestion is to accept that patient's interpretations of surgeons' performance data will be biased, and encourage patients to rely on expert testimony about comparative surgeons' performance ability, when deciding whether or not to consent to be operated on by a particular surgeon.

A third response is to accept that patients will employ System 1 processing, when incorporating surgeons' performance information into their decisions to consent and to seek to avoid bias by translating the relevant statistical information into ordinary language, before presenting it to patients. A fourth option is to accept that patients will employ System 1 processing, when incorporating surgeons' performance information into their decisions to consent and to try to present that statistical information in such a way as to minimise the potential for error. In this section I consider these options in turn. I will argue that the first three are impractical and that option four is the most feasible course of action.

The first option is currently impractical because the level of statistical education amongst patients is low (Lloyd, 2001). Many will not be capable of applying System 2 reasoning to the problem of calculating how the performance ability of a particular surgeon modifies the level of risk associated with a particular operation. It would take a major overhaul of education systems in most countries to improve the statistical education of the general public to the level where most are capable of performing such calculations. While improving statistical education is a worthy aim, it is not a viable solution to our problem in the short or even medium term. But, even if we could improve statistical education to the desired level, it would still not ensure that most people would employ System 2 processing to incorporate surgeons' performance information into their decisions to provide informed consent for surgery. Even people who are statistically educated tend to employ System 1 processing to 'extract the gist' of risk information, rather than utilize System 2 processing, when attempting to understand risk information (Lloyd *et al.*, 2001).[7]

It can be surprisingly difficult to convince people that their use of reasoning based on System 1 processing has biased their decisions. Although people are able to recognize that others are frequently the victims of cognitive bias, they are often oblivious to the possibility that they themselves may be victims of bias. Furthermore, there is no guarantee, even if they are convinced, that they will not slide back into System 1 modes of reasoning as Steven Jay Gould repeatedly did, when faced with the Linda example. Wilson and Brekke (1994, pp. 119–20) argue that, for a person to successfully avoid biased reasoning, four conditions must be met. Firstly, they must be aware of the presence of a biased mental process. Secondly, they must be motivated to correct any error that the biased mental process has caused. Thirdly, they must be aware of the direction and the magnitude of the error. An over-correction or under-correction of an error results only in further error. Fourthly, even if the first three conditions are satisfied, they must be able to exert sufficient control over their mental processes to correct the error. Wilson and Brekke (1994) argue that it is exceedingly difficult for all four of these conditions to be met.

Asking patients to rely on expert testimony, our second option, would be vigorously resisted by orthodox interpreters of the doctrine of informed consent, such as Faden and Beauchamp (1986), who emphasize the importance of comprehensive disclosures in the informed consent process. I am not opposed to the utilization of expert testimony, as a part of the informed consent process, for reasons that are set out in Clarke (2001). However, the appeal to expert testimony as a substitute for comprehension may be impractical to implement in this context. Doctors are the standard providers of disclosure of relevant information. Doctors are generally somewhat better educated about the interpretation of statistics than lay folk and can play a part in helping patients to understand basic statistics (Paling, 2003). Nevertheless, like patients, doctors are often in the grip of cognitive biases, in virtue of the fact that they typically apply System 1 processing to the interpretation of statistical information (Schwartz, 1994). So, relying on doctors' testimony would not solve the problem of System 1 processing-induced bias in the interpretation of statistics. It might be possible to involve trained statisticians and experts in behavioural decision-making in the informed consent process, but given how few of these there currently are, who could reasonably be expected to be available, and give the expenses involved in employing such experts this seems a very utopian solution to our general problem;[8] so it is one that will not be investigated here.

The third option, translation into ordinary language, also turns out to be impractical because of the vagueness of ordinary language. When people are asked to quantify ordinary probabilistic terminology, they typically provide a very broad range of answers (Mosteller and Youtz, 1990). This is not only true of lay interpreters. Mosteller and Youtz (1990, p. 3) discuss a case in which four experts were asked to quantify the phrase 'a very real possibility'. Their respective answers were 2%, 10%, 35% and 'less than even'. But, even if conventions could be established about the translation of statistics into lay terminology, there is not much reason to believe that the biases that plague the interpretation of statistics would thereby be avoided. The failure of lay interpreters to understand the effect of conjunction, in the 'Linda' study, was not a consequence of the information being presented in a statistical format. Rather, it was a consequence of their failure to employ elementary logical considerations, in circumstances where it seems that elementary logical considerations should have been employed. Shifting into ordinary language format does not obviate the need for the employment of logical considerations when reasoning about the Linda case, but there is no reason to suppose that such a shift would prompt people to employ ordinary logical considerations in their deliberations. The biases in question are, it seems, a by-product of System 1 processing, which is highly likely to be operative in manipulations of information, regardless of how that information is presented.[9] So it seems that there is little reason to hope that the use of ordinary language can provide a way to avoid cognitive biases, in the processing of information about risk.

Given the propensity of people to employ System 1 processing to interpret statistics and make decisions based on statistics, it seems best to investigate our fourth option and accept that patients will typically employ System 1 processing when interpreting surgeons' performance information and incorporating this information into their decision making processes. For the purposes of obtaining informed consent, we should ensure that surgeons' performance data are presented in such a way as to enable people to make the best decisions that they can, using System 1 processing. For the benefit of those patients who are willing and able to make consenting decisions incorporating surgeons' performance information, on the basis of System 2 processing, we should make surgeons' performance information available in a second format, suitable for System 2 processing.[10] However, the initial presentation of information, which forms a part of the informed consent process, should be tailored to System 1 processing.

Presentation of data

For the purposes of enabling accurate System 1 processing, we should present individual surgeons' performance information to patients in a simple and clear format that does not prompt the application of unnecessary System 1 heuristics, which may lead to error. The OMR and the EMR, presented in the New York State report cards, are unnecessary for the purposes of patient decision making and may prompt erroneous inferences. Patients' tendencies to 'extract the gist' of risk information (Lloyd *et al.*, 2001), means that they are liable to make decisions on the basis of a mix of OMR, EMR and RAMR (or RASR), instead of focussing solely on RAMR (or RASR). So we should only present RAMR, or RASR, as is now done in the United Kingdom. Of course there is no objection to including OMR and the EMR in a System 2 format report card.

Explicit rankings of individual surgeons, such as those that occur in the New York State report cards, are also unhelpful to patients in circumstances where there is considerable overlap in the 95% confidence intervals of those individuals (as there is in our earlier excerpt from the New York State report cards). Many patients will not understand the concept of a 95% confidence interval and may be liable to draw the erroneous conclusion that, if one surgeon has a lower RAMR than a second, then he or she is definitely a superior surgeon to the second surgeon, even if there is considerable overlap between the 95%

confidence intervals for their respective RAMRs. A better alternative for patients is an easy-to-comprehend broad banding system of ranking individuals.[11]

The three-point scale, which was used to rank the performance ability of cardiac surgeons in the United Kingdom from 2004 to 2006, before percentile performance data for individual surgeons was first provided in April 2006, was an easy-to-comprehend broad-banding system of ranking individuals. However, it was probably too coarse-grained for the purposes of enabling surgeons' performance information to be fully incorporated into the informed consent process. If we are warranted in being confident that, for a given type of operation, one surgeon is a better performing surgeon than a second, then it is important that that information be presented to patients, for the purposes of enabling effective informed consent. It may well be that, within a given performance band, there were some British cardiac surgeons whose performance ability was demonstrably superior to other British cardiac surgeons, who were listed as being within the same performance band. If some surgeons are demonstrably superior performers to other surgeons within the same band, then it seems that we should provide finer-grained information to patients for the purposes of better enabling effective informed consent. In such circumstances, the provision of finer-grained information would not introduce any new interpretive biases, or increase the magnitude of existing biases. However, it will enable patients to decide more effectively when choosing between surgeons, and when choosing between surgery and non-surgical alternatives.[12]

Notes

1. The choice of presenting surgeons' performance information in terms of survival rather than mortality rates can be expected to have a significant effect on the behaviour of prospective patients, in virtue of the influence of 'framing effects'. In general, we can expect that the presentation of such data in terms of mortality rates will encourage more risk-averse behaviour in prospective patients than will presentation in terms of survival rates (see Kahneman and Tversky, 1984). Although different frames will promote different values, in general there is no one correct way to frame data, any more than there is a correct way to frame a picture. Framing does not typically involve a distortion from accuracy and there are not generally any correct frames. So, framing is conceptually distinct from bias. Discussion of the various philosophical issues raised by framing is beyond the scope of this chapter.
2. I am not alone in arguing for the importance of consideration of psychological biases, in the articulation of the informed consent process. See also Thompson (1996) and Lloyd et al. (2001).
3. I have focused specifically on issues of presentation of comparative surgeons' performance data to patients. There is a growing body of literature that addresses

more general issues of information presentation, for the purpose of informing patient choice. See, for example, Hibbard *et al.* (1997); Hibbard (2003).

4. For more on the relations between autonomy, informed consent and deliberation, see Beauchamp and Childress (2001, pp. 57–98).

5. Some of the heuristics that Gigerenzer *et al.* (2002) discuss may not be instances of System 1 processing, but consciously applied 'rules of thumb', which look more like special cases of System 2 reasoning.

6. For a discussion of these and other lines of criticisms of the 'heuristics and biases' research program, see Gilovich and Griffin (2002).

7. For a discussion of when it is appropriate to employ System 1 processing, and when it is appropriate to employ System 2 processing, see Kleinmuntz (1990).

8. I do not wish to deny that our second option could be used on an *ad hoc* basis. My claim is it is impractical to apply it systematically and it will remain impractical to do so for the foreseeable future.

9. It is sometimes suggested that the presentation of risk information in a frequency format can eliminate bias. However, see Gilovich and Griffin (2002, pp. 14–15).

10. Thanks to Justin Oakley for this suggestion.

11. Note that a broad-banding system still requires representation of a measure of uncertainty (Royal Statistical Society Working Party on Performance Monitoring in the Public Services, 2005).

12. Thanks to Justin Oakley, Steve Matthews and audiences at the Centre for Applied Philosophy and Public Ethics, Canberra and Wagga Wagga divisions, and at 'Publicising Performance Data on Individual Surgeons: the Ethical Issues', a workshop sponsored by the *Academy of the Social Sciences in Australia*, held in Melbourne 2004. This research was supported by National Health and Medical Research Council Project Grant 236877.

References

Beauchamp, T. L. and Childress, J. F. (2001). *Principles of Biomedical Ethics*, 5th edn. New York: Oxford University Press.

Clarke, S. (2001). Informed consent in medicine in comparison with consent in other areas of human activity. *The Southern Journal of Philosophy*, **39**, 169–87.

Clarke, S. and Oakley, J. (2004). Informed consent and surgeons' performance. *The Journal of Medicine and Philosophy*, **29**, 11–35.

Faden, R. R. and Beauchamp, T. L. (1986). *A History and Theory of Informed Consent*. New York: Oxford University Press.

Gigerenzer, G. and Todd, P. M. (1999). Fast and frugal heuristics: the adaptive toolbox. In *Simple Heuristics that Make Us Smart*, ed. G. Gigerenzer, P. M. Todd and the ABC Research Group. New York: Oxford University Press, pp. 3–34.

Gilovich, T. and Griffin, D. (2002). Introduction – heuristics and biases: then and now. In *Heuristics and Biases: the Psychology of Intuitive Judgement*, ed. T. Gilovich, D. Griffin and D. Kahneman. Cambridge: Cambridge University Press, pp. 1–18.

Gould, S. J. (1991). *Bully for Brontosaurus: Reflections in Natural History*. London: Penguin.

Healthcare Commission (2006). Press release: patients have access to rates of survival for heart surgery for the first time. http://www.healthcarecommission.org.uk/news-andevents/pressreleases.cfm?cit_id=3785&FAArea1=customWidgets.content_view_1&usecache=false.

Hibbard, J. H. (2003). Engaging health care consumers to improve the quality of care. *Medical Care*, **41**, Supplement I.61–I.70.

Hibbard, J. H., Slovic, P. and Jewett, J. J. (1997). Informing consumer decisions in health care: implications from decision-making research. *The Millbank Quarterly*, **75**, 395–414.

Kahneman, D. and Frederick, S. (2002). Representativeness revisited: attribute substitution in intuitive judgement. In *Heuristics and Biases: The Psychology of Intuitive Judgement*, ed. T. Gilovich, D. Griffin and D. Kahneman. Cambridge: Cambridge University Press, pp. 49–81.

Kahneman, D. and Tversky, A. (1984). Choices, values and frames. *American Psychologist*, **39**, 341–50.

Kleinmuntz, B. (1990). Why we still use our heads instead of formulas: toward an integrative approach. *Psychological Bulletin*, **107**, 296–310.

Lloyd, A. (2001). The extent of patients' understanding of the risk of treatments. *Quality in Health Care*, **10**, (Suppl. 1), i14–i18.

Lloyd, A., Hayes, P., Bell, P. R. F. and Ross Naylor, A. (2001). The role of risk and benefit perception in informed consent for surgery. *Medical Decision Making*, **21**, 141–9.

Marshall, M., Shekelle, P., Brook, R. and Leatherman, S. (2000). *Dying to Know: Public Release of Information about Quality of Health Care*. Santa Monica: RAND Corporation and The Nuffield Trust. www.rand.org/publications/MR/MR1255/.

Moskowitz, G. B., Skurnik, I. and Galinsey, A. D. (1999). The history of dual-process notions, and the future of preconscious control. In *Dual-Process Theories in Social Psychology*, ed. S. Chaiken and Y. Trope, New York: The Guilford Press, pp. 12–36.

Mosteller, F. and Youtz, C. (1990). Quantifying probabilistic expressions. *Statistical Science*, **5**, 2–34.

Neil, D., Clarke, S. and Oakley, J. (2004). Public reporting of individual surgeon performance information: United Kingdom developments and Australian issues. *Medical Journal of Australia*, **181**, 266–8.

New York State Department of Health (2005). *Adult Cardiac Surgery in New York State 2001–2003*. http://www.health.state.ny.us/nysdoh/heart/pdf/2001-2003_cabg.pdf.

Paling, J. (2003). Strategies to help patients understand risks. *British Medical Journal*, **327**, 745–8.

Royal Statistical Society Working Party on Performance Monitoring in the Public Services (2005). Performance indicators: good, bad and ugly. *Journal of the Royal Statistical Society, Series A*, **168**, Part 1, 1–27.

Schwartz, S. (1994). Heuristics and biases in medical judgement and decision making. In *Applications of Heuristics and Biases to Social Issues*, ed. L. Heath, R. Scott Tindale, J. Edwards *et al.* New York: Plenum Press, pp. 45–72.

Slovic, P., Finucane, M., Peters, E. and MacGregor, D. G. (2002). The affect heuristic. In *Heuristics and Biases: the Psychology of Intuitive Judgement*, ed. T. Gilovich, D. Griffin and D. Kahneman. Cambridge: Cambridge University Press, pp. 397–420.

Stanovich, K. and West, R. (2002). Individual differences in reasoning: implications for the rationality debate. In *Heuristics and Biases: the Psychology of Intuitive Judgement*, ed. T. Gilovich, D. Griffin and D. Kahneman. Cambridge: Cambridge University Press, pp. 421–40.

Thompson, W. C. (1996). Research on human judgement and decision making: implications for informed consent and institutional review. In *Research Ethics: A Psychological Approach*, ed. B. H. Stanley, J. E. Sieber and G. B. Melton. Lincoln: University of Nebraska Press, pp. 37–72.

Tversky, A. and Kahneman, D. (1974). Judgement under uncertainty: heuristics and biases. *Science*, **185**, 1124–31.

Tversky, A. and Kahneman, D. (1983). Extensional versus intuitive reasoning: the conjunction fallacy in probability judgement. *Psychological Review*, **90**, 293–315.

Wilson, T. D. and Brekke, N. (1994). Mental contamination and mental correction: unwanted influences on judgements and evaluations. *Psychological Bulletin*, **116**, 117–42.

Yamagishi, K. (1997). When a 12.86% mortality is more dangerous than 24.14%: implications for risk communication. *Applied Cognitive Psychology*, **11**, 495–506.

12

Report cards, informed consent and market forces

Adrian J. Walsh

University of New England, Australia

Introduction

What ethical ramifications might the commercial context of much modern medicine have for the report card movement? We live in a world in which medicine in general is increasingly subject to market forces; not only are more and more goods and services commodified, and hence able to be procured on the open market, but within the public sphere, market-like accountability processes are increasingly set in place. We need to consider what implications this social context might have for the ethical status of report cards. Perhaps what is morally permissible in the context of public provision might transmogrify into the morally pernicious in a commercial environment. What difference, if any, might market forces make?

In examining this question, I shall assume that the market and market forces are here to stay and provide a background context for any public policy decisions in this area. My focus will be upon the moral legitimacy of report cards in a market context. In pursuing this agenda I identify three morally salient features of markets, that concern (1) the market as an information system, (2) the market as a distributive mechanism and (3) the market as an incentive system. I subsequently argue that close examination of these features provides genuine grounds for caution. The first worry involves the distributive consequences of report cards. In so far as report cards increase the levels of distributive inequality, this is a *pro tanto* reason against them. The second worry involves the transformation of our incentive structures. In so far as report cards increase the prevalence of perverse incentives or increase the tendency for the profit motive to undermine altruism, then this again provides a mark against them in our all-things-considered judgements. We should note, at the outset, that the focus here is ethical rather than economic, so in considering the effects of market forces it is the *moral ramifications* rather than the likely economic effects of reports cards in which I am interested.

Informed Consent and Clinician Accountability: The Ethics of Report Cards on Surgeon Performance. Steve Clarke and Justin Oakley (eds.). Published by Cambridge University Press. © Cambridge University Press 2007.

Market: what market?

Before proceeding, it is important to clarify what we mean by 'market' and 'market forces'. This kind of talk can be misleading, for there are a variety of social practices that might be said to be examples of market forces in play. In some cases we are talking about *genuine markets*. In this sense a market is that social sphere which emerges from the interactions of many buyers and sellers. It is an 'area over which buyers and sellers negotiate the exchange of a well-defined commodity' (Lipsey, 1972, p. 69). So, when medicine is fully subject to market forces, medical services are bought and sold on a market with prices reflecting the relative supply and demand of the commodities in question. Access to medical goods and services are determined by one's financial wherewithal.

In other cases, in speaking of market forces, we are really talking about *quasi-markets* (Marginson, 1997, pp. 37–8). Here, medical services are not bought and sold on an open market and access is not determined by one's wealth. Rather, 'market-like' procedures are put in place within a system of public provision with the explicit aim (or hope) of increasing 'efficiency' or facilitating genuine accountability. So, for example, one might expect doctors working for a wage in a public system to charge a nominal fee for each patient they see. At the end of the week, the doctor would be expected to have treated enough patients as to have 'made' so many dollars within the week. Market forces are often said to be in operation here.

Between genuine markets and these quasi-markets, there will be a range of institutional arrangements in which buying and selling occurs to lesser and greater extents with differing degrees of government intervention. The term 'market forces' is used to cover all of these. Given the variance in institutional forms, there will be morally significant differences in the way they operate. Some morally relevant consequences will arise in some of these contexts while not in others. At the same time, there will also be some features of markets that are common to all.

The second point is that there is considerable disagreement about the moral standing of markets amongst political economists and philosophers of economics. These arguments concern the *legitimacy* of market relations. In one corner are those who laud the virtues of the market. *Ex hypothesi*, the market furnishes us with a cornucopia of goods, is efficient and provides, through the price mechanism, a system for informing producers of the wants of consumers. This is the position espoused by many proponents of neo-classical economics, a position which is articulated through an examination of the market under conditions of perfect competition. This ideal market of perfect competition is one in which, amongst other things, there are no barriers to entry for producers, all consumers have perfect knowledge of what it is that they are buying, there is neither monopoly nor monopsony and the goods sold are homogenous (Stilwell, 2002, pp. 176–7). It is not that such econo-mists think that this is an accurate description of actually existing markets. Instead, it is said to provide a convenient theoretical benchmark (Stiglitz, 1997, pp. 29–30).

In another corner, are those more circumspect about the virtues of so-called free markets. There is an extensive body of literature that focuses on the ways markets may fail to account for the social costs of many economic activities and to realise the maximum social benefit (Coase, 1960, pp. 1–44). These concerns are captured in two ideas, *externalities* and *market failure*. An 'exter-nality' refers to a third-party side effect to a transaction; it is a cost or benefit of production or consumption not experienced by the transacting agents (Dahlman, 1979, pp. 141–62; Cornes and Sandler, 1986; Eatwell *et al.*, 1987, p. 265). Where there are *negative externalities* (i.e. there are social costs to production or consumption), even though the parties to the transaction may individually benefit, the transactions do not lead to social efficiency. Accordingly, given the way markets operate, such costs and benefits are not internalized within the price mechanism. This raises questions about the moral status of the market since the price system is meant to allow us to maximize social efficiency. *Coase's Theorem* is a response to this problem, according to which with appropriately designed property rights, markets could take care of externalities without direct government intervention. But, equally, many economists take externalities to be an insoluble within the market (Stiglitz, 1997, p. 509).

A criticism of the market to which it is even harder for the free marketer to respond involves what is sometimes called 'market failure' (Cowan, 1988). This is a more general notion – of which the existence of externalities amongst other things might be an explanation – that concerns the failure of markets to achieve an optimal resource allocation. Market failure might, for instance, be thought to be the result of externalities, or a product of monopoly (Stilwell, 2002, pp. 200–3). One thing we do know is that *actually existing markets* are not always optimal and often generate unnecessary social costs (Stiglitz, 1997, pp. 160–3).

There is another ground of criticism that one might sheet home to market forces, yet which – unsurprisingly given the consequentialist orientation of economic theory – one rarely finds discussed in the standard economic literature. This concerns the quality of the motivations one finds in interac-tions subject to market forces. The claim is that, within social arrangements subject to market forces, the motivations of those engaging in any activity become instrumentalist and any other-regarding component is driven out by the profit motive (Sloman and Norris, 1999, p. 21). If one believes that medical activity should be undertaken in part for other-regarding motives, then the instrumentalism of much profit-driven market activity might well be a reason for criticizing untrammeled market forces.

What should we take from these debates? The central point is that 'actually existing' markets do have various morally deleterious elements and it is those upon which I shall now focus.

Information systems and consumer sovereignty justifications

Among other things, markets function as *information systems* for the allocation of resources. Social resources move, via the price mechanism, in response to the signals of the market. Prices respond to shortages and surpluses. Shortages cause prices to rise and surpluses cause prices to fall (Lipsey, 1972, p. 41). Obviously, this provision of automatic signals for determining allocation occurs without any systematic and conscious coordination. It operates through an 'invisible hand' since no one intends these particular outcomes.

This account of the market as an information system that is both automatic and efficient, is seen by many as providing a *legitimation* or *defence* of the market itself (O'Neill, 1998, pp. 12–21). More radical defenders of the free-market claim that because under conditions of perfect competition markets provide an optimal allocation, in actual imperfect conditions, they also provide us with an optimal (rather than just better) resource allocation. More circumspect defenders acknowledge that the oligopolistic world we live in is a long way from the conditions required for optimality, arguing that the market provides a method for decentralized decision-taking that is *moderately* well co-ordinated and, as it turns out, *better* coordinated than any available or feasible alternatives (Lipsey, 1972, p. 412).

Further, the information content of this system is sometimes said to favour the consumer. Some economists argue that, within the price system, the consumer, rather than the producer, is king, queen or sovereign. This is the idea of '*consumer sovereignty*' that describes a situation wherein firms respond to changes in consumer demand, without being in a position in the long run to charge a price above average cost (Keat, Whitely and Abercrombie, 1994; Sloman and Norris, 1999, p. 544). Paul Samuelson, whose textbook was the standard for orthodox economics in the second half of the twentieth century, writes that 'the consumer is, so to speak, the king ... each is a voter who uses his money to get the things done he wants done' (Samuelson, 1964, p. 56).

Unsurprisingly, not all economists agree with this, some wanting to say that producers have more control than writers like Samuelson suppose. More radical critics focus on the way that the market shapes, through advertising and related processes, the tastes and wants of consumers. Leaving these issues to one side, for our purposes, there is a more important point regarding consumer sovereignty. The idea of consumer sovereignty also has, in addition to its descriptive functions, a *justificatory function* that is of great interest to the report card movement. Although standard justifications of the market are utilitarian (focusing on optimal efficiency and the like), there is a strand of political philosophy, often associated with the Austrian school (which would include thinkers such as von Mises and Hayek), that is concerned with the market as an expression of human freedom. Markets are morally justified according to this strand of thought because their outcomes are the products of sovereign agents exercising their autonomy or freedom – although this is a view about which there are many critics (Sen, 1993). It is the very sovereignty of consumers that makes markets morally valuable.

Analogies are made here with democracy; market outcomes are, *mutatis mutandis*, like democratic ones, but with consumers exercising their vote through their purchasing choices. The choices of informed consumers are *ex hypothesi* to be treated as being of paramount importance. Thus consumers should be free to choose market products on the basis of full information about those products. Perhaps, instead of focusing on democratic values, a better way of explicating the view is through a connection with informed consent. The notion of consumer sovereignty might well be rebadged as the idea of informed consent applied to the context of the market; and to do so would be no grave injustice to the idea of informed consent since there is no reason to think it applies only in a medical context (Faden and Beauchamp, 1986; Clarke, 2001, pp. 169–87). This justification of the market requires that consumers be fully, or at least adequately, informed. And, if we take this requirement seriously, then it has implications for the publication of performance indicators. Report cards seem to be a necessary condition for the realization of consumer sovereignty. Just as a commitment to the publication of performance indicators follows from a commitment to informed consent, so too advocacy of this normative account of consumer sovereignty entails a commitment to report cards.

If information about performances is published and we allow it to affect fees for surgeons, then the rates surgeons are able to charge will reflect their relative standings on the performance indicators. In this case, prices will typically convey information to medical consumers about the relative competencies of the surgeons in question.

There are considerable objections to 'normative' consumer sovereignty, and to the justificatory use of the notion. After all, one might argue that the information to which consumers have access is, as a matter of fact, so limited that their choices cannot really be said to be fully informed. This criticism is underpinned by the 'authenticity model' of autonomy that views various internal barriers to full personal autonomy as restricting the possibility of any individual actually realizing this value (Clarke, 2001, p. 170). Alternatively, one might argue that the influence of advertising is so powerful that the consumers' wants cannot be said to be fully autonomous. Or, if consumers are faced with monopoly producers, then there will arguably be no need for the producer to respond to the wishes of the consumer. Again, consumer sovereignty is undermined. However, the status of normative consumer sovereignty is not really what is at issue. My point is not whether consumers really are sovereign, but rather that, *if one believes* that the market is justified because it reflects the wishes of sovereign consumers, then one should be in favour of report cards. What implications might this final claim have for proponents of the publication of performance indicators? Does the connection between informed consent and normative consumer sovereignty mean that defenders of the report card movement must be in favour of free markets for the provision of health services? The answer here is 'no'. One might believe that markets do not provide sufficient information and, given the power of capitalist industry, they are unlikely ever to do so.

There are three conclusions to draw from the preceding discussion. If one adheres to the notion of consumer sovereignty as a justificatory ground of markets, then there is a *pro tanto* case that one should be a defender of report cards. Secondly, given what we are told about markets and the transfer of information is true, then in the market context the price mechanism will provide information that reflects the relative standings of surgeons and hence the market itself will function as a further information device. Finally, there is no reason to think that proponents of report cards need be proponents of the free market.

Let us turn now from questions of our intellectual commitments to the moral implications for report cards of market forces.

Markets as distributive mechanisms

Markets also function as distributive mechanisms. In markets resources are bought and sold as commodities and so allocated across society in an 'unpatterned' manner (Nozick, 1974, pp. 155–60). Financial resources and the strength of one's wants determine the pattern of distribution. In the medical context, this means that medical goods and services are allocated to those who have the financial resources and a desire for these commodities. Conversely, if medical goods are primarily distributed within a fully marketised environment, those without financial resources are not able to access medical goods and services. This is to be contrasted with a public system of provision where (in principle at least) it is the perception of relative need that determines how resources are distributed.

What should we make of these distributive possibilities? We need to acknowledge that markets have many virtues in the distributive realm; they provide an automatic mechanism for distributing goods and services that is often more efficient than other systems. Such considerations of efficiency and overall utility need to be balanced against those of justice. If the goods in question answer to fundamental human needs – as can plausibly be claimed for medical goods – then the fact that some, because of their lack of financial resources, might miss out on these goods appears to be an injustice. There are real issues concerning the fundamental failure of market allocations to be distributively just, a point which many economists have noted by classifying distributive inequities as one form of market failure (Stiglitz, 1997, pp. 152–7).

What is the import of this for the report card movement? Assume that we are talking about genuine markets where access is determined by one's relative financial standing. What is now morally salient? If we have genuine markets for surgery and surgeons' performance indicators are published, this will affect the rates that surgeons charge. It is hard to see how it wouldn't. Their relative prices will become reflections of the relative standing of surgeons on the scales provided by the report cards. (And, if we allow doctors to advertise their performances on such comparative scales, then such differential charges will presumably be increased.) Such price differentiation will have *distributive consequences*. Those who rank higher on the report cards will be treating the wealthier, rather than the poorer, members of society. Assuming that these performance indicators track something meaningful, then the differential rates will *systematically* ensure that the rich enjoy the services of more skilled surgeons than the less well-off. In effect, we would increase the disadvantage of the poor. This seems undesirable, for there is enough discrimination and disadvantage in the world without providing information that would systematically ensure that the disadvantaged have access only to the least capable surgeons.

It might be argued that, in fact, these processes occur already without the presence of report cards. Top surgeons charge top dollar and, as a consequence, only the wealthy can afford their services. But there is a difference in this case – and not just a *bare difference* – in that there currently is no systematic method for the wealthy to ensure that the surgeons they hire are in fact the best. Their prices may be hefty but there is no exact method for checking that the prices they pay reflect anything about the quality of the surgeons. With the publication of performance data, such checking would be possible.

One concern then is with the possible distributive consequences of report cards within a free market system. But this is not the end of the story. There are various mechanisms involving government intervention, which might be put in place within the market to avoid such consequences. For example, we might set standard rates for surgeons and then have bonuses paid by the government to those surgeons with good report cards. In this way, there would be no differential rates for surgeons whilst rewarding those surgeons who do well.

On the other side, we might well wonder about the distributive consequences for doctors themselves. In a market context, report cards could lead to some doctors being penalised for poor results. Whether or not this is unfair will depend upon what it is that the performance indicators measure and how accurate they are. If report cards are organized so as to indicate what counts as a threshold competency and some doctors fail to reach those required levels of competency, then it does not seem inappropriate that they receive lower levels of remuneration than those who do reach such thresholds. This is not to suggest that threshold competencies should be published instead of perform-ance indicators – an idea which Clarke and Oakley explore in some detail (Clarke and Oakley, 2004, p. 15). Instead, it is simply to make the claim that the data should indicate what counts as a threshold of competency.

However, if the scales do not indicate threshold competencies, then prob-lems might arise. Imagine surgeons' performances are scaled on a bell-curve, so that some will necessarily be on the bottom end of the scale, even when they achieve requisite levels of competency. For such scaling to lead to large differ-ence in remuneration would be unfair, since the scale may not be measuring large degrees of difference in competency.

Moreover, if the tests fail to differentiate between the degrees of difficulty of some surgical operations then there may be a grave injustice being done to those who take on more difficult operations. This again would be a distributive injustice. But as Clarke and Oakley indicate it is possible to publish risk-adjusted mortality rates; and indeed the New York State Department, for one, has done so (Clarke and Oakley, 2004, p. 15). So, the point is not that it will necessarily give rise to undesirable distributive outcomes, but that such distributive injustice is a danger that sometimes comes with the territory and against which we should be vigilant.

The transformation of our incentive structures

In unleashing market forces we also transform the *incentive structures* of economic agents. When a sphere of social life is subjected to market forces, the pursuit of profit becomes a central motivating feature for social agents *qua* social agents. Many think that this is not only a constitutive feature of market-ization, but it is its very point since this is the 'engine' which fosters the production of social benefits within market-based societies. Because people are driven to increase their profits, they search for more efficient and more attractive ways of producing goods for consumption as well as new ways of satisfying needs and wants. In *quasi*-markets some kind of approximation to profit that involves *pro rata* benefits will typically be introduced to attempt to mimic the market and hence reap the positive outcomes of markets.

There has been a great deal of discussion about the moral status of the profit motive. While it has been common since the advent of Adam Smith and Bernard Mandeville's contributions to political philosophy to sing hymns of praise to the myriad ways in which the 'vice' of self-interest leads us to the 'virtue' of social plenty, equally there is a long tradition of moral criticism of the profit motive in which it is argued that financial incentives bring with them moral corruption. Given that report cards will often be employed in commercial contexts, let us now consider two elements of the criticism of the profit motive, the first of which concerns what we might call 'perverse incentives'. The search for profit often leads to the production of considerable social benefits, through *inter alia* the increase in levels and efficiency of production. But profit can be achieved through means that are not socially beneficial. Think of the asset-stripping of companies. What we have here are perverse incentives at play. Such cases involve circumstances where the desire for advancement can be satisfied or realised in ways that are socially costly rather than beneficial.

With respect to report cards, there are a number of ways in which markets might furnish medical practitioners with perverse incentives. The publication of performance indicators might provide surgeons with an incentive to manipulate their results. Thus, we might find surgeons refusing to take on difficult cases if those were to affect their results, or surgeons might engage in 'gaming' the system, whereby data on outcomes are manipulated through surgeons misreporting or misclassifying patient details, an outcome that would not be good for the health system as a whole. As Clarke and Oakley note: 'It has been claimed that the more widespread use of public report cards will result in surgeons becoming much more reluctant to operate on patients who require relatively complex procedures' (2004, p. 13). Or else they might fail to disclose some information where it is possible to conceal it. To be sure, incentives to manipulate such report card data will also be present in a non-market environment. For instance, motivations deriving from a desire to maintain or enhance one's professional reputation will be enough to create such outcomes. However, these are likely to be intensified in a market context where one's professional standing has a direct effect on one's level of remuneration.

The second criticism concerns the *quality* of the motives that animate agents who operate in markets. It concerns the way in which, in the market, commercial considerations can come to dominate more altruistic ones. Underpinning this is the thought that the market and altruism are, in some deep sense, incompatible. The strongest version of this thesis holds that altruism and the profit motive are mutually exclusive and therefore adoption of the profit motive *necessarily* evacuates any altruistic aims from one's motivational set (Walsh, 2001, pp. 525–30). However, there are readily available counterexamples. Think of the goals and aims of a traditional family doctor in general practice. That she is a private contractor who charges consultancy fees for each patient she sees, and hence can be said to be animated by the profit motive, does not mean that she is animated *only* by the profit motive (Flew, 1976, pp. 312–22). It is not implausible to suggest that such a doctor is also motivated by benevolent other-regarding motives.

There is a more moderate version of the thesis according to which a commercial orientation, while compatible with benevolent motives will, often, as a matter of fact, lead to the *gradual evacuation* of such motives. This seems a far more plausible way of putting the objection. The idea is that market forces can corrode our attitudes towards our work and, in particular, corrode its other-regarding content. There is no suggestion here that the *mere presence* of commercial motives is enough to evacuate an action of any moral content.

Report cards may well lead surgeons to concentrate more on the commercial element of their profession than the altruistic element. In this way the altruistic element may be corroded to oblivion. Of course, in a commercial environment, such pressures towards an exclusively commercial orientation – as opposed to an orientation characterized by an admixture of commercial and altruistic motives – will always be present. But report cards, in so far as they increase the commercial pressure on surgeons and thus make the commercial consequences of any particular operation evident to them, might well worsen such processes.The dangers of this corrosion of surgeons' motives – dangers that exist in any commercial environment – are likely to be increased with the advent of report cards. If we think that surgeons should be motivated in part by other-regarding benevolent motives, then any social phenomenon that deepens the corrosion of such motivations is of concern. In so far as report cards exacerbate such corrosion of the proper goals of medicine, then they are matters of concern.

Concluding remarks: informed consent as a fundamental value?

What difference does the increasingly marketized environment in which medicine is practised have for the moral status of the publication of performance indicators? My first point concerned the consequences for the moral status *of a certain style of market justification*. In so far as one adopts an autonomy-based justification of the market, in which the notion of consumer sovereignty is central, then it would seem that this provides strong reasons for supporting the publication of performance indicators.

But this does not end matters. I considered the implications or consequences of *market forces themselves* for the moral status of the report cards. The first of these involved the distributive consequences of report cards. If report cards increase distributive inequality, then this counts as a mark against them. The second feature of market forces I examined concerned the transformation of our incentive structures with the spread of the profit motive as a primary motivation of medical practitioners. Here there were two lines of criticism. In so far as report cards increase any perverse incentives that might exist in a commercial medical environment, then this is morally undesirable.

Furthermore, in so far as report cards magnify the tendency for the profit motive to corrode the altruistic quality of medical practitioners' motivations, then this too is a mark against the publication of performance indicators.

It is important to stress that none of the morally pathological features identified is *fatal* for the report card movement. Whilst it might make us a little more circumspect about how we implement any policy, the fact that report cards will be published in a commercial and commercializing environment does not provide grounds for rejecting the movement, since there are various ways in which government policy might be enacted to constrain those pathologies.

The discussion does have ramifications for informed consent understood as the primary and fundamental value of medicine. Much of the debate over the moral status of report cards involves a clash between the competing values of informed consent and privacy. How do we weigh the need of medical patients for all relevant information regarding any procedures they are to undergo against the doctors' right to privacy? Herein the debate is between informed consent and social costs (albeit broadly defined, if a decline in the quality of our motives is to count as a social cost). In cases where the social costs of report cards are sufficiently high, then we might well take those social costs to trump concerns with informed consent (Chassin, Hannan and DeBuono, 1996; Neil, Clarke and Oakley, 2004). If this is correct, then whatever else is true, informed consent no longer stands as the single fundamental value. This is not to say that informed consent is not an important value, indeed this line of reasoning fits with the idea that 'all-things being equal, we ought to provide more fine-grained information where it is available' (Clarke and Oakley, 2004, p. 14). It is to say that, in the formation of public policy for health-related matters, informed consent is but one value amongst a number that we are to weigh in our all-things-considered judgements.

References

Chassin, M. R., Hannan E. L. and DeBuono, B. A. (1996). Benefits and hazards of reporting medical outcomes publicly. *New England Journal of Medicine*, **334**, 394–8.

Clarke, S. (2001). Informed consent in medicine in comparison with consent in other areas of human activity. *Southern Journal of Philosophy*, **39**, 169–87.

Clarke, S. and Oakley, J. (2004). Informed consent and surgeons' performance. *Journal of Medicine and Philosophy*, **29**, 11–35.

Coase, R. W. (1960). The problem of social cost. *Journal of Law and Economics*, **3**, 1–44.

Cornes, R. and Sandler, T. (1986). *The Theory of Externalities, Public Goods and Club Goods*. Cambridge: Cambridge University Press.

Cowan, T. (ed.) (1988). *The Theory of Market Failure: A Critical Examination*. Fairfax, Virginia: George Mason University Press.

Dahlman, C. J. (1979). The problem of externality. *Journal of Law and Economics*, **22**, 141–62.

Eatwell, J., Milgate, M. and Newman, P. (1987). *The New Palgrave: A Dictionary of Economics*. London: MacMillan, Vol. 2.

Faden, R. and Beauchamp, T. L. (1986). *A History and Theory of Informed Consent*. New York: Oxford University Press.

Flew, A. (1976). The profit motive. *Ethics*, **86**, 312–22.

Keat, R., Whitely, N. and Abercrombie, N. (1994). *The Authority of the Consumer*. London: Routledge.

Keogh, B., Spiegelhalter, D., Bailey, A., Roxburgh, J., Magee, P. and Hilton, C. (2004). The legacy of Bristol: public disclosure of individual surgeons' results. *British Medical Journal*, **329**, 450–4.

Lipsey, R. G. (1972). *An Introduction to Positive Economics*. 3rd edn. London: Weidenfeld and Nicolson.

Marginson, S. (1997). *Markets in Education*. Melbourne: Allen and Unwin.

Neil, D., Clarke, S. and Oakley, J. G. (2004). Public reporting of individual surgeon performance information: United Kingdom developments and Australian issues. *Medical Journal of Australia*, **181**, 266–8.

Nozick, R. (1974). *Anarchy, State and Utopia*. New York: Basic Books.

O'Neill, J. (1998). *The Market: Ethics, Knowledge and Politics*. London: Routledge.

Samuelson, P. (1964). *Economics: An Introductory Analysis*. 6th edn. New York: McGraw-Hill.

Sen, A. (1993). Markets and freedom: achievements and limitations of the market mechanism in promoting individual freedom. *Oxford Economic Papers*, **45**, 519–41.

Sloman, J. and Norris, K. (1999). *Economics*. New York: Addison-Wesley.

Stiglitz, J. (1997). *Economics*, 2nd edn. New York: Norton.

Stilwell, F. (2002). *Political Economy: The Contest of Economics Ideas*. Oxford: Oxford University Press.

Walsh, A. (2001). Are market norms and intrinsic valuation mutually exclusive? *Australasian Journal of Philosophy*, **79**, 525–43.

Part III

Reporting performance
information

Part introduction

Reporting performance information

Surgeon performance information has been collected, tabulated and publicly reported since the early 1990s, first in New York State and then in other American States, and now in the United Kingdom. Performance information on surgical units and on hospitals has been collected for some time before this, but the public release of such information is a relatively recent phenomenon, as are report cards on the performance of individual surgeons and certain other clinicians. In this final section of the collection we turn our attention to the 'report cards movement' itself, with chapters examining a variety of issues that have emerged in studies of the impact of report cards on the performance of hospitals, units and individual surgeons.

Our first chapter in the section, by Silvana Marasco and Joseph Ibrahim, examines the impact of public reporting of surgeons' performance on patient care. The authors consider, in some detail, the impact of cardiac surgeon report cards on the quality of cardiac surgery, on cardiac patients and on cardiac surgeons and other stakeholders, particularly in light of the US experience with report cards on individual cardiac surgeons. Rachel Werner and David Asch also examine evidence of the impact of public reporting on the quality of health care services. They argue that existing US public reporting initiatives have not been conclusively shown to improve healthcare quality, and indeed, that there is some evidence that public reporting has various unintended negative consequences for patient care. Werner and Asch suggest that much is to be done if report card systems are to fulfil the promise of enabling substantial improvements to the quality of care provided. Our next contributor, Paul Aylin, takes a step back from debates about what the report card movement has, or has not, achieved and asks us to consider what hospital and clinician data could tell us, whether or not such data is publicly reported. He considers issues of data quality and a variety of statistical issues, before surveying available methods of data presentation and intepretation.

The following two chapters in the section concern the 'defensive surgery objection' to publicizing surgeon performance information. This objection has it that public reporting of surgeon performance information motivates surgeons to avoid taking on high-risk patients. Proponents of the defensive surgery objection usually concede that risk-adjustment of surgeon performance information can reduce the motivation of surgeons to practise 'defensive surgery'; however, they are not convinced that it can fully remove it. Justin Oakley looks at the actual evidence for defensive surgery and finds that the available evidence is inconclusive. Provocatively, he argues that, even if report cards have led to the conduct of defensive surgery, they may nevertheless be ethically justified, all things considered. Yujin Nagasawa also considers the defensive surgery objection and identifies a new form of this objection that has not hitherto been explicitly articulated, arising from surgeons' anxieties regarding malpractice suits. Nevertheless, he argues that the solution to this form of the defensive surgery objection is to be found in careful risk adjustment of surgeon performance data.

Tony Eyers attends to another well-known concern about surgeon report cards, which is that they may make it difficult for surgical trainees to receive appropriate training. He also points out that they may make it difficult for surgical innovations to take place. Eyers argues, however, that, if properly used, surgeon report cards can have a positive impact on both training and innovation. The final chapter in the section is by Ian Freckelton, who brings a legal perspective to the report cards movement. He examines legal developments with regard to surgeon report cards in the United States, Canada, the United Kingdom and Australia, and argues that report cards must be designed in such a way that patients and courts remain aware of their limitations as measures of clinician performance and do not use them uncritically.

13

Is the reporting of an individual surgeon's clinical performance doing more harm than good for patient care?

Silvana F. Marasco

The Alfred Hospital, Prahan, Australia

Joseph E. Ibrahim

Monash University, Melbourne, Australia

Introduction

Report cards, also known as league tables, allow publication of outcome data that can reflect the performance of a particular hospital, clinical unit, or an individual doctor. Increasing interest is being focused on clinical report cards, particularly on their use in monitoring the performance of individual doctors and in making that data public. Report cards do have a number of possible roles including self-audit, accountability and to demonstrate safety and industry regulation. Almost 10 per cent of Australia's Gross National Product is devoted to healthcare, so it is an extremely important sector of government (www.aihw. gov.au). Other industries spending this level of tax payers' funds are accountable to the community and it certainly seems appropriate that healthcare is also kept under scrutiny. However, how far should that scrutiny extend and in what form should outcomes be made available to the community? Should the outcomes of individual doctors be made available or should this level of outcome data be retained within the craft groups for self-regulation and audit, leaving unit-based and hospital-based data available for publication and dissemination to the public. What other industries are subject to public distribution of the results of individuals within that industry?

In this chapter we explore the issue of report cards, specifically with regard to cardiac surgeons, who are currently at the forefront of this debate. We will explore the events in the United States of America and the United Kingdom which have preceded the debate in Australia, and will then explore the real and potential consequences of the introduction of report cards in this country.

Informed Consent and Clinician Accountability: The Ethics of Report Cards on Surgeon Performance. Steve Clarke and Justin Oakley (eds.). Published by Cambridge University Press. © Cambridge University Press 2007.

Report cards on cardiac surgeons

In many ways, cardiac surgery has become the focal point for the debate about clinical performance reporting of individual surgeons. Possible reasons why this has occurred are outlined below.

Firstly, cardiac surgery, in particular coronary artery bypass grafting (CABG) is one of the most commonly performed operative procedures in the western world today and has been for a number of years. Large international databases exist, which allow hospital units and individual surgeons to compare their results to the international surgical community. As such, cardiac surgery lends itself to comparisons of outcomes both internationally and within countries.

Secondly, cardiac surgical procedures can be clearly and easily defined. There are only a few different cardiac surgical operations and the numbers of each of these particular operations that are performed is large. This is not the case with many other surgical specialties, where small numbers of very different operations are performed.

Thirdly, patient groups that present for CABG surgery are relatively homogeneous, in comparison with other clinical conditions, and therefore lend themselves to risk stratification more readily.

Fourthly, there are numerous outcomes, which can be easily and accurately defined after cardiac surgery, such as mortality. Such definitive endpoints can be accurately monitored and verified allowing reliable comparisons to be made.

Fifthly, cardiac surgery is costly and it consumes a substantial proportion of government healthcare budgets. This generates questions about resource allocation and access to surgery, and naturally focuses attention on this specialty.

Finally, cardiac surgery is a major event in patients' lives. It is usually the biggest operation they will ever have and there is generally an understanding and acceptance that the stakes are high. The enormous stress felt by most patients upon realizing they need cardiac surgery, as well as the fact that it is a time where they have to face their own mortality, makes it a highly emotive issue.

Thus, we can explain why the debate regarding report cards is so inextricably linked to cardiac surgery. However, in producing report cards detailing the results of individual cardiac surgeons, we are placing the entire responsibility for that patient's outcome on one individual. Is this a realistic expectation? It is undeniable that a patient's post-operative course hinges on the technical expertise of the surgery. However, the entire team who take part in the patient's care all bear some responsibility for that patient's recovery. There are many cardiac patients who have complicated medical problems, which lie outside the expertise of cardiac surgeons. Other clinicians within the hospital are relied upon to assess, advise and manage these conditions. However, from the point of view of the patient, the surgeon is seen as the face of the team. The patient will not even meet many of the members of the team, such as the scrub nurses in the operating room and the perfusionists who run the heart–lung bypass machine. This explains why from the consumer's point of view, it is the surgeon who bears responsibility for their outcome. The reality, however, is that the patient's outcome is dependent on a myriad of inter-related factors for which each member of the team bears some responsibility.

International experience with report cards on cardiac surgeons

Report cards on cardiac surgeons in the United States of America and United Kingdom

The initial catalyst for the debate on publicly disclosed report cards came with the publication of cardiac surgeons' results in New York State in 1991. Although initially developed as a hospital-specific dataset which was published with the hospitals de-identified (Hannan, 1990), the media discovered that surgeon-specific data existed and successfully sued under the *Freedom of Information Act* for access to these data. In 1991 New York *Newsday* published a list of all cardiac surgeons in New York who had performed coronary bypass surgery over the preceding 2 years, along with the surgeons' case load numbers and risk-adjusted mortality.

The impact of the *Newsday* publication has been extensive. Hospitals and surgeons performing low-volume cardiac surgery were found to have significantly higher mortality rates than high-volume centres, leading to further investigation of those centres. Twenty-seven cardiac surgeons who were identified as low-volume providers with higher mortality figures either left New York State or ceased performing cardiac surgery over the 1989–1992 period (Hannan, 1995; Chassin, 2002). As a result of these figures, wide-ranging changes to the delivery of care to these patients were also implemented, including changes in pre-operative management and stabilisation, further training of staff and creation of dedicated intensive care beds. Thus, not all of the changes which led to improvements in outcomes were directly as the result of changes in surgeons' practices.

Interestingly, risk-adjusted mortality in New York State fell by 41% over the 3 years following the first publicly released report cards. This has been applauded by some as the result of a successful programme. However, others have been critical of the perceived effects. Critics have argued that surgeon-specific report cards lead surgeons to avoid operating on high-risk patients. This alleged avoidance behaviour is purported to be because these patients are more likely to have unsuccessful outcomes, and such outcomes would have a negative impact on the surgeon's report card. A recent study suggested a phenomenon of 'out-migration' of high-risk cardiac patients from New York State during 1989–1993, after reviewing the mortality rates in a neighbouring state (Omoigui *et al.*, 1996). However, the findings in this study have been challenged by others (Chassin *et al.*, 1996; Peterson, 1998). More recently, another unintended consequence of report cards has also been identified. Over the period of the introduction of report cards in New York state, the disparity in CABG use between white patients and black or Hispanic patients increased significantly, indicating that surgeons perceived black and Hispanic patients as being higher risk (Werner *et al.*, 2005). Data on surgeons in New York State continue to be collated annually and are available to the public on the internet: http://www.health.state.ny.us/. Other states have since started collecting data and are also providing surgeon-specific results to the public: www.phc4.org; www.state.nj.us/health. However, not all states agree with this type of reporting. Massachusetts has elected to publish hospital-specific results, while conducting a confidential, legislatively protected review process for individual surgeons (Shahian, 2005).

In the United Kingdom, the strongest stimulus for the development of report cards came on the heels of the highly publicized Bristol Royal Infirmary Inquiry into paediatric cardiac deaths. The Royal College of Surgeons immediately commenced review and audit processes, which included the development of an internet-based report card system. In March 2005, the Secretary of State for Health announced that fully risk-adjusted CABG mortality rates for every cardiac surgeon working in the NHS would be available on a publicly accessible website by the end of the year. This announcement was made after publication of surgeon-specific CABG mortality rates (not all of them risk-adjusted), which a British newspaper, *The Guardian*, had obtained through the *Freedom of Information Act* (as had *Newsday* with the 1991 New York surgeon data). The website showing most British cardiac surgeons' risk-adjusted survival rates for CABG was subsequently launched by the UK Healthcare Commission in April 2006.

A more detailed description of the sequence of events and ramifications in the USA and UK can be found elsewhere (Marasco *et al.*, 2005). Review of these international events is particularly instructive, as it appears that the development of report cards has spread well in advance of our understanding of them. Despite almost 15 years of experience with report cards in New York State, there remain many questions as to their usefulness, and most states in the USA have still to develop some type of publicly accessible reporting system. In particular, there has been very little focus on the ethical aspects of this type of reporting and the effects that it may have on the doctor–patient relationship.

The status of cardiac surgery report cards in Australia

Self-directed audit is a mandatory activity for all surgical specialties in Australia at both a unit and individual level. Participation in audit activities is stipulated and monitored by the Royal Australasian College of Surgeons

(RACS) for all surgeons. In 1999, the Australian Society of Cardiothoracic Surgeons (ASCTS) established a state-wide database collecting cardiac surgery data from all Victorian public hospitals, with the aim of eventually making the database nation-wide. At much the same time, the Victorian Health Services Policy Review recommended that comparative performance data of specific procedures from all public hospitals be collected and made available. The unit-based data is published yearly, and is made available to cardiac surgeons and the Victorian Department of Human Services in a de-identified form. A report summarising these unit-based data is publicly available on the Department website: www.health.vic.gov.au/cardiacsurgery. Individual surgeon data exists and will be used by the ASCTS council to conduct confidential reviews of outliers. These data are, however, protected by law against access by the media or publication.

Real and potential impact of report cards

The course of events in the USA and UK with regard to report cards has been closely observed, particularly by cardiac surgeons in Australia. There are concerns about the impact these developments may have on surgeons, patients, other key stakeholders and the health system overall.

Effects on surgeons

The potential effects on the surgeon include changing their practice to avoid high-risk patients, disengagement and disenchantment from healthcare and a potential negative impact on surgical training.

Surgery, and cardiac surgery in particular, is a specialty requiring exceptional technical skills in addition to the knowledge and experience required to treat these very sick patients. Report cards therefore, place a judgement on the technical ability of the surgeon as well as on other facets of the surgeon's abilities. This makes the introduction of report cards very personal. Not only do report cards have the potential to affect the livelihood of surgeons, but they also have the potential to diminish a surgeon's belief in his or her ability, and confidence in his or her skills. This judgement of technical ability is a facet of report cards to which other clinicians will not be subjected.

There are clearly concerns about the impact of report cards on the surgeon's willingness to accept and care for higher-risk patients. There are strong arguments that proper risk-adjustment of data would overcome this problem. However, because risk-adjustment models are fallible, the use of different models on the same set of data can produce different results (Shahian *et al.*, 2001). Other 'gaming' behaviours such as up-coding of co-morbidities to increase the risk adjustment have also been reported (Shahian, 2005).

In contrast, collection of unit-based data is unlikely to generate the level of anxiety that leads to the avoidance behaviours noted above. There is a concern that direct focus on individual surgeons is likely to create an atmosphere where surgeons become disenchanted and disengage from health care. If report cards specify the performance of individual surgeons, rather than teams, it could be argued that cardiac surgeons carry the professional, psychological and emotional burden and responsibility for the patient outcome. This is clearly not an accurate and fair reflection. Unit-based data, however, would take into account the performance of the entire team, giving a better idea of the risk of surgery for a patient in a particular hospital.

The observed association of volume of work with outcomes, both with regard to individual surgeons and hospitals, has been extensively investigated (Hannan *et al.*, 2003; Shahian and Normand, 2003; Peterson *et al.*, 2004). It appears that volume is important, although the lower limit at which it becomes significant is still unknown. The most consistent observation is that low-volume surgeons in low-volume hospitals tend to have higher mortalities than high-volume surgeons in high-volume hospitals. Interestingly, low-volume surgeons in high-volume hospitals tend to have good results. This is likely to be as the result of superior processes and post-operative care in these centres, reinforcing the impact of the entire team on outcomes (Shahian, 2005). The impact of low volumes on outcomes may become even more important in coming years, as cardiothoracic workloads diminish. Numbers of CABG operations (the mainstay of cardiac surgeons workloads) performed in the western world have dropped 25% since 1997, and look set to drop even further due to increasing intervention with stents by cardiologists; www.sts.org. Cardiac surgery has been identified by the Royal Australasian College of Surgeons as one of only two surgical specialties in Australia which does not need to increase workforce numbers to cope with the current workload.

All of the debates regarding report cards have centred on the publication of surgical results. However, part of a surgeon's job in assessing the potential pre-operative patient is to decide whether that patient is even suitable for surgery. There are patients who have so many co-existing medical conditions that the risk of surgery outweighs the risks of continuing with medical management alone for that condition. Making such assessments is not without risk in itself, and calls on a surgeon's clinical acumen and experience. Should report cards also include this type of information? Obviously, this information becomes more challenging to collect and collate, but it does take into account a very important facet of the surgeon's job. Would such data change the information presented in report cards? It may be that greater institutional rather than individual differences are seen. Surgeons working in a transplant centre may be more likely to take on high-risk cardiac failure patients, thus leaving a much smaller group of patients in the non-operative group. The reason for this is because transplant centres also provide services such as mechanical assist devices for the heart, which other cardiac surgery centres do not provide. Thus a surgeon in a transplant centre may take on a very high-risk case knowing that, if the patient's heart fails after the operation, then a mechanical assist device is available to implant into the patient and save his/her life. This is not a back-up plan available to most cardiac surgery centres, and in those centres such a patient would most likely die of heart failure, despite maximal medical therapy in that hospital. The willingness of a transplant surgeon to take on these high-risk cases, then, may adversely affect results both in the non-operative group and in the operative group, because of the higher risk nature of the patients on whom they agree to operate.

Concerns have been expressed about the potential negative impact of publication of report cards particularly on junior surgeons. Collation of individual surgeon data from a single year is unlikely to provide statistically meaningful results. Data from several consecutive years will be required for accurate analysis. However, this may not accurately reflect a given individual surgeon's practice, due to evolving practice and technique over that time. This is especially applicable to junior surgeons, where case numbers may be lower and techniques evolving rapidly.

However, the junior surgeon may also benefit from report cards. Referral patterns tend to favour more senior surgeons who have been practising for many years. However, technical skills do deteriorate with age, and there are many cases where senior surgeons whose abilities are waning are still receiving a large proportion of the market share based on their history, rather than on their recent results. Publication of report cards may actually show some interesting results whereby more junior surgeons are, in fact, performing better than some of their more senior counterparts.

Another group who may be particularly susceptible to a negative impact of report cards are trainee surgeons. Cardiac surgery is a challenging specialty to teach and train the next generation of surgeons. Not only does the surgery require skilled technical ability, but there is also a time imperative to complete the surgery without unduly prolonging the time that the heart is stopped and attached to the heart-lung machine. Will the introduction of report cards lead surgeons to become more reluctant to allow trainees to operate? How, given such a high level of scrutiny, is the next generation of surgeons to be taught? If surgeon-specific report cards were to be used in Australia, will the results of operations performed by trainees be included in their supervising surgeons' figures?

Effects on patients

One very important aspect of a possible future practice in an era of unit-based or individual-based outcome reporting is the attitude of the consumer (patient) to the available information. The effect report cards will have for patients is the most difficult to predict. There exist many assumptions about what patients want or how they will use this information.

Amazingly, it seems that patients are the consumer group least influenced by report cards (Schneider and Epstein, 1998; Schneider and Lieberman, 2001). This may be due to the complexity of the information presented, and the general lack of experience patients and surgeons have in using this information for decision-making. Further questioning reveals that many patients are more concerned with convenience and access to healthcare than reported outcomes (Bodenheimer, 1999). Emphasis is also placed on costs and medical insurance coverage in cases of privately insured patients (Bodenheimer, 1999). Most patients want their surgery as soon as possible, and they want it to take place as close to home as possible. Patients are also very much influenced by previous personal or family experience, and by media treatment of a particular hospital. Privately insured patients rely on their referring doctor to choose a surgeon who has an acceptable track record and who has previously serviced the doctors' patients well. In the case of public patients, they seem to be content with the knowledge that the hospital and the governing doctors' board or college is monitoring surgeon performance and taking appropriate steps if that performance falls short of acceptable standards.

It is unknown how much weight patients place on numerical data in making their decision, and how much on their rapport with the surgeon when they consent to an operation. Informed consent requires that the patient understands the need for the operation, possible alternative treatment options, the nature of the operation, and the potential adverse consequences or complications. Given the amount and complexity of this information, it is debatable whether consent to any operation is fully informed. It could be argued that no patient can ever be fully informed as to all the possible consequences of a major procedure, especially with heart surgery where the possible complications are almost limitless. Most patients have difficulty grasping the details of the operative procedure itself, let alone all the possible complications. Also, when complications of an operation or procedure are presented as numerical information as 'percentages of risk' this is often misunderstood by patients. It is doubtful whether report cards *per se* will add to a patient's ability to give informed consent for a procedure. It is more likely that they will add another layer of confusion. Other reasons for a patient's lack of interest in mortality rates include difficulty understanding the information, disinterest in the nature of the information, lack of trust in the data, problems with timely access to the information, and lack of choice (Marshall *et al.*, 2000).

Many patients express more interest in the risk of complications such as stroke rather than the risk of death *per se*. Generally, cardiac surgical patients have faced the prospect of death as a direct consequence of their underlying disease process. They realize that cardiac surgery is a major undertaking and accept that there is a risk of death. However, many patients are less accepting of debilitating complications such as stroke, which lead to significant loss of quality of life.

It is not obvious that patients have the ability to look at league tables of risk-adjusted mortality figures and draw reasonable inferences from these data. However, it is likely that many patients will be satisfied with the knowledge that internal audit will be performed, and that mechanisms have been put in place to identify outliers and institute appropriate changes. Most importantly, public reporting of such data ensures practitioners remain accountable to the community overall, thus helping to maintain public trust in the profession. As the events at Bristol, UK, and more recently in Bundaberg, Australia, demonstrated, when poor surgical results come to the public's attention only through the revelations of a whistleblower colleague, the resulting crisis of trust in the profession is almost irreparable.

Patients are also affected as a consequence of physician attitude to the release of report cards. As mentioned earlier, there has been an observation of avoidance of high-risk patients by surgeons unwilling to expose themselves to likely poorer outcomes. This, in turn, has led to changing patterns in the provision of service. A recent study identified that among patients admitted to hospital with a heart attack, outcomes were worse for patients in states with CABG report cards than in those states without such report cards (Dranove *et al.*, 2003). Presumably this was as a result of delays in operation or avoidance of operating on these patients.

Other stakeholders

In the United States, employers are the largest purchasers of healthcare, either as large corporations or as coalitions. Surprisingly, the vast majority of these organisations have not implemented available league tables in their decision-making of which healthcare organization to use (Marshall *et al.*, 2000). In contrast, there is some evidence that hospitals are taking note of their standing in league tables, and making changes to their own services in an attempt to bolster their standing in a very competitive market (Longo *et al.*, 1997).

Whether or not the publication of league tables alters the referral practices of cardiologists – who could look for better-performing surgeons to whom to refer patients – is a matter of much speculation. A survey of cardiologists in Pennsylvania reported that the majority of cardiologists have not changed their referral practice in the light of such report cards, although they did report having more difficulty in finding a surgeon to accept the higher risk cases (Schneider and Epstein, 1996). Others suggest that cardiologists are sceptical of the veracity of information contained in league tables (Marshall *et al.*, 2000).

Effects on the health system

There is limited information about how introducing report cards may alter the healthcare system. Specifically, what happens if patients exercise their rights to act on information provided in the report cards?

In the public hospital health system in Australia, each patient presenting for cardiac surgery is assigned to the surgeon on call at the time the patient presented. The patient has no choice of surgeon, the workload being distributed between all surgeons on a unit in an equitable manner. If a system of individual surgeon report cards was to be implemented, how do we cater for the patient who wants to change their surgeon? The logistics of swapping patients on a waiting list are not too complex. However, if the patient is too ill to be discharged home and is waiting for surgery in hospital, then the concept of changing patients from one surgeon's list to another and then perhaps waiting longer in hospital until that surgeon has an operating day are clearly going to create havoc with the running of an operating schedule. If all the patients decide they want surgeon X, then the problem would rapidly escalate.

Variations in patient populations between hospitals are another factor which needs to be considered. For example, heart failure patients tend to cluster in the transplant centres of which there are fewer than one per state in Australia. The expertise gained at these centres in looking after these patients is not going to be reflected in a league table, because the patient group will not be comparable to any other hospital in that state.

Implementation of report cards into practice

How to present the information

An issue that deserves consideration, in light of the US experience, is the ways in which surgeon-specific report cards are presented. The New York State league tables are published in a risk-adjusted format. This method of presenting data poses problems for patients who may have difficulty making reasonable inferences from these data. Research indicates that this is also difficult for trained health professionals (Burack *et al.*, 1999). Performance information is often rank ordered, and this can be a cause of ill-informed decisions because of the commonly made false assumption that the rank order equates to order of merit. Decision-making is strongly influenced by the way in which information is presented. Further analysis of report cards available on the internet, comparing care by hospitals in the USA of patients presenting with heart attacks, showed that the hospital ratings as published discriminated poorly between hospitals, and may well lead to misperceptions of standards of care (Krumholz *et al.*, 2002).

Who should present the information?

If we assume that patients with heart disease will be provided clinical performance data to assist their decision-making about the risks and benefits of surgery, who will present the information? Who will assist in ensuring patients comprehend the data? Is it appropriate for the cardiac surgeon to present their own performance data to patients? Will patients accept the veracity of the information, and will they be willing to question the surgeon about their performance and ask about alternatives? And should the cardiac surgeon then be expected to explain that surgeon X has a mortality rate 0.2% lower and perhaps the patient would like to see that surgeon? Surely, such a discussion will undermine the patient's confidence in the surgeon and alter the patient–doctor relationship to a degree not encountered by other craft groups. To date, there has been no suggestion that intensivists or respiratory physicians, for example, discuss their outcomes with patients they are about to treat.

The referral to the cardiac surgeon generally comes from the cardiologist who has diagnosed the patient's heart condition. The cardiologist is in the ideal position to make the patient aware of league table results and their importance. However, cardiologists already base their referral patterns on their perception of good results and good service. Studies have shown that cardiologists are unlikely to change their referral patterns on the basis of information in league tables (Schneider and Epstein, 1996). It therefore seems unlikely that they would be interested in spending their time explaining league tables to patients.

Evaluation of report cards

It has been assumed that report cards improve the delivery of healthcare, but this has in no way been definitively proven. As has been mentioned earlier, few patients utilize report cards to choose their physician, and those patients who are even aware of the existence of report cards are in the minority (Schneider and Epstein, 1998). Referring physicians' practices have not been markedly altered by the publication of report cards (Schneider and Epstein, 1996). Finally, there is little evidence that report cards have significantly changed the market share of high-quality hospitals or surgeons (Chassin, 2002).

The ethical boundaries of reporting on a group of health professionals also needs to be explored. The concept of public reporting of individual surgeon results has generated significant anxiety and defensiveness by a group of highly skilled individuals. The fundamental aim of report cards is to improve quality of care, and this is the same aim of surgeons. Do report cards improve quality of care? This is by no means certain. Within Australia, all specialists are subject to credentialing, certification and registration requirements that mandate ongoing learning and training. Many specialist groups are already taking part in audit activities that define acceptable practice, identify outliers, and action changes to improve results. Thus, specialist groups are constantly striving to improve the service they provide.

Do report cards provide patients with informed understanding? It is questionable whether a patient can ever completely give informed consent. In a specialist area such as cardiac surgery, where the procedure is so complex and the possible complications are almost limitless, it is difficult to expect any patient to comprehend more than a very small part of what they are about to undergo. Whether report cards will add to this process is doubtful. In fact, they may make it even more difficult for a patient to comprehend the procedure they are about to have.

How will report cards be disseminated so as to maintain transparency and equity? The very publication of this information provides transparency to the public. If report cards are disseminated to the public, then all members of the public must have equal access to this information. Most cardiac surgery patients are elderly and do not have access to the internet, so other modes of publication will need to be found. Transparency is essential to support the legitimacy and public accountability of this tool. As such, the public should be involved in the formulation of appropriate ways to present this data.

How can we claim equity amongst patients if they are not all provided with the ability to access, understand and act on the information in report cards? This is a complex area that requires substantial thought. We seek only to highlight the need for further work in this area, and for debate about what is equity in health – for example, is it access or is it the ability to choose? Some of the complexities that need exploration are the diversity and setting of the different patient groups, which include those in metropolitan or rural health settings, differing educational backgrounds that impact on understanding of numerical information, culturally and linguistically diverse groups, as well as private or public sector patients.

How the private or public sector patients may use the information in report cards highlights the need to consider the equity issue. At present, public patients remain bound by the organizational and government policy that does not readily allow choice of surgeon, however, it is more likely that performance information from publicly-funded health care will be available. In contrast, private patients are able to choose their surgeon and so are able to act on information in report cards; however, it may be difficult to get this information because some would argue the data is owned by the surgeon or the private practice.

What will we tell the public patients about the merit of report cards? Perhaps we can argue that although they have no power to act on the information when their health is at stake, the report cards will highlight the real and potential inequities in health for society and so lead to necessary reforms. If this is the answer then, where does that leave the patient and their surgeon in the clinic when they are discussing the risks and benefits for each individual case?

Conclusions

Currently, in Australia, no comparative data on individual performance of any doctors is publicly available. The momentum towards the use of comparative data on surgeons' performance appears to be increasing more rapidly than our understanding of the consequences of publishing this information. The potential ramifications of publicly available report cards which we have explored include changes in the doctor–patient relationship, changes in the surgeon's behaviour, career choice and market share, changes in future training and service provision and changes to organizational behaviour policy and requirements. Perhaps the most important of these is the possible shift in the doctor–patient relationship. If publication of individual report cards does occur, it will be important to protect the doctor–patient relationship and not jeopardise that for one craft group alone.

From the consumers' point of view, report cards will provide accountability of the profession, which the public have the right to expect. The public have supported the training and development of specialty groups and hold these groups in a privileged position. Surely, we have a duty to disclose our results and reassure the community that their interests are being served. But the method and form in which this should take place is by no means clear. There seems to be little gain in exposing individual surgeons to the detrimental effects of public reporting of results when there is clearly an entire team involved in and responsible for the patient's care.

While the practical, philosophical and ethical ramifications of report cards provide an interesting and intellectual debate, it is essential that we remain focused on our first and foremost concern, which is to improve patient care. It seems appropriate therefore to finish with a reminder of the mantra that all doctors must work by – first do no harm.

References

Bodenheimer, T. (1999). The American health care system: the movement for improved quality in health care. *New England Journal of Medicine*, **340**, 488–92.

Burack, J. H., Impellizzeri, P., Homel, P. and Cunningham, J. N. Jr. (1999). Public reporting of surgical mortality: a survey of New York State cardiothoracic surgeons. *Annals of Thoracic Surgery*, **68**, 1195–200.

Chassin, M. R. (2002). Achieving and sustaining improved quality: lessons from New York State and cardiac surgery. *Health Affairs*, **21**, 40–51.

Chassin, M. R., Hannan, E. L. and DeBuono, B. A. (1996). Benefits and hazards of reporting medical outcomes publicly. *New England Journal of Medicine*, **334**, 394–8.

Commonwealth Law Report (1998). 232 199 *Chappel v Hart*. High Court of Australia, HCA 55, 2 September 1998, 195.

Dranove, D., Kessler, D., McClellan, M. and Satterthwaite, M. (2003). Is more information better? The effects of 'report cards' on health care providers. *Journal of Political Economy*, **11**, 555–88.

Freckelton, I. (1999). Materiality of risk and proficiency assessment: the onset of report cards? *Journal of Law and Medicine*, **6**, 313–18.

Hannan, E. L., Kilburn, H. Jr., O'Donnell, J. F., Lukacik, G. and Shields, E. P. (1990). Adult open heart surgery in New York State. An analysis of risk factors and hospital mortality rates. *Journal of the American Medical Association*, **264**, 2768–74.

Hannan, E. L., Siu, A. L., Kumar, D., Kilburn, H. and Chassin, M. R. (1995). The decline in coronary artery bypass graft mortality in New York State. *Journal of the American Medical Association*, **273**, 209–13.

Hannan, E. L., Wu, C., Ryan, T. J. *et al.* (2003). Do hospitals and surgeons with higher coronary artery bypass graft surgery volumes still have lower risk-adjusted mortality rates? *Circulation*, **108**, 795–801.

Krumholz, H. M., Rathore, S. S., Chen, J., Wang, Y. and Radford, M. J. (2002). Evaluation of a consumer-oriented internet health care report card. The risk of quality ratings based on mortality data. *Journal of the American Medical Association*, **287**, 1277–87.

Longo, D. R., Land, G., Schramm, W., Fraas, J., Hoskins, B. and Howell, V. (1997). Consumer reports in health care. *Journal of the American Medical Association*, **278**, 1579–84.

Marasco, S. F., Ibrahim, J. E. and Oakley, J. (2005). Public disclosure of surgeon specific report cards – current status of the debate. *Australian and New Zealand Journal of Surgery*, **75**, 1000–4.

Marshall, M. N., Shekelle, P. J., Leatherman, S. and Brook, R. H. (2000). The public release of performance data. What do we expect to gain? A review of the evidence. *Journal of the American Medical Association*, **283**, 1866–74.

Omoigui, N. A., Miller, D. P., Brown, K. J., Annan, K., Cosgrove, D. and Lytle, B. (1996). Outmigration for coronary bypass surgery in an era of public dissemination of clinical outcomes. *Circulation*, **93**, 27–33.

Peterson, E. D., De Long, E. R., Jollis, J. G., Muhlbaier, L. H. and Mark, D. B. (1998). The effects of New York's bypass surgery provider profiling on access to care and patient outcomes in the elderly. *Journal of the American College of Cardiology*, **32**, 993–9.

Peterson, E. D., Coombs, L. P., DeLong, E. R., Haan, C. K. and Ferguson, T. B. (2004). Procedural volume as a marker of quality for CABG surgery. *Journal of the American Medical Association*, **291**, 195–201.

Schneider, E. C. and Epstein, A. M. (1996). Influence of cardiac-surgery performance reports on referral practices and access to care. *New England Journal of Medicine*, **335**, 251–6.

Schneider, E. C. and Epstein, A. M. (1998). Use of public performance reports: a survey of patients undergoing cardiac surgery. *Journal of the American Medical Association*, **279**, 1638–42.

Schneider, E. C. and Lieberman, T. (2001). Publicly disclosed information about the quality of health care: response of the US public. *Quality Health Care*, **10**, 96–103.

Shahian, D. M. (2005). Improving cardiac surgery quality – volume, outcome, process? *Journal of the American Medical Association*, **291**, 246–8.

Shahian, D. M. and Normand, S. L. (2003). The volume-outcome relationship: from Luft to Leapfrog. *Annals of Thoracic Surgery*, **75**, 1048–58.

Shahian, D. M., Normand, S.-L. T., Torchiana, D. F. *et al.* (2001). Cardiac surgery report cards: comprehensive review and statistical critique. *Annals of Thoracic Surgery*, **72**, 2155–68.

Shahian, D. M., Torchiana, D. F. and Normand, S.-L. T. (2005). Implementation of a cardiac surgery report card: Lessons from the Massachusetts experience. *Annals of Thoracic Surgery*, **80**, 1146–50.

Werner, R. M., Asch, D. A. and Polsky, D. (2005). Racial profiling: the unintended consequences of coronary artery bypass graft reports cards. *Circulation*, **111**, 1257–63.

www.aihw.gov.au/mediacentre/2004/mr20040929.cfm Australian Institute of Health and Welfare Media Release. Health spending grows to $72.2 billion. Canberra, 29 September 2004.

www.health.state.ny.us/nysdoh/heart/heart_disease.htm#cardiovascular New York State Cardiac Advisory Committee. Adult cardiac surgery in New York State 2000–2002, October 2004, New York State Department of Health, Albany, NY.

www.health.vic.gov.au/cardiacsurgery/ Australasian Society of Cardiac and Thoracic Surgeons Database Project Steering Committee. Cardiac surgery in Victorian public hospitals – Report to the public 2002. August 2003, Victorian Government Department of Human Services, Melbourne.

www.phc4.org Pennsylvania Health Care Cost Containment Council, Pennsylvania's Guide to Coronary Artery Bypass Graft (CABG) Surgery 2003, Commonwealth of Pennsylvania, Harrisburg, PA.

www.state.nj.us/health Office of Health Care Quality Asessment. Cardiac Surgery in New Jersey 2001 – A Consumer Report. November 2004, New Jersey Department of Health and Senior Services, Trenton, NJ.

www.sts.org Society of Thoracic Surgeons. Spring 2005 Report – Executive Summary. Duke Clinical Research Institute, Duke University Medical Centre, NC.

14

Examining the link between publicly reporting healthcare quality and quality improvement

Rachel M. Werner

Philadelphia Veterans Affairs Medical Center, University of Pennsylvania, USA

David A. Asch

Philadelphia Veterans Affairs Medical Center, University of Pennsylvania, USA

Public reporting of comparative information on healthcare quality of physicians and hospitals through 'report cards' is hailed as a plausible way to improve health care (Arrow, 1963; Akerlof, 1970; Stiglitz *et al.*, 1989). Without this information, patients may choose their physicians based on more measurable characteristics (such as cost) or by word-of-mouth or other informal referral practices not obviously related to their needs.

There are two general types of healthcare report cards: those that measure outcomes and those that measure process. Reports of cardiac surgeons' and hospitals' risk-adjusted mortality rates following coronary artery bypass graft (CABG) surgery are examples of outcomes-based reporting (Pennsylvania Health Care Cost Containment Council, 1992; New York State Department of Health, 1993; California CABG Mortality Reporting Program, 2001; New Jersey Department of Health and Senior Services, 2003). Process-based report cards, often called quality indicators, report on rates of medical interventions, such as screening tests and medication usage, which are assumed to be related to outcomes. The Centers for Medicare and Medicaid Services (CMS) nursing homes report card, reporting on quality of care in nursing homes nationwide (2003), the Agency for Healthcare Research and Quality's congressionally mandated National Healthcare Quality Report, reporting on 150 measures of quality (2003), and the National Committee for Quality Assurance Health Plan Employer Data and Information Set (HEDIS), which includes quality indicators on health plan performance (2004) are examples of report cards that use process measures.

Although much of what is known about public report cards comes from research on CABG report cards, both process and outcomes report cards are published based on the same critical premise – only by making quality

Informed Consent and Clinician Accountability: The Ethics of Report Cards on Surgeon Performance. Steve Clarke and Justin Oakley (eds.). Published by Cambridge University Press. © Cambridge University Press 2007.

information publicly available can one make it influential in improving health-care quality. For this reason, publicly reporting quality and quality improvement are often seen hand-in-hand.

Nevertheless, this reasoning has two shortcomings. Firstly, public reporting is assumed to improve healthcare quality, but this has not been demonstrated. Despite the enthusiastic support for the public release of performance measures (Chassin et al., 1996; Berwick, 2002; Steinberg, 2003) and extensive adoption of quality measurement and reporting (Pennsylvania Health Care Cost Containment Council, 1992; New York State Department of Health, 1993; California CABG Mortality Reporting Program, 2001; Agency for Health Care Research and Quality, 2003; Centers for Medicare and Medicaid, 2003; New Jersey Department of Health and Senior Services, 2003; National Committee for quality assurance, 2004), little research examines the effect of public reporting on the delivery of healthcare (Marshall et al., 2000; Leatherman et al., 2003) and even less examines how report cards may improve care (Longo et al., 1997; Berwick et al., 2003; Leatherman et al., 2003). Secondly, the potential unintended and negative consequences of public reporting are largely unexplored.

Collecting measures of provider performance and using that information to improve practice by providing private feedback to physicians, hospitals, and health plans are by now established mechanisms for improving healthcare quality (Ferguson et al., 2003; Jencks et al., 2003; Jha et al., 2003). In this chapter, our aim is not to challenge those practices, but to critically examine the role of publicly reporting this information on healthcare quality.

How might reporting of healthcare quality improve the quality of healthcare?

Patients and referring physicians might use public report cards to help them select high-quality providers. Rated physicians might respond to report cards by improving the quality of care they deliver. Either of these two processes might explain how reports cards enhance delivered quality, if indeed they do. Less directly, report cards may also provide a mechanism to convey a sense of trust among patients, or to hold health care providers accountable for quality.

Selection of high-quality providers by patients

Although the idea that patients will use public report cards to select the best clinical providers is plausible, this process requires several intermediate steps that are not so assured: (1) report cards must exist; (2) patients must know about the report cards and have access to them; (3) patients must be able to understand the quality rankings and believe them; and (4) patients must act on the report card information.

Public report cards have become a prominent part of the quality improvement landscape over the last quarter-century (Pennsylvania Health Care Cost Containment Council, 1992; New York State Department of Health, 1993; California CABG Mortality Reporting Program, 2001; Agency for Health Care Research and Quality, 2003; Centers for Medicare and Medicaid, 2003; New Jersey Department of Health and Senior Services, 2003; National Committee for Quality Assurance, 2004). While initial reports suggested that the majority of patients did not know that this comparative quality information is publicly available, the number of people who have seen quality information in the past year has slowly increased to from 27% in 2000 to 35% in 2004 (Schneider and Epstein, 1998; Kaiser Family Foundation and Agency for Health Care Research and Quality, 2000, 2004). Among the minority of patients who *are* aware of quality information, many do not understand it, trust it or view it as useful. Patients report misunderstanding the language and terms used in report cards, what an indicator is supposed to reveal about quality of care, and whether high or low rates of an indicator reflect good performance (Jewett and Hibbard, 1996; Kaiser Family Foundation and Agency for Health Care Research and Quality, 2000, 2004). Misunderstanding is more common among patients of lower socioeconomic status (Jewett and Hibbard, 1996).

Patients also report not trusting the information in report cards. Most patients think that friends and relatives are highly credible, and they prefer these sources to published information (Gibbs *et al.*, 1996). Consumers also continue to report that they value information on health choices from friends, family, and personal physicians much more than information from governmental sources (Kaiser Family Foundation and Agency for Health Care Research and Quality, 2004).

A minority of patients actually use quality information when they make healthcare decisions. In 2000, a national survey found that 12% of respondents reported using any information they saw comparing quality among health plans, hospitals, or physicians in the past year (Kaiser Family Foundation and Agency for Health Care Research and Quality, 2000). Four years later, that number increased to 19% (Kaiser Family Foundation and Agency for Health Care Research and Quality, 2004). Another survey of patients in Pennsylvania who had undergone CABG surgery, reported that only 1 to 2 per cent of patients said the CABG report card was a major or moderate influence in their choice of a hospital or surgeon (Schneider and Epstein, 1998). Whether from lack of awareness, lack of trust, misunderstanding or relative inattention, few patients use report cards to select providers. These circumstances may change, but report cards' potential for helping patients select providers has not yet been realized.

Selection of high-quality providers by physicians

Even if patients do not use public report cards for provider selection, other physicians might use them in their choice of referrals, so patients may benefit from report cards through the more informed choices of their referring physicians (Schneider and Epstein, 1996; Hannan *et al.*, 1997).

The majority of physicians report being aware that public report cards exist; however, many do not trust the information. In one survey, 82 per cent of Pennsylvania cardiologists knew of the state's CABG report card, but many of these physicians thought the risk adjustment was inadequate and that the ratings could be manipulated by the surgeons and hospitals who were being rated. Sixty-two per cent responded that the report card had no influence on their referral recommendations, and only 13 per cent responded that the report card had a moderate or substantial influence on their referral recommendations (Schneider and Epstein, 1996). Although limited, the available evidence suggests that public report cards have a minor influence on physician referral patterns.

Selection of high-quality providers by purchasers

Even if the majority of patients and referring physicians do not use report cards for provider selection, purchasers might use public report card information in establishing provider contracts. Hospital administrators say that report cards are useful in negotiating with health plans, however, less than one-quarter of health plans say that quality rankings in report cards were a major factor in their decision to contract with surgeons (Romano *et al.*, 1999; Mukamel *et al.*, 2000). More objective evidence of whether report cards have caused insurers to contract with higher-quality providers is mixed. Mukamel *et al.* found that while purchasers are paying attention to quality report cards, the impact is small (2000, 2002). More recently, Erickson *et al.* found that New York health plans do not use performance data to choose high-performance centres for CABG surgery (2000).

Provider response to report cards

Public report cards' effect on physician selection is diminished at each of the necessary steps required to make report cards work, attenuating the ultimate impact of report cards in directing patients to higher-quality providers. This might be corrected over time, as consumers become more aware of report cards' availability and are more willing and able to use them in physician selection.

While waiting for greater uptake of public report cards by consumers, it is still possible for report cards to provide value if they lead physicians to improve their practices. Were physicians to respond to report cards by improving their quality, the population distribution of quality might improve, and even patients who do not select physicians based on quality would receive higher quality of care.

Public report cards might lead to an improvement in physician quality in three general ways: (1) remediation (report cards cause providers to change their practices to improve quality); (2) restriction (report cards lead to restriction or limitation of physicians' practices so that they no longer provide care for which they rated poorly); and (3) removal (report cards cause low quality physicians to exit the health care market). These three responses to report cards could occur in several ways.

Report cards might remediate lower quality practices by providing benchmarking and feedback to physicians. Educating physicians about practice guidelines can influence the ways physicians practice, especially when such activities are targeted at opinion leaders (Billi *et al.*, 1992; Berner *et al.*, 2003). Informing individual physicians about their quality rankings affects physicians in a similar way to educating physicians about practice guidelines. It may cause these physicians to pay more attention to standards of care and thus improve the care they provide.

Report cards might also give providers the necessary information to start formal quality improvement programmes. There is some evidence that providers respond to public report cards with quality improvement initiatives. For example, the committee overseeing New York's CABG report card advises the State's Department of Health which hospitals and surgeons may need special attention and recommends that some hospitals obtain outside consultants to design quality improvements for their programmes (New York State Department of Health, 1996; Chassin, 2002). The report card has also been credited with removing low-volume cardiac surgeons in New York, after 27 low-volume surgeons ceased performing CABG surgery in the state between 1989 and 1992 (Chassin, 2002).

The positive impact of report cards on quality improvement may be larger when the quality reports are publicly reported rather than privately reported. In a recent study on reporting hospital quality in Wisconsin, hospitals were randomly assigned to receive publicly reported quality information, privately reported quality information or no quality information. The investigators found that the hospitals that had their quality information released publicly engaged in a higher number of quality improvement activities compared to the other two groups of hospitals. This was particularly true for hospitals that had received low-quality scores (Hibbard *et al.*, 2003).

Public report cards might also improve quality by stimulating quality competition, causing healthcare providers to compete on quality in order to maintain or improve their market share. However, given the apparently limited effect of report cards on consumer choice, the indirect effects on provider behaviour might be even more limited. Research on the effect of reporting quality on market share suggests that report cards *may* encourage hospitals and physicians to compete on quality, but studies have been contradictory (Mukamel and Mushlin, 1998; Chassin, 2002; Baker *et al.*, 2003).

Report cards provide accountability and may enhance trust

Even if public report cards have a limited impact on improving healthcare quality, they fill another important need. By publicly reporting on the quality of healthcare, report cards allow the public to hold the healthcare providers accountable for the quality of care they deliver. Recent surveys have revealed that public accountability in quality is important to the public. In one study, 92 per cent of Americans said that reporting of serious medical errors should be required (Kaiser Family Foundation and Agency for Health Care Research and Quality, 2004) and over 60 per cent wanted this information released publicly (Blendon *et al.*, 2002; Kaiser Family Foundation and Agency for Health Care Research and Quality, 2004). Despite the public's strong preference for the public reporting of medical errors, only 6 per cent of the public identified medical errors as a top problem facing health and medicine (Blendon *et al.*, 2002).

Has public reporting of healthcare quality improved the quality of healthcare?

After New York began releasing its CABG report card, CABG risk-adjusted mortality rates in New York dropped from 4.17 per cent to 2.45 per cent, a decrease of 41 per cent (Hannan *et al.*, 1994). There was a larger decline in CABG-associated mortality rates in New York than in other states at the same time (Peterson *et al.*, 1998) and the decline persisted through the 1990s (Hannan *et al.*, 2003). As a result, many hailed the CABG report card as a successful quality improvement initiative.

However, this enthusiasm has been curbed by simultaneous reports of cardiac surgeons turning away the sickest and most severely ill patients in states with CABG report cards in an effort to avoid poor outcomes and lower publicly reported ratings. Omoigui *et al.* noted that the number of patients transferred to the Cleveland Clinic from New York hospitals rose by 31% after the release of CABG report cards in New York, and that these patients who were transferred generally had higher risk profiles than patients transferred to Cleveland Clinic from other states (1996). In Pennsylvania, which also introduced CABG report cards, 63 per cent of cardiac surgeons admit to being reluctant to operate on high-risk patients, and 59 per cent of cardiologists report having increased difficulty in finding a surgeon for high-risk patients with coronary artery disease since the release of report cards (Schneider and Epstein, 1996). New York had a similar experience after the release of report cards, with 67 per cent of cardiac surgeons refusing to treat at least one patient in the preceding year who was perceived to be high risk (Burack et al., 1999).

Moreover, patients undergoing bypass surgery in Pennsylvania and New York were less severely ill than patients in states that did not publicly release the information. This was particularly true for patients of surgeons who were rated as low quality (Dranove et al., 2003). Furthermore, the release of New York's CABG report card was associated with an increase in racial disparities in CABG use, suggesting that surgeons also may have responded to CABG report cards by avoiding patients perceived to be at risk for having a bad outcome, such as blacks and Hispanics (Werner et al., 2005). Although some prior studies have noted improvements in CABG mortality rates after the release of CABG report cards (Hannan et al., 1994; Peterson et al., 1998; Hannan et al., 2003), if quality report cards cause physicians to 'cherry pick' their patients, the quality of care and outcomes of people eligible for CABG may worsen even as mortality rates among those who receive CABG improves.

Other public report cards have also been hailed for improving healthcare quality. The National Committee on Quality Assurance publishes its HEDIS measures of health plan performance annually and, over the past 5 years, has reported that performance on key measures of clinical quality improved from the preceding year (2004). These improvements should be interpreted with caution. Public disclosure of the HEDIS measures is voluntary and in past years less than one-third of health plans chose to disclose their quality scores (Farley et al., 1998). Evidence suggests that health plans that have a low-score are more likely to stop disclosing their quality data in future years (McCormick et al., 2002). Biased dropout rates among poorer performers may falsely inflate the apparent performance of the health plans as a whole.

The nursing home quality reports published by CMS have thus far had mixed results on nursing home quality. The Boston Globe recently reported that fewer nursing home residents experience untreated pain or are placed in restraints since the report card was first published in 2002. However, there has been no significant change in other areas of nursing home quality such as the occurrence of pressure sores among residents, or the ability of residents to walk or feed themselves (Dembner and Dedman, 2004).

There have been some noteworthy quality improvements following perform-ance measurement without public profiling. Both the Department of Veterans Affairs (VA) and Medicare have instituted performance-evaluation pro-grammes that provide feedback to hospitals on the quality of care they deliver, but do not make the performance information publicly available. Notably, both the VA and Medicare report improvements in quality since performance evaluation was initiated (Jencks *et al.*, 2003; Jha *et al.*, 2003; Asch *et al.*, 2004).

Others have noted there may be downsides to using quality indicators to rate performance (Walter *et al.*, 2004). Quality indicators may cause physicians to screen or treat all patients, regardless of whether they are appropriate for the intervention. Quality indicators are based on practice guidelines derived from evidence linking treatment to outcomes. Practice guidelines are meant to offer clinicians guidance to help improve patient care. However, translating practice guidelines into publicly reported quality measures shifts their emphasis away from providing guidance and toward achieving target rates. Because these quality measures assume that higher levels of compliance with practice guidelines always translates into higher quality care, report cards may lead to unnecessary interventions, discounting clinician judgment and patient preferences.

A recent study by Walter *et al.* examined the use of performance evaluation using quality indicators at the VA. Examining rates for colorectal cancer (CRC) screening at a centre noted for failing to meet the target rate for CRC screening, the researchers found that among patients who did not undergo CRC screening 47 per cent had declined screening, 12 per cent failed to complete or show up for screening, and, in 31 per cent of patients, testing was not medically indicated or the patient had high levels of co-morbid illnesses (Walter *et al.*, 2004). The hospital in question may have failed to meet the VA's target rate of CRC screening. However, it seems that 90 per cent of unscreened patients were appropriately unscreened. If quality indicators push healthcare providers to meet target rates, they may fail to reward physicians for appropriately incorporating their clinical judgement and patient preferences into their decision-making. Thus, quality indicators may result in inappropriately high rates of screening tests, medications usage or other items being measured.

Implications

Public reporting of healthcare quality may represent an important step in improving openness and accountability among the health professions. Public reporting has also been hailed as a critical step in improving healthcare quality. Principle supports the first of these goals, but the evidence supporting success with the second goal is mixed. Moreover, some evidence suggests that public reporting reduces overall healthcare quality.

Is it worth revisiting whether public reporting should continue? The number of public report cards has grown tremendously over the past several decades. Enthusiasm for the practice stems from the idea that publicly reporting quality information allows consumers to make informed choices. Yet, there is limited evidence that public report cards improve quality through this mechanism and there is some evidence that they paradoxically reduce quality. Instead of publicly reporting quality, report cards might be more constructively used to give private feedback to the providers who are being rated, as is done in Medicare and the VA. Such an approach might limit physicians' negative response to report cards, while retaining incentives to improve. Just as distancing system participants from blame may encourage an open environment that reduces medical errors and enhances patient safety, the most constructive audience for report cards may be physicians alone.

However, keeping quality information private may appear conspiratorial. It may reduce patient trust, damage the profession's credibility, and hinder future efforts at quality improvement. The Institute of Medicine has suggested that what is really needed to improve quality is a culture that encourages sharing rather than hiding errors (2003). Leaders in healthcare have suggested that the principal obstacle to broader action on quality improvement is a lack of consensus on publicly reporting quality measures (Altman *et al.*, 2004), and the public is unambiguously positive about the accountability provided by public reporting (Blendon *et al.*, 2002). Because public reporting provides this important mechanism for accountability, its perceived value is hard to challenge. If this is the case, what can be done to help public reporting achieve its goals in reality?

Firstly, if publicly reporting quality measures is to facilitate the selection of high-quality physicians, those measures must be promoted widely, understandably and credibly. An emerging literature suggests that the design format and type of information presented in report cards affects its interpretation and use (McGee *et al.*, 1999; Spranca *et al.*, 2000). Other work has extensively explored ways to link reported quality information to specific decisions made by consumers to increase the likelihood that consumers will use the information in report cards to select high-quality physicians (Hibbard *et al.*, 2001; Hibbard *et al.*, 2002; Hibbard, 2003; Hibbard *et al.*, 2004). As quality information is presented in more comprehensible and useful ways, its uptake and use may increase.

Secondly, publicly reported quality measures should decrease physicians' incentive to select patients to improve their rankings. With outcomes-based report cards, decreasing the incentive to avoid patients who are at high-risk for having adverse outcomes is best achieved through detailed and credible risk adjustment. New York State's CABG report card set the standard over a decade ago for adjusting rankings based on detailed clinical information (New York State Department of Health, 1996). However, detailed risk adjustment does little to mitigate physicians' incentive to migrate toward healthy patients for whom treatment may provide fewer benefits. One way to decrease this unintended consequence of public reporting is to include measures of the appropriateness of care. In the case of CABG report cards, appropriateness criteria might diminish surgeons' incentive to substitute potentially less appropriate low-risk patients for potentially more appropriate high-risk patients.

Taking case-mix into account may be relevant not only for outcomes-based measures, but also for process-based measures. As Walter *et al.* (2004) found in the case of CRC screening, the reason some patients do not undergo screening is because of a high level of comorbid illnesses. When adjusting screening rates for severity, it is critical to make sure that patients receiving primary prevention are those who will benefit the most from it. Other factors, such as patients' socioeconomic status and race, may also confound the measurement of quality through indicators. Quality indicators such as satisfaction with care are correlated with race and socioeconomic status (Harpole *et al.*, 1996). Performance measures that fail to account for these factors may penalize physicians who care for minority patients or patients of low socioeconomic status (Fiscella and Franks, 1999). Race and socioeconomic status may also affect a physician's perception of whether a patient will follow recommendations for screening or treatment (van Ryn and Burke, 2000). If the race, socioeconomic status, and illness severity of patients are not accounted for, physicians may shy away from treating some groups of patients out of fear of being penalized in their report card rankings.

Finally, if public report cards are to improve the quality of care, participation must be mandatory and quality measurement and reporting must be universally adopted. Otherwise, providers who receive low-quality scores face incentives to avoid reporting and the sickest patients will be shifted from rated to unrated providers.

Public reporting of healthcare quality information is well intentioned. But we should not allow our enthusiasm for public reporting to let us lose sight of our ultimate goal – which is to improve the care received by patients and populations. That goal seems within reach, but we will need to improve our processes if we are to get there.[1]

Note

1. This is a slightly revised version of an article, 'The unintended consequences of publicly reporting quality information', originally published in the *Journal of the American Medical Association*, **293**, (10)(2005), pp. 1239–44. Copyright © 2005, American Medical Association. All rights reserved.

References

Agency for Health Care Research and Quality (2003). National health care quality report. Accessed 08/26/2003. Available at: http://www.ahrq.org/qual/nhqr02/nhqrprelim.htm.

Akerlof, G. (1970). The market for lemons. *Quarterly Journal of Economics*, **84**, 488–94.

Altman, D. E., Clancy, C. and Blendon, R. J. (2004). Improving patient safety – five years after the IOM report. *New England Journal of Medicine*, **351**, 2041–3.

Arrow, K. J. (1963). Uncertainty and the welfare economics of medical care. *American Economic Review*, **53**, 941–73.

Asch, S. M., McGlynn, E. A., Hogan, M. M. *et al.* (2004). Comparison of quality of care for patients in the Veterans Health Administration and patients in a national sample. *Annals of Internal Medicine*, **141**, 938–45.

Baker, D. W., Einstadter, D., Thomas, C., Husak, S., Gordon, N. H. and Cebul, R. D. (2003). The effect of publicly reporting hospital performance on market share and risk-adjusted mortality at high-mortality hospitals. *Medical Care*, **41**, 729–40.

Berner, E. S., Baker, C. S., Funkhouser, E. *et al.* (2003). Do local opinion leaders augment hospital quality improvement efforts? A randomized trial to promote adherence to unstable angina guidelines. *Medical Care*, **41**, 420–31.

Berwick, D. M. (2002). Public performance reports and the will for change. *Journal of the American Medical Association*, **288**, 1523–4.

Berwick, D. M., James, B. and Coye, M. J. (2003). Connections between quality measurement and improvement. *Medical Care*, **41**, I-30–8.

Billi, J. E., Duran-Arenas, L., Wise, C. G., Bernard, A. M., McQuillan, M. and Stross, J. K. (1992). The effects of a low-cost intervention program on hospital costs. *Journal of General Internal Medicine*, **7**, 411–17.

Blendon, R. J., DesRoches, C. M., Brodie, M. *et al.* (2002). Views of practicing physicians and the public on medical errors. *New England Journal of Medicine*, **347**, 1933–40.

Burack, J. H., Impellizzeri, P., Homel, P. and Cunningham, J. N. (1999). Public reporting of surgical mortality: a survey of New York State cardiothoracic surgeons. *Annals of Thoracic Surgery*, **68**, 1195–200.

California CABG Mortality Reporting Program (2001). The California report on coronary artery bypass graft surgery: 1997–1998 hospital data. Summary report. Accessed 08/26/2003. Available at: http://www.oshpd.cahwnet.gov/HQAD/HIRC/Outcomes/CABG/Archives/ccmrp_summary.pdf.

Centers for Medicare and Medicaid (2003). Nursing home compare. Accessed 08/26/2003. Available at: http://www.medicare.gov/Nhcompare/Home.asp.

Chassin, M. R. (2002). Achieving and sustaining improved quality: lessons from New York State and cardiac surgery. *Health Affairs*, **21**, 40–51.

Chassin, M. R., Hannan, E. L. and DeBuono, B. A. (1996). Benefits and hazards of reporting medical outcomes publicly. *New England Journal of Medicine*, **334**, 394–8.

Dembner, A. and Dedman, B. (2004). Nursing homes show uneven gains: national effort at grading has mixed results. *Boston Globe*, December 13, A1.

Dranove, D., Kessler, D., McClellan, M. and Satterthwaite, M. (2003). Is more information better? The effects of 'report cards' on health care providers. *Journal of Political Economy*, **111**, 555–88.

Erickson, L. C., Torchiana, D. F., Schneider, E. C., Newburger, J. W. and Hannan, E. L. (2000). The relationship between managed care insurance and use of lower-mortality hospitals for CABG surgery. *Journal of the American Medical Association*, **283**, 1976–82.

Farley, D. O., McGlynn, E. A. and Klein, D. (1998). *Assessing Quality in Managed Care: Health Plans Reporting of HEDIS Performance Measures*. New York: The Commonwealth Fund.

Ferguson, T. B., Peterson, E. D., Coombs, L. P. *et al.* (2003). Use of continuous quality improvement to increase use of process measures in patients undergoing coronary artery bypass graft surgery: a randomized controlled trial. *Journal of the American Medical Association*, **290**, 49–56.

Fiscella, K. and Franks, P. (1999). Influence of patient education on profiles of physician practices. *Annals of Internal Medicine*, **131**, 745–51.

Gibbs, D. A., Sangl, J. A. and Burrus, B. (1996). Consumer perspectives on information needs for health plan choice. *Health Care Financing Review*, **18**, 55–74.

Hannan, E. L., Kilburn Jr, H., Racz, M., Shields, E. and Chassin, M. R. (1994). Improving the outcomes of coronary bypass surgery in New York State. *Journal of the American Medical Association*, **271**, 761–6.

Hannan, E. L., Stone, C. C., Biddle, T. L. and DeBuono, B. A. (1997). Public release of cardiac surgery outcomes data in New York: what do New York State cardiologists think of it? *American Heart Journal*, **134**, 55–61.

Hannan, E. L., Vaughn Sarrazin, M. S., Doran, D. R. and Rosenthal, G. E. (2003). Provider profiling and quality improvement efforts in coronary artery bypass graft surgery: The effect on short-term mortality among Medicare beneficiaries. *Medical Care*, **41**, 1164–72.

Harpole, L. H., Orav, E. J., Hickey, M., Posther, K. E. and Brennan, T. A. (1996). Patient satisfaction in the ambulatory setting. Influence of data collection methods and sociodemographic factors. *Journal of General Internal Medicine*, **11**, 431–4.

Hibbard, J. H. (2003). Engaging health care consumers to improve the quality of care. *Medical Care*, **41**, 161–70.

Hibbard, J. H., Slovic, P., Peters, E., Finucane, M. L. and Tusler, M. (2001). Is the informed-choice policy approach appropriate for Medicare beneficiaries? *Health Affairs*, **20**, 199–203.

Hibbard, J. H., Slovic, P., Peters, E. and Finucane, M. L. (2002). Strategies for reporting health plan performance information to consumers: evidence from controlled studies. *Health Services Research*, **37**, 291–313.

Hibbard, J. H., Stockard, J. and Tusler, M. (2003). Does publicizing hospital performance stimulate quality improvement efforts? *Health Affairs*, **22**, 84–94.

Hibbard, J. H., Stockard, J., Mahoney, E. R. and Tusler, M. (2004). Development of the Patient Activation Measure (PAM): conceptualizing and measuring activation in patients and consumers. *Health Services Research*, **39**, 1005–26.

Institute of Medicine (2003). *Patient Safety: Achieving a New Standard of Care*. Washington, DC, National Academy Press.

Jencks, S. F., Huff, E. D. and Cuerdon, T. (2003). Change in the quality of care delivered to Medicare beneficiaries, 1998–1999 to 2000–2001. *Journal of the American Medical Association*, **289**, 305–12.

Jewett, J. J. and Hibbard, J. H. (1996). Comprehension of quality care indicators: differences among privately insured, publicly insured, and uninsured. *Health Care Financing Review*, **18**, 75–94.

Jha, A. K., Perlin, J. B., Kizer, K. W. and Dudley, R. A. (2003). Effect of the transformation of the veterans affairs health care system on the quality of care. *New England Journal of Medicine*, **348**, 2218–27.

Kaiser Family Foundation and Agency for Health Care Research and Quality (2000). *Americans as Health Care Consumers: An Update on the Role of Quality Information.* Washington, DC, Kaiser Family Foundation.

Kaiser Family Foundation and Agency for Health Care Research and Quality (2004). *National Survey on Consumers' Experiences with Patient Safety and Quality Information.* Washington, DC: Kaiser Family Foundation.

Leatherman, S. T., Hibbard, J. H. and McGlynn, E. A. (2003). A research agenda to advance quality measurement and improvement. *Medical Care*, **41**, I-80–6.

Longo, D. R., Land, G., Schramm, W., Fraas, J., Hoskins, B. and Howell, V. (1997). Consumer reports in health care: do they make a difference in patient care? *Journal of the American Medical Association*, **278**, 1579–84.

Marshall, M. N., Shekelle, P. G., Leatherman, S. and Brook, R. H. (2000). The public release of performance data: what do we expect to gain? A review of the evidence. *Journal of the American Medical Association*, **283**, 1866–74.

McCormick, D., Himmelstein, D. U., Woolhandler, S., Wolfe, S. M. and Bor, D. H. (2002). Relationship between low quality-of-care scores and HMOs' subsequent public disclosure of quality-of-care scores. *Journal of the American Medical Association*, **288**, 1484–90.

McGee, J., Kanouse, D. E., Sofaer, S., Hargraves, J. L., Hoy, E. and Kleimann, S. (1999). Making survey results easy to report to consumers: how reporting needs guided survey design in CAHPS. Consumer Assessment of Health Plans Study. *Medical Care*, **37**, MS32–40.

Mukamel, D. B. and Mushlin, A. I. (1998). Quality of care information makes a difference: an analysis of market share and price changes after publication of the New York State cardiac surgery mortality reports. *Medical Care*, **36**, 945–54.

Mukamel, D. B., Mushlin, A. I., Weimer, D., Zwanziger, J., Parker, T. and Indridason, I. (2000). Do quality report cards play a role in HMOs' contracting practices? Evidence from New York State. *Health Services Research*, **35**, 319–32.

Mukamel, D. B., Weimer, D. L., Zwanziger, J. and Mushlin, A. I. (2002). Quality of cardiac surgeons and managed care contracting practices. *Health Services Research*, **37**, 1129–44.

National Committee for Quality Assurance (2004). The state of health care quality: 2004. National Committee for Quality Assurance. Accessed 12/28/2004. Available at: http://www.ncqa.org/communications/SOMC/SOHC2004.pdf.

New Jersey Department of Health and Senior Services (2003). Cardiac surgery in New Jersey: consumer report. Accessed 08/26/2003. Available at: http://www.state.nj.us/health/hcsa/cabgs01/cabg_consumer01.pdf.

New York State Department of Health (1993). Coronary artery bypass surgery in New York State 1990–1992. New York State Department of Health.

New York State Department of Health (1996). Coronary artery bypass surgery in New York State 1992–1994. Accessed 08/26/2003. Available at: http://www.health.state.ny.us/nysdoh/heart/1992-94cabg.pdf.

Omoigui, N. A., Miller, D. P., Brown, K. J. *et al.* (1996). Outmigration for coronary bypass surgery in an era of public dissemination of clinical outcomes. *Circulation*, **93**, 27–33.

Pennsylvania Health Care Cost Containment Council (1992). *A consumer guide to coronary artery bypass graft surgery.* Harrisburg, PA, Pennsylvania Health Care Cost Containment Council.

Peterson, E. D., DeLong, E. R., Jollis, J. G., Muhlbaier, L. H. and Mark, D. B. (1998). The effects of New York's bypass surgery provider profiling on access to care and patient outcomes in the elderly. *Journal of the American College of Cardiology*, **32**, 993–9.

Romano, P. S., Rainwater, J. A. and Antonius, D. (1999). Grading the graders: how hospitals in California and New York perceive and interpret their report cards. *Medical Care*, **37**, 295–305.

Schneider, E. C. and Epstein, A. M. (1996). Influence of cardiac-surgery performance reports on referral practices and access to care: a survey of cardiovascular specialists. *New England Journal of Medicine*, **335**, 251–6.

Schneider, E. C. and Epstein, A. M. (1998). Use of public performance reports: a survey of patients undergoing cardiac surgery. *Journal of the American Medical Association*, **279**, 1638–42.

Spranca, M., Kanouse, D. E., Elliott, M., Short, P. F., Farley, D. O. and Hays, R. D. (2000). Do consumer reports of health plan quality affect health plan selection? *Health Services Research*, **35**, 933–47.

Steinberg, E. P. (2003). Improving the quality of care – can we practice what we preach? *New England Journal of Medicine*, **348**, 2681–3.

Stiglitz, J. E., Schmalensee, R. and Willig, R. D. (1989). Imperfect information in the product market. In *Handbook of Industrial Organization*, vol. 1. New York: Elsevier Science Publishers B.V., pp. 769–847.

Van Ryn, M. and Burke, J. (2000). The effect of patient race and socio-economic status on physicians' perceptions of patients. *Social Science and Medicine*, **50**, 813–28.

Walter, L. C., Davidowitz, N. P., Heineken, P. A. and Covinsky, K. E. (2004). Pitfalls of converting practice guidelines into quality measures: lessons learned from a VA performance measure. *Journal of the American Medical Association*, **291**, 2466–70.

Werner, R. M., Asch, D. A. and Polsky, D. (2005). Racial profiling: the unintended consequences of coronary artery bypass graft report cards. *Circulation*, **111**, 1257–60.

15

Hospital and clinician performance data: what it can and cannot tell us

Paul Aylin

Imperial College London, UK

Introduction

The monitoring of healthcare performance has a surprisingly long history, going back to the work of Florence Nightingale, who produced analyses of mortality outcome measures and campaigned for uniform hospital and surgical statistics (Spiegelhalter, 1999). More recently, there has been a renewed focus on monitoring clinical standards in many countries' health services, particularly in the UK in light of high-profile cases like Bristol (The Bristol Royal Infirmary Inquiry, 2001) and Shipman (Baker, 2001; Aylin *et al.*, 2003a) and in the US with the Agency for Healthcare Research and Quality's Patient Safety Initiative (Agency for Healthcare Research and Quality, 2003) and the Institute for Healthcare Improvement's 100 000 Lives Campaign (Institute for Healthcare Improvement).

Monitoring of performance data is not straightforward, with many pitfalls and it is important to get it right. A recent report from the Royal Statistical Society noted that: 'Performance monitoring done well is broadly productive for those concerned. Done badly, it can be very costly and not merely ineffective but harmful and indeed destructive' (The Royal Statistical Society Working Party on Performance Monitoring of Public Services, 2003).

This chapter looks at:
- Sources of data, both administrative and clinical, and their quality
- Statistical issues around performance monitoring
- Methods and presentation of data
- How to deal with analyses suggesting poor performance

Sources of data

The Bristol Inquiry report concluded that 'Bristol was awash with data' (The Bristol Royal Infirmary Inquiry, 2001). Many sources of data were identified including returns submitted to the UK Cardiac Surgical register, Hospital

Informed Consent and Clinician Accountability: The Ethics of Report Cards on Surgeon Performance. Steve Clarke and Justin Oakley (eds.). Published by Cambridge University Press. © Cambridge University Press 2007.

Episode Statistics (HES), the surgeons' own logs, the local patient administration system, the perfusionists' logs, and a local Congenital Heart Register
(Spiegelhalter *et al.*, 2000). However, little of this information was available to
parents or the rest of the public and certainly did not help in the identification,
prior to the Inquiry, of the problems brewing there. There are a multitude of
clinical databases in existence within the UK. An exercise to look at the utility
of electronic health data to assess new health technologies identified around
270 databases at the level of UK, England and Wales or England (Raftery,
Roderick and Stevens, 2005). A recent survey of multicentre clinical databases
documented at least 105 clinical databases, in all areas of UK healthcare. Two-
thirds of these databases have approval from at least one clinical or professional
body and almost all have doctors on the management teams. It found that their
distribution was uneven and their scope and the quality of the data varied
(Black, Barker and Payne, 2004).

Hospital activity data have been collected since 1949 from all NHS hospitals
in the UK (Rowe, 1972). Initially these were based on paper returns, which did
not record age, sex or diagnosis. Hospital Episode Statistics (HES), introduced
in 1987, is the most recent system in England and originated from the work of
Edith Körner, an economist. The HES system attempts to measure all hospital
inpatient activity for England. The basic unit of the database is the Finished
Consultant Episode (FCE), covering the period during which a patient is under
the care of one consultant. Every NHS hospital in England has to submit data
items of HES electronically for each FCE in every patient's stay in that hospital.
The data items are entered onto the hospital's Patient Administration Systems
from the medical notes by trained clinical coders. The items include date of
birth, sex, postcode of residence and clinical data such as primary and secondary
diagnoses and dates and details of any operations performed during the
patient's stay. Diagnoses are coded using the International Classification of
Diseases (ICD 10), often with the help of computer software. Clinical coding
is not subject to any external audit, and there is potential for inter-coder
variation (Walshe, Harrison and Renshaw, 1993; Dixon *et al.*, 1998). Since
1991, HES has been used for contracting in an internal market, where providers
of care were split from purchasers or commissioners of care. HES now contains
some 14 million records per financial year.

Data quality

There are three principal quality issues to consider around the quality of health
data: coverage, completeness and accuracy. Coverage refers to the proportion
of the total activity actually recorded by a system; completeness refers to the
proportion of records that have an entry in any specified field; accuracy refers
to how far completed records reflect what actually happened.

Hospital activity data are regarded as unreliable by clinicians, and attempts to use HES data for monitoring clinical performance have been met with claims by clinicians that they are not suitable for monitoring performance. Although quality has improved greatly in recent years, HES data need careful interpretation (Hansell *et al.*, 2001). A recent comparison of counts of episodes generated through HES and paper returns provided by each hospital trust suggests that the administrative database is capturing 98.9 per cent of all activity (Data Quality Index, 2003–4). One study suggested that paper returns are 'considered to yield the more reliable total number of episodes within a district' but rarely found substantial deviation from the HES totals (Sheldon *et al.*, 1994).

The quality of clinical databases varies. An analysis of the UK Central Cardiac Audit Database (CCAD) for 2000–1 in paediatric cardiac surgery suggested that hospital episode statistics data under-reported the total number of procedures by 10 per cent (Gibbs, 2004). The same analysis revealed, however, that 22 per cent of deaths were missed through voluntary reporting. Reporting of outcomes such as out of hospital death within administrative datasets is also lacking, limiting analysis of HES data to in-hospital deaths only. Within the CCAD, these deaths were later recovered through a central tracking process linking death certificates to clinical records. A similar exercise has now been carried out for HES allowing analysis of out of hospital mortality. A comparison of HES and the National Adult Cardiac Surgical Database concluded that statistical correlation was good, although counts of operations were consistently lower within HES. This was likely to be due to a stricter definition of what constitutes an isolated CABG (The Society of Cardiothoracic Surgeons of Great Britain and Ireland, 2004). Conversely, comparing numbers of procedures carried out to repair abdominal aortic aneurysms within HES and the National Vascular Database for 2003/4 (4102 vs. 1083) suggests substantial under-reporting within this particular clinical database (Department of Health, 2003/04; Fourth National Vascular Database Report, 2004).

Completeness of records is easier to determine, and within HES, 99.6 per cent of records have a valid date of birth, a valid postcode and sex. 97.5 per cent of records have a valid primary diagnosis (HES Data Quality Indicators, 2003–4). Within adult cardiac surgery, risk adjusted mortality by unit or surgeon was not published by the Society of Cardiothoracic Surgeons in their 2003 annual report because the information required for adequate risk adjustment was missing in 30 per cent of records (The Society of Cardiothoracic Surgeons of Great Britain and Ireland, 2004).

McKee summed up the poor reputation of routine data: 'Many clinicians have concluded that, despite a massive investment in technology, routinely collected data still fail ... and that separate systems are still required'. Many clinical departments have acquired their own Clinical Information Systems and medical staff use these systems to produce discharge letters, to manage waiting lists and for other clinical office functions (McKee, Dixon and Chenet, 1994). Such duplication of effort (by clinicians on Clinical Information Systems and medical records staff on Patient Administration Systems) is widespread (Walshe, Harrison and Renshaw, 1993). The Bristol Inquiry report criticized the current 'dual' system of collecting data in the health service in separate administrative and multiple clinical systems as 'wasteful and anachronistic' (The Bristol Royal Infirmary Inquiry, 2001).

In terms of data quality there seem to be strengths and weaknesses to both types of data. Within the UK, Hospital Episode Statistics appear to be relatively complete, and most patients admitted within the NHS will appear somewhere in the database, but there may be problems with accuracy of coding. Some clinical databases may have the same or better coverage than HES, but others fall very short of recording every case. Because the submission of data is voluntary, information is not necessarily collected from every unit or even every relevant clinician within a unit. Clinical datasets have the potential to collect more useful data for case-mix adjustment, but this may be hampered by incomplete recording. Recent research suggests, however, that in some cases, creative use of administrative data, using variables as proxy for clinical complexity, results in models for case-mix adjustment comparable to that derived from clinical datasets (Ugolini, 2004). Other work has suggested that simplified models of risk prediction might be just as effective in predicting outcome as some complex models currently in use (Jenkins, 2002; Sutton *et al.*, 2002). These simpler models have potential for use for administrative data sets for case-mix adjustment.

Clinical databases are expensive to maintain compared to routine administrative systems. The cost for HES has been put at around US$1.75 per record, whereas clinical databases range from around US$20 (UK Cardiac Surgical Register) to US$100 (Scottish Hip Fracture Audit) per record (Raftery, Roderick and Stevens, 2005).

High-quality administrative data is essential for a healthcare system based on the reimbursement for providers of healthcare for each individual case treated. This system of reimbursement is used in many countries such as Australia, Norway and the United States and there is evidence of better recording of secondary diagnoses and complications where there is some financial incentive to record diagnoses more thoroughly (McKee, 1993; Carter, Newhouse and Relles, 1990). Within the NHS, 'Payment by results' may help to drive up coverage and coding accuracy (Dixon, 2004). Routine administrative data are increasingly being used for performance monitoring (The Healthcare Commission; Dr Foster Intelligence) as they are relatively comprehensive and increasing in quality.

Administrative data and clinical databases each have their strengths, with the former often achieving better coverage, and the latter containing more detailed clinical information required for audit and some clinical governance issues. It has been suggested that, ideally, clinical and administrative datasets should function as one. With the increasing emphasis on performance monitoring and systems like 'Payment by results', a strong case can be made for all clinicians to be prepared to take a role in institutional data collection (Keogh, 2005). Incorporating more detailed clinical data within an administrative information system and involving clinicians in the recording of data would appear to be a sensible way forward. I suspect, however, that clinicians might be resistant to this idea, having already invested heavily in their own systems, being mistrustful of administrative data and perhaps unwilling to give up control of potentially sensitive information on performance.

Statistical issues

It is important to be clear about the aim of any analysis of performance data. Is it to investigate suspected poor or good performance (of a unit or individual) within a particular pre-selected clinical specialty, typified by the *post-hoc* analysis commissioned by the Bristol Inquiry (Aylin *et al.*, 1999) or, alternatively, is it to carry out prospective surveillance of health statistics in order to detect areas of concern about clinical performance? This former approach shares problems similar to the investigation of a putative disease cluster, where the reason for the investigation (i.e. the fact that the risk in the area appears high) is generated by the data themselves and so the lack of prior hypothesis may invalidate conventional statistical testing procedures (Elliott *et al.*, 2000). The latter is analogous to prospective disease cluster detection. Both approaches have problems including sensitivity, specificity and multiple significance testing (Elliott *et al.*, 2000; Aylin *et al.*, 2001).

Variation

Performance outcomes will vary either from one time point to the next for a given unit and/or for different units at the same time point. It is important to understand how performance varies within and between units. This then allows assessment of whether performance outcomes observed in one unit fit into the pattern of variation seen for the other units.

The pattern of variation between units or over time takes the form of a *distribution* giving the relative probability of possible 'true' values for the typical outcome measure. It is helpful to think of these 'true' values as being the outcomes that would be observed for each unit if an infinitely large amount of data were available (Christiansen and Morris, 1997). Since the true outcomes are unknown, they must be estimated from the data. The distribution referred to above reflects the statistical uncertainty about these true quantities due to variation in the observed outcomes from which they are estimated. There are a number of explanations for variation in outcomes.

Random fluctuations

These reflect the normal variation predicted due to chance and can be quantified using a variety of statistical techniques.

Known sources of variation

In the context of surgical mortality, this might represent differences in patient-specific pre-operative risk. These factors are often referred to as case-mix. It may also include known seasonal variation. As an example, seasonal temperatures are known to influence mortality, while epidemics or particularly severe winters may act to increase annual mortality rates across some or all units and would manifest as 'spikes' in the underlying temporal process.

Inevitable between-unit variability due to unmeasured factors

These may reflect differences in hospital admissions policies, unmeasured differences in patient case-mix, etc. The outcome measures for most units are likely to be influenced by such factors; although the individual impact of any particular factor may be small, the combined effect of many small unmeasured factors can lead to an excess variability among units (otherwise known as over-dispersion). Depending on the purpose of any monitoring exercise, this can be thought of as 'acceptable' variation, and if not taken account of, can lead to a number of units being unjustifiably identified as having unacceptable performance (Marshall *et al.*, 2004).

Systematic unknown sources of variation

Systematic unknown sources of variation may only be associated with one or a handful of units, but may also lead to unusual outcomes for those units. In general, this is the type of variation that is relevant in terms of monitoring performance, as it may reflect quality of care, or, in the extreme case of Harold Shipman, homicide. In the context of Bristol Royal Infirmary, no factor was singled out as the explanation for the excess mortality seen there, but systematic differences between Bristol and other centres, such as the timing of surgery in infants under one year old, were identified as possible contributory factors which would fall into this category.

Analyses of outcome data typically involve a comparison between observed outcome rates and those expected, under the assumption that the unit's performance is acceptable. Interest lies, therefore, either in monitoring the process and detecting the exact point at which it shifts, if at all, from being acceptable to unacceptable (prospective surveillance) or ascertaining whether the process has been running at an unacceptable level for the time interval of interest (retrospective analysis).

It is usual to adjust the expected outcome rate of each unit for variation due to the first of the above two kinds of variation, chance variation and any known risk factors (including any observed temporal trends common to all units). This can be achieved by setting up a statistical model for the underlying process which assumes an appropriate sampling (probability) distribution for the random variations in observed outcome, and accounts for the effects of known risk factors and common seasonal trends by covariate-adjustment using regression or standardisation. Identifying differences between units due to the latter two types of variation (both the inevitable between-unit variability and more systematic sources of variation) will usually be the focus of any monitoring exercise.

Adjusting for case-mix

Case-mix adjustment requires careful consideration. Florence Nightingale herself recognized the limitations of naïve calculations of surgical mortality rates 'without reference to age, sex or cause of operation' (Spiegelhalter, 1999). However, care must be taken not to adjust for every available factor. For example, it has been argued that when comparing whole surgical systems in units, you should ideally concentrate on case-mix stratification, i.e. factors beyond all influence of the organization (Spiegelhalter *et al.*, 2000). In contrast, if surgical performance alone were being compared, then a full 'operative-risk stratification' exercise may be appropriate, taking into account the precise clinical state and previous history of the patient just prior to their operation. However, this is not appropriate methodology when comparing the whole surgical system, since many features at operation may be influenced by early care, age at referral, timing of operation, etc. For example, it is arguable in some circumstances that you should not adjust for age at operation since the process of care could influence this factor (Spiegelhalter *et al.*, 2002). Within the analysis of HES for the Bristol Inquiry, examination of age in months at operation showed a peak of activity in Bristol in month 11 in open procedures, contrasting with a steady decline in activity with increasing age seen in other centres. The pattern for timing of surgery suggested that operations carried out just before an infant's first birthday were delayed, a factor which was within the control of the unit and which accounted for about 25% of excess deaths there.

Examples of retrospective analyses of performance outcomes where adjustment has been made for patient case-mix include the New York State Department of Health (New York State Department of Health, 2001), who adjust mortality rates for coronary artery bypass surgery for a range of demographic and clinical patient-specific characteristics, and the standard severity index used by Normand *et al.*, which is based on 34 patient characteristics at admission, to adjust 30-day hospital-specific mortality rates for patients with acute myocardial infarction (Normand, Clickman and Gatsonis, 1997). Other scoring systems have been developed with specific surgical outcomes in mind (EuroSCORE – European System for Cardiac Operative Risk Evaluation; Parsonnet, Dean and Bernstein, 1989).

Adjusting for over-dispersion

Over-dispersion is excess variation due to the impact of unmeasured covariates not taken into account in any risk-adjustment method. You can think of it as 'acceptable' excess variation, and if it is not taken into account there will be an inappropriate number of units identified as poor performers (and good performers). It is helpful to think of extreme units as those for which the net effect of many small sources of variation leads to outcomes in the tails of the between-unit distribution of true outcomes. If interest focuses on identifying units with systematic sources of variation, then a method for detecting *divergent* outcomes (i.e. outcomes beyond the tails of the between-unit distribution) is needed. Unfortunately, disentangling these systematic effects from the combined effect of the many small unmeasured factors is a difficult statistical problem. Hierarchical models can be used to estimate the between-unit distribution of true outcomes. If it is accepted that there will be some inevitable between-unit variation, but the sort of systematic variation occurring, for example, at Bristol and with Shipman only arises in unusual circumstances, then systematic differences in units that are beyond what would be reasonable under inevitable between-unit variation alone can be detected. The cross-validation approach adopted by the statistical experts for the Bristol Royal Infirmary Inquiry used this strategy (Aylin *et al.*, 1999; Aylin *et al.*, 2001). The approach involved excluding the data for one unit at a time, and fitting a hierarchical model to the remaining units. The resulting between-unit distribution of true outcome rates represents the predictive distribution for the outcome rate expected at the excluded unit if it belongs to the same distribution as the other units. Since the observed outcome rate in the unit of interest exhibits random chance variation, statistical uncertainty about the 'true' rate in this unit is also represented by a probability distribution. The extent to which the distribution of mortality rates in the unit differs from the predicted distribution reflects the extent to which it can be viewed as divergent.

A further approach to dealing with over-dispersion used in statistical process control charts is to change the definition of what is acceptable performance (often corresponding to standard deviation intervals), inflating limits beyond which an outcome measure for a particular unit is deemed to be unacceptable, to take into account this over-dispersion (Spiegelhalter, 2005).

Multiple statistical testing

Issues of multiple statistical testing must also be taken into account when considering the analysis of performance outcomes. Multiple testing refers to the problem of rising false positive rates with increasing number of statistical tests, each of which will have, independently, a known probability, say 5 per cent, of resulting in a false alarm. The problem is exacerbated in the case of routine performance assessment as, potentially, outcome rates at multiple units, for multiple subgroups and over multiple time periods will be examined simultaneously. Some statistical process control charts (described in more detail later), are designed to address the problem of multiple testing of a single unit over time and may be extended to multiple statistical testing over multiple units and time points (Marshall *et al.*, 2004).

Extreme and divergent units

When considering the goal of identifying 'poorly performing outlier organisations, teams and individuals', it is helpful to distinguish between the identification of outliers that are *extreme* and those that are truly *divergent*.

Extreme units fit into the pattern of variation seen for the other units but are either in the tails of the associated distribution or are unusual relative to a clinically acceptable threshold. Their identification may be interesting if the aim is either to provide early warning of a possible problem, or to feed back information regarding practice at units both substantially above and below average, with a view to facilitating the perpetual improvement of outcome rates across *all* units. In contrast, divergent units cannot be assumed to be drawn from the same distribution as that of their peers and lie *beyond* these tails. It is convenient to think about extreme units as being those with poor performance due to an extreme combination of many sources of variation, while divergent units are those with systematic factors leading to variation. The latter may be indicative of a specific problem that warrants immediate investigation.

Methods

League tables

League tables are a common and popular means of presenting performance data. They are an intuitively appealing and easily understood summary of relative performance. However, it is widely accepted that simple rankings are a very imprecise measure of 'true' performance and that comparing institutional performance can be highly misleading, since one unit will always be ranked worst, and tables generally take no account of chance variations in mortality rates between units (Goldstein and Spiegelhalter, 1996; Howell *et al.*, 2002). It is true that 'even if all surgeons are equally good, about half will have below average results, one will have the worst results, and the worst results will be a long way below average' (Poloniecki, 1998). A point estimate of rank will be deceptively over-precise and this is particularly relevant when observed rates are based on small numbers. There are statistical methods which can be used to minimise the problem of spurious rankings in 'league tables'. These provide confidence intervals around the ranks and can attach a probability that a particular unit ranks highest or that it is in the top n per cent (Marshall and Spiegelhalter, 1998). These methods therefore acknowledge the full uncertainty in the ranks due to the underlying uncertainty in the true outcome estimates.

Statistical process control charts

Statistical process control (SPC) charts were developed within the context of industry and quality control. Walter Shewhart pioneered the development of the control chart. He devised a simple graphical method for identifying what he termed 'special cause variation'. He defined this as variation caused by factors extrinsic to the underlying process. A data point falling outside a given control limit (by convention, equivalent to 3 standard deviations from the mean), means that the process is deemed to be 'out of control' and merits further investigation. Several researchers have proposed their use in monitoring healthcare outcomes (Mohammed *et al.*, 2001).

A variety of other SPC charts have been suggested in the context of monitoring health care but they all share the following common features.

Definition of what is in-control and out-of-control
Based on historical performance, some sort of average based on comparison units or independently determined benchmarks defined through other means.

Test statistic
The test statistic is a function of the difference between the observed outcome and that expected from the benchmark performance.

Pre-defined alarm threshold
Set to minimize false alarms but remain sensitive to true signals.

Measures of chart performance (sensitivity and specificity)
The chart's ability to detect when the underlying process is truly in and out of control must be measured, akin to the percentage of false positives and false negatives calculated for screening tests.

Funnel plots

Funnel plots provide a simple and easily understandable way to plot institutional comparisons. Outcome data are plotted against a measure of its precision, so that the control limits form a funnel around the benchmark (Spiegelhalter, 2005) (see

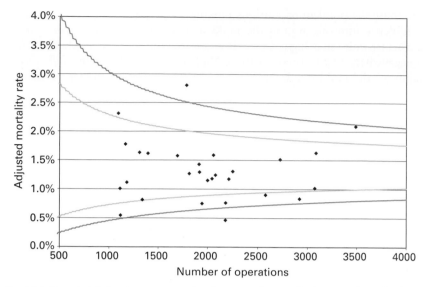

Fig. 15.1 Funnel plot showing coronary artery bypass graft mortality by centre in England (3 years' data up to May 2005), adjusted by age, sex, year, elective/non-elective with 95% and 99.9% control limits.

Fig. 15.1). These have been used to plot anonymized mortality rates by surgeon for paediatric cardiac surgery (Stark *et al.*, 2002) and have been promoted as providing a strong visual indication of divergent performance with the advantage of displaying actual event rates and allowing an informal check of a relationship between outcome and volume of cases (Spiegelhalter, 2002).

Cumulative sum plots

Although Shewhart charts and funnel plots are generally used to compare outcomes at a particular point in time, they are designed as 'one-off' tests to be carried out only after all the data have been collected. They are looking back in time to discover problems that have already occurred and are not ideally suited to monitoring or prospective surveillance, where the purpose is to detect a problem as soon as possible, and to potentially minimize its impact. The distinctive feature of a prospective monitoring system is that data are accumulating over time and the analysis is repeated at every time point. This is known as sequential analysis, and there is a large literature on the subject in the context both of industrial quality control (Page, 1954) and in healthcare.

A number of different cumulative sum (CUSUM) charts have been used in applications of routine health surveillance, the exponentially weighted moving average chart (EWMA) (Hunter, 1986), the log-likelihood CUSUM chart

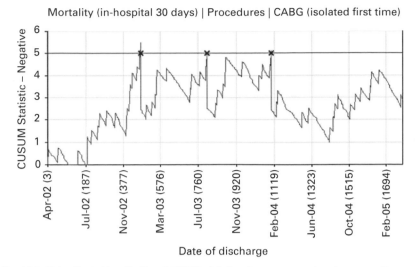

Fig. 15.2 Risk adjusted log-likelihood CUSUM plot showing coronary artery bypass graft mortality in one centre in England (3 years' data up to March 2005), adjusted by age, sex, year, elective/non-elective. (*Note*: Each point on the graph represents a single patient outcome. The chart is reset to half the value of the alarm threshold after signalling.)

(Steiner *et al.*, 2002) and the sequential probability ratio test (SPRT) (Wald, 1947). What distinguishes the various methods is the way in which the test statistic is derived. The log-likelihood CUSUM chart has been put forward as the most appropriate when the aim is to detect small shifts or gradual trends in the underlying process, but it can also be tuned to detect larger shifts by specification of the *out of control* rate to be detected (Marshall *et al.*, 2004) (see Fig. 15.2).

Investigating an alert

Assuming there are good-quality data out there, appropriate measures are taken to control for case-mix and suitable methods are applied in the analysis of performance outcomes, what further investigation is required following the identification of a potentially poorly performing unit?

A useful model has been put forward by Lilford *et al.* suggesting a staged investigation of such an alert starting with data and ending with individuals (Lilford *et al.*, 2004). The first stage is to determine whether the apparent poor performance is due to an artefact of the data. This could either be due to inaccuracies in the data, through problems in coding diagnoses or procedures, or in the grouping and selection of these codes for analysis. Comparisons of admissions and outcomes within the analysis, firstly, to the hospital's electronic records and, secondly, to the patient notes may help to resolve this issue.

The next explanation to consider is case-mix. Although models mentioned above do exist for case-mix adjustment, they will never be perfect. There will inevitably be some residual confounding, which could affect outcomes. To some extent, the effect of many small sources of variation as discussed earlier can be taken into account through adjusting for over-dispersion.

The next consideration is how the structure of the organization might affect outcomes. For example, if a hospital has a palliative care unit attached to it, then it is not unreasonable to expect that that unit might justifiably have a higher mortality rate than a comparison hospital without such a unit. A unit with low mortality might have been discharging or transferring many of its patients to another unit, rather than keeping them on an acute ward.

Only after excluding these other explanations can you then consider whether quality of care might be a possible explanation. Even then, you ought to consider the whole process of care before narrowing down the explanation to an individual.

Conclusions

It is clear that there are a number of matters to consider in generating and interpreting performance data. There are a variety of different data sources out there, with the two main types routinely collected being administrative data and clinical data sets. There are advantages and disadvantages to both, although administrative data collected in the NHS has good coverage and is increasingly used in performance monitoring. There are statistical issues that should be accounted for before more systematic variation due to quality of care can be identified. There is also a choice in methodology and how data should be presented. Finally, there is the question of what to do with an analysis that highlights a particular unit as performing outside what is considered as acceptable performance. What is apparent is that hospital and clinician performance data are only part of the process of improving quality of healthcare. Taken in isolation, they are unlikely to provide an explanation for why a particular unit is an outlier, and should not be used as the sole basis to judge how a unit or clinician is performing. Performance monitoring can act as a focus for further investigation and clinical audit with potential to spot both problems and potential good practice.[1]

Note

1. The section on statistical issues was based to a large extent on a discussion paper (Aylin *et al.*, 2003b) prepared for the Office for Information on Healthcare Performance at the Commission for Health Improvement (now the Healthcare

Commission) with the assistance of Nicky Best, Alex Bottle and Clare Marshall from Imperial College London.

References

100k lives Campaign. Institute for Healthcare Improvement. Available from: URL; http://www.ihi.org/IHI/Programs/Campaign/.

AHRQ's Patient Safety Initiative: Building Foundations, Reducing Risk. 'Interim report to the Senate Committee on appropriations.' AHRQ Publication 04-RG005, December 2003. Agency for Healthcare Research and Quality, Rockville, MD. Available from: URL; http://www.ahrq.gov/qual/pscongrpt/.

Aylin, P., Alves, B., Cook, A. *et al.* Analysis of hospital episode statistics for the Bristol Royal Infirmary inquiry. (1999). Available from: URL: http://www.bristol-inquiry. org.uk/Documents/hes_(Aylin).pdf.

Aylin, P., Alves, B., Best, N. *et al.* (2001). Comparison of UK paediatric cardiac surgical performance by analysis of routinely collected data 1984–96: was Bristol an outlier? *The Lancet*, **358**, 181–7.

Aylin, P., Best, N. G., Bottle, A. and Marshall, C. (2003a). Following Shipman: a pilot system for monitoring mortality rates in primary care. *The Lancet*, **362**, 485–91.

Aylin, P., Best, N., Bottle, A. and Marshall, C. (2003b). Methodological issues in the analysis of performance data. A discussion paper produced for the Office for Information on Healthcare Performance.

Baker, R. (2001). *Harold Shipman's Clinical Practice 1974–1998*. London: Stationery Office.

Black, N., Barker, M. and Payne, M. (2004). Cross sectional survey of multicentre clinical databases in the United Kingdom. *British Medical Journal*, **328**, 1478.

The Bristol Royal Infirmary Inquiry (2001). Learning from Bristol: the report of the public inquiry into children's heart surgery at the Bristol Royal Infirmary 1984–1995. Available from: URL; http://www.bristol-inquiry.org.uk/.

Carter, G. M., Newhouse, J. P. and Relles, D. A. (1990). How much change in the case mix index is DRG creep? *Journal of Health Economics*, **9**, 411–28.

Christiansen, C. and Morris, C. (1997). Improving the statistical approach to health care provider profiling. *Annals of Internal Medicine*, **127**, 764–8.

Commission for Health Improvement (2001). Report on the investigation into heart and lung transplantation at St George's Healthcare NHS Trust. http://www.chi.gov. uk/eng/organisations/london/st_georges/2001/st_georges.pdf.

Department of Health (England) (2003/4). Hospital Episode Statistics (2003/4). Available at: http://www.hesonline.nhs.uk/Ease/servlet/AttachmentRetriever?site_id= 1802&file_name=:\efmfiles\1802\A Free Data Jane\Tables-21\Tb 21 03-04.xls&short_ name=Tb 21 03-04.xls&u_id=2460.

Dixon, J. (2004). Payment by results – new financial flows in the NHS. *British Medical Journal*, **328**, 969–70.

Dixon, J., Sanderson, C., Elliot, P., Walls, P., Jones, J. and Petticrew, M. (1998). Assessment of the reproducibility of clinical coding in routinely collected hospital activity data: a study of two hospitals. *Journal of Public Health Medicine*, **20**, 63–9.

Dr Foster Intelligence. Available from URL: http://www.drfoster.co.uk/.

Elliott, P. and Wakefield, J. C. (2000). Bias and confounding in spatial epidemiology. In *Spatial Epidemiology – Methods and Applications*, ed. P. Elliott, J. C. Wakefield, N. G. Best and D. J. Briggs. Oxford: Oxford University Press, pp. 68–84.

European System for cardiac operative risk evaluation. Available from: URL; http://www.euroscore.org/.

Fourth National Vascular Database Report. Vascular Surgical Society of Great Britain and Ireland. (2004). Available: http://www.vascularsociety.org.uk/Docs/nvdr2004.pdf.

Gibbs, J. L., Monro, J. L., Cunningham, D. and Rickards, A. (2004). Survival after surgery or therapeutic catheterisation for congenital heart disease in children in the United Kingdom: analysis of the central cardiac audit database for 2000–1. *British Medical Journal*, **328**, 611–15.

Goldstein, H. and Spiegelhalter, D. J. (1996). League tables and their limitations: statistical issues in comparisons of institutional performance. *Journal of the Royal Statistical Society, Series A*, **159**, 385–443.

Hansell, A., Bottle, A., Shurlock, L. and Aylin, P. (2001). Accessing and using hospital activity data. *Journal of Public Health Medicine*, **21**, 51–6.

The Healthcare Commission (2005). 2005 Performance Ratings. Available from URL: http://www.healthcarecommission.org.uk/.

HES Data Quality Indicator (DQI) reports for 2003–04. Available from: URL; http://www.hesonline.nhs.uk/Ease/servlet/DynamicPageBuild?siteID=1802&categoryID=405&catName=DQI%20Reports%20for%202003-04.

Howell, J., Shiu, M. F., Bridgewater, B. *et al.* (2002). Performance league tables – letters. *British Medical Journal*, **324**, 542.

Hunter, S. J. (1986). The exponentially weighted moving average. *Journal of Quality Technology*, **18**, 203–10.

Jenkins, J., Gauvrau, K., Newburger, J., Spray, T., Moller, J. and Lezzoni, L. (2002). Consensus-based method for risk adjustment for surgery for congenital heart disease. *Journal of Thoracic and Cardiovascular Surgery*, **123**, 110–18.

Keogh, B. (2005). Surgery for congenital heart conditions in Oxford. *British Medical Journal*, **330**, 319–20.

Lilford, R., Mohammed, M. A., Spiegelhalter, D. and Thomson, R. (2004). Use and misuse of process and outcome data in managing performance of acute medical care: avoiding institutional stigma. *The Lancet*, **363**, 1147–54.

Lovegrove, J., Valencia, O., Treasure, T., Sherlaw-Johnson, C. and Gallivan, S. (1997). Monitoring the results of cardiac surgery by variable life-adjusted display. *The Lancet*, **350**, 1128–30.

Marshall, E. C. and Spiegelhalter, D. J. (1998). League tables of *in vitro* fertilisation clinics: how confident can we be about the rankings? *British Medical Journal*, **316**, 1701–4.

Marshall, E. C., Best, N. G., Bottle, A. and Aylin, P. (2004). Statistical issues in the prospective monitoring of health outcomes at multiple units. *Journal of the Royal Statistical Society*, Series A, **167**(3), 541–59.

McKee, M. (1993). Routine data: a resource for clinical audit? *Quality Health Care*, **2**, 104–11.

McKee, M., Dixon, J. and Chenet, L. (1994). Making routine data adequate to support clinical audit. *British Medical Journal*, **309**, 1246–7.

Mohammed, M., Cheng, K., Riyse, A. and Marshall, T. (2001). Bristol, Shipman, and clinical governance: Shewhart's forgotten lessons. *The Lancet*, **357**, 463–7.

New York State Department of Health (2001). Coronary Artery Bypass Graft Surgery in New York State 1996–1998, New York State Department of Health. Available from: URL: http://www.health.state.ny.us/nysdoh/consumer/heart/1996-98cabg.pdf.

Normand, S-L., Clickman, M. E. and Gatsonis, C. A. (1997). Statistical methods for profiling providers of medical care: issues and applications. *Journal of the American Statistical Association*, **92**, 803–14.

Page, E. S. (1954). Continuous inspection schemes. *Biometrika*, **41**, 100–15.

Parsonnet, V., Dean, D. and Bernstein, A. D. (1989). A method of uniform stratification of risk for evaluating the results of surgery in acquired heart disease. *Circulation*, **79**, I3–I12.

Poloniecki, J. (1998). Half of all doctors are below average. *British Medical Journal*, **316**, 1734–6.

Poloniecki, J., Valencia, O. and Littlejohns, P. (1998). Cumulative risk adjusted mortality chart for detecting changes in death rate: observational study of heart surgery. *British Medical Journal*, **316**, 1697–700.

Raftery, J., Roderick, P. and Stevens, A. (2005). Potential use of routine databases in health technology assessment. *Health Technology Assessment*, **9**(20). Available from: URL; http://www.hta.nhsweb.nhs.uk/fullmono/mon920.pdf.

Rowe, B. (1972). *Computers in Medicine Series: Hospital Activity Analysis*. London: Butterworths.

The Royal Statistical Society Working Party on Performance Monitoring of Public Services (2003). Performance indicators: good, bad and ugly. Available from:URL; http://www.rss.org.uk.

Sheldon, T. A., Smith, P., Borowitz, B., Martin, S. and Carr-Hill, R. (1994). Attempt at deriving a formula for setting general practitioner fundholding budgets. *British Medical Journal*, **309**, 1059–64.

The Society of Cardiothoracic Surgeons of Great Britain and Ireland Fifth National Adult Cardiac Surgical Database Report 2003. (2004). Dendrite clinical systems. Henley-upon-Thames: The Society of Cardiothoracic Surgeons of Great Britain and Ireland.

Spiegelhalter, D. (1999). Surgical audit: statistical lessons from Nightingale and Codman. *Journal of the Royal Statistical Society*, **162**, 45–58.

Spiegelhalter, D. (2002). Funnel plots for institutional comparison. *Quality and Safety in Health Care*, **11**, 390–1.

Spiegelhalter, D. (2005). Funnel plots for comparing institutional performance. *Statistics in Medicine*, **24**, 1185–202.

Spiegelhalter, D., Evans, S. J. W., Aylin, P. and Murray, G. (2000). Overview of statistical evidence presented to the Bristol Royal Infirmary Inquiry concerning the nature and outcomes of paediatric cardiac surgical services at Bristol relative to other specialist centres from 1984 to 1995. Available from: URL; http://www.bristol-inquiry.org.uk/Documents/statistical overview report.pdf.

Spiegelhalter, D. J., Aylin, P., Best, N., Evans, S. J. W. and Murray, G. D. (2002). Commissioned analysis of surgical performance using routine data: lessons from the Bristol Inquiry. *Journal of the Royal Statistical Society, Series A*, **165**, (2), 1–31.

Stark, J., Galliavan, S., Lovegrove, J. *et al.* (2002). Mortality rates after surgery for congenital heart defects in children and surgeon's performance. *The Lancet*, **355**, 1004–7.

Steiner, S., Cook, R., Farewell, V. and Treasure, T. (2002). Monitoring surgical performance using risk-adjusted cumulative sum charts. *Biostatistics*, **1**(4), 441–52.

Sutton, R., Bann, S., Brooks, M. and Sarin, S. (2002). The Surgical Risk Scale as an improved tool for risk-adjusted analysis in comparative surgical audit. *British Journal of Statistics*, **89**, 763–8.

Terje Lie, R., Heuch, I. and Irgens, L. M. (1993). A sequential procedure for surveillance of Down's syndrome. *Statistics in Medicine*, **12**, 13–25.

Ugolini, C. (2004). Risk adjustment for coronary artery bypass graft surgery: an administrative approach versus EuroSCORE. *International Journal for Quality in Health Care*, **16**, 157.

Vanbrackle, L. and Williamson, G. D. (1999). A study of the average run length characteristics of the national notifiable disease surveillance system. *Statistics in Medicine*, **18**, 3309–19.

Wald, A. (1947). *Sequential Analysis*. Chapman and Hall: London.

Walshe, K., Harrison, N. and Renshaw, M. (1993). Comparison of the quality of patient data collected by hospital and departmental computer systems. *Health Trends*, **25**, 105–8.

16

An ethical analysis of the defensive surgery objection to individual surgeon report cards[1]

Justin Oakley

Monash University, Centre for Human Bioethics, Australia

The public reporting of individual surgeon performance information encounters a variety of objections, from medical, economic and ethical perspectives. The most common ethical argument against publicizing surgeon-specific performance data is that the use of individual surgeon report cards leads surgeons to avoid operating on high-risk patients, because these patients are more likely to have unsuccessful outcomes, and such outcomes would have a negative impact on the surgeon's report card. In their discussion of report cards in the US, Green and Wintfeld (1995) write that:

Anecdotal reports suggest that some surgeons may have declined to operate on severely ill patients for fear that to do so could have lowered their standing in the mortality report. (p. 1230)

The former President of the UK Society of Cardiothoracic Surgeons, Bruce Keogh made a similar comment in relation to the introduction of surgeon report cards in the UK:

We ... are concerned that publishing data could lead to the practice of defensive surgery, where high-risk cases are avoided. Surgeons have already begun to avoid high-risk cases. (Keogh, quoted in Vass 2002, p. 189)

And these comments are echoed by the President of the Royal Australasian College of Surgeons, Dr Russell Stitz:

In the United States, the surgeons are practising defensive medicine, because the surgeons are now avoiding the more difficult cases if they're exposed to public risk. ... [A]s soon as you actually expose surgeons to public risk, they're going to change their practice, and that's the sad thing, because then the patient suffers. [ABC Radio, *The Health Report*, 27/9/04]

If these concerns prove to be well founded, patients for whom surgery carries higher risks would be seriously disadvantaged in their access to surgical care,

Informed Consent and Clinician Accountability: The Ethics of Report Cards on Surgeon Performance. Steve Clarke and Justin Oakley (eds.). Published by Cambridge University Press. © Cambridge University Press 2007.

for such patients may then experience great difficulties in finding a surgeon who is prepared to operate upon them. In many developed countries, the highest-risk patients tend to be operated on by the most skilled surgeons (thus increasing the probability of a successful outcome);[2] but if these surgeons are led to avoid taking on such patients, due to concerns about ending up with an unduly negative report card, then high-risk patients will find themselves unable to access the sort of surgeon that they need most.[3] If individual surgeon report cards do lead surgeons to practice this kind of defensive medicine, then report cards face important ethical objections on grounds of justice in access to surgical care, and from the point of view of the overall quality of surgical care provided to the community. It should be noted that some who put this objection do not seem opposed to greater transparency and public account-ability in healthcare, and may support the publicizing of cardiac surgery out-comes at the level of cardiac units (rather than for individual surgeons). This indicates how convinced the proponents of this objection are of the deleterious outcomes of individual surgeon report cards in particular.[4]

In this chapter I evaluate this objection, which I call the 'defensive surgery objection'. I look at the evidence in favour of the empirical claim on which this objection depends, and I examine what moral weight the objection plausibly carries, if its empirical claim were well founded. I argue that the evidence in support of this claim is not conclusive, but that it cannot be dismissed as unfounded. I also argue that the moral significance of the defensive surgery objection is often overstated. The defensive surgery objection relies impor-tantly on the empirical claim that report cards on surgeons lead them to avoid operating on high-risk patients (such as those aged over 65 with acute myo-cardial infarction), so I begin my evaluation of this objection by investigating whether or not this claim is supported by the available empirical evidence on this matter. In the second part of the chapter I consider the ethical significance of this objection, should the empirical claim turn out to be well founded, for the overall ethical justifiability of individual surgeon report cards.

What evidence is there of defensive surgery as a response to report cards?

What does the available empirical research tell us about whether providing public access to surgeon-specific performance information leads surgeons to avoid operating on high-risk patients? I will concentrate primarily on cardiac surgeons, the focus of the longest-running public reporting schemes (pio-neered by the New York State Department of Health in 1991), and the subject of most empirical research on this question. Surveys of cardiac surgeons in two US states provide some empirical support for the defensive surgery objection. Burack *et al.*'s (1999) survey of the 150 cardiac surgeons practising in

New York State in 1997 asked surgeons about any changes they made to their practice due to the advent of report cards. Of the 104 cardiac surgeons who responded, 62 per cent said that they had turned away at least one high-risk cardiac patient during the previous year because of public reporting. Similar results were found in Schneider and Epstein's (1996) influential survey of cardiac surgeons and cardiologists in Pennsylvania, where half of the 171 cardiac surgeons practising in Pennsylvania were randomly selected and sent a questionnaire asking about their responses to the publication of surgeon-specific performance data, which began in that state in 1992. Of the 58 cardiac surgeon respondents, 63 per cent said that they were now (3 years after report cards began) less willing to perform CABG surgery on the most severely ill patients, following the public release of individual surgeon performance data. Also, 59 per cent of the cardiologists who responded 'reported increased difficulty in finding surgeons willing to perform CABG surgery in severely ill patients who required it' (p. 251).[5] These studies do provide some cause for concern, if high-risk patients were in fact disadvantaged by delays in finding a surgeon willing to operate on them. Nevertheless, 38 per cent of New York cardiac surgeon respondents and 37 per cent of Pennsylvania cardiac surgeon respondents said they were *no* less willing to take on high-risk patients, following the introduction of surgeon report cards, so these studies do not support a general claim (in the extreme version of the defensive surgery objection) that high-risk patients cannot find a surgeon prepared to take them on.[6]

Another consideration relevant to determining how these studies bear on the defensive surgery objection is that higher risk-adjusted mortality rates tend to be more common amongst surgeons who perform relatively low numbers of CABG operations each year (cf. Marshall *et al.*, 2000, p. 70; Chassin, 2002), and some New York cardiac surgeons with low patient volumes and high risk-adjusted mortality rates reacted to the introduction of report cards by ceasing to perform CABG surgery altogether (cf. Hannan *et al.*, 1995). (Indeed, in many such cases, this decision seems to have been made for them by their hospital employers, as Hannan *et al.* explain: 'Several hospitals report that [following the introduction of report cards in New York in December 1991] they took action to restrict the surgical privileges of some low-volume surgeons, in many cases no longer permitting them to perform CABG surgery' [p. 212].) Thus, when high-risk patients have CABG surgery within an environment where surgeon report cards exist, it may be less likely that this procedure will be carried out by a surgeon who performs low numbers of CABG operations, and so (the evidence suggests) these patients may well have an increased chance of a successful outcome. If responses similar to those in the New York and Pennsylvania surveys were found elsewhere, such that report cards resulted in fewer surgeons willing to treat high-risk patients, it is possible that at least some such patients may actually be *better off*, as their chances of surviving the procedure (once a surgeon has taken them on) would usually be improved.[7] So, the fact that some surgeons seem to become more reluctant to operate on high-risk patients in a report card environment does not establish that such patients are disadvantaged – if the surgeons who begin practising more defensively are also the surgeons who are least proficient at the procedure in question, then it may actually be to the advantage of high-risk patients that those surgeons are now avoiding them.[8] At the very least, negative inferences about the overall plight of high-risk patients cannot justifiably be made from surveys such as those in New York and Pennsylvania, until we know more about the skills of those surgeons who do react to report cards by practising defensively, so that we can then compare these with the skills of surgeons who do not react to report cards in this way. High-risk patients would indeed be seriously disadvantaged if report cards led the most skilled surgeons to practise defensively, but I am aware of no systematic evidence that supports that claim.[9]

Another empirical study often used to support the defensive surgery objection looked at the 'out-migration' of high-risk cardiac patients from New York State to other states, during 1989–1993 (Omoigui et al., 1996). This was not a comprehensive study of high-risk cardiac patient out-migration from New York State as a whole, but rather focused only on the Cleveland Clinic (in nearby Ohio). The study reported that the period 1989–1993 saw an increase in the average number of high-risk patients from New York undergoing CABG surgery at Cleveland Clinic each year from 61 per annum in the previous 8 years, to 96 per annum from 1989–1993. The authors hypothesize that this increase may indicate that the introduction of surgeon report cards in New York State resulted in surgeons and hospitals in that state transferring more of their high-risk cardiac patients to hospitals in other states, where surgeon report cards did not exist.

However, as Chassin et al. (1996) point out, generalizations about defensive surgery cannot be reliably drawn from this study, for several reasons. Firstly, the increase in high-risk patients undergoing CABG surgery at Cleveland Clinic occurred 2 years before the introduction of report cards in New York State. Secondly, there was little change in the expected mortality of the high-risk cardiac patients referred from New York State to Cleveland Clinic during the whole period 1989–1993, even though report cards were introduced in the middle of this period. Thirdly, there is reason to believe that this increase in out-migration is a local phenomenon, reflecting long-established patterns of referral from the Western corner of New York State (around Buffalo) to nearby Cleveland, rather than demonstrating any general referral practices with high-risk cardiac patients across the whole of New York State. Indeed, a subsequent comprehensive study (Peterson et al., 1998) of high-risk cardiac patient out-migration across the whole of New York State from 1987–1992 found that there was *no* increase in out-of-state CABG referrals during this period, and that the percentage of New Yorkers over 65 who underwent CABG surgery in another state actually *decreased* from 12.5 per cent to 11.3 per cent in this period. Further, Peterson *et al.* found that older high-risk cardiac patients in New York were *more* likely to receive CABG surgery during 1987–1992 (which was consistent with trends across the US), and that mortality rates had decreased during this time. This study therefore suggests that high-risk cardiac patients in New York who required CABG surgery were overall *better off* after the introduction of cardiac surgeon report cards, than they were previously.

Another point worth mentioning here is that some New York hospitals and surgeons soon realized that the particular risk-adjustment process used in the New York report cards could actually provide something of a *disincentive* to turn away high-risk patients, because achieving above-average results with high-risk patients would lead to a greater decline in one's risk-adjusted mortality rate than would achieving above-average results with low-risk patients. And, if one ceased surgery with high-risk patients altogether, one's risk-adjusted mortality rate would typically *increase*.[10] Putting this point about the risk-adjustment process together with Peterson *et al.*'s observation of an increase in CABG surgery with high-risk patients in New York State after report cards were introduced there, the empirical evidence would seem to suggest that, contrary to the defensive surgery objection, high-risk cardiac patients are not *generally* being avoided by surgeons, and that, in fact, such patients may in some cases actually be welcomed by hospitals and surgeons. In summary then, the available empirical evidence does not conclusively support the claim that publicizing surgeon-specific performance information leads to a general avoidance of high-risk patients by surgeons, and this danger seems to be overstated by proponents of the defensive surgery objection.[11]

Nevertheless, the defensive surgery objection cannot be dismissed as unfounded. Apart from the studies mentioned above, there is a good deal of anecdotal evidence from both the US and the UK that some highly skilled cardiac surgeons have responded to the advent of report cards by turning away high-risk patients that they would have previously taken on. For example, from 1997 onwards, when the collection of surgeon-specific data started in the UK, a substantial number of cardiac surgeons apparently began refusing to perform CABG surgery on high-risk patients, due to concerns about how their mortality rates would be perceived when these data were to be released to the public (see Keogh and Kinsman, 2002; and BBC TV programme *Newsnight*, 18/7/2001). And, even in Australia, where there has been no official government commitment to introduce surgeon report cards, some cardiac surgeons have reportedly become reluctant to take on certain high-risk cases, apparently because of concerns that overseas developments and the tragic recent surgical deaths at Bundaberg Base Hospital[12] may make surgeon report cards inevitable in this country.[13] So, the absence of conclusive evidence that report cards lead skilled surgeons generally to avoid high-risk patients, should not make us complacent about this concern. And, in any case, even though the worry

expressed in the defensive surgery objection currently seems somewhat speculative (causal claims are, after all, notoriously difficult to substantiate empiri-
cally), we should still consider what moral force this objection has against the
ethical justifiability of surgeon report cards, should the empirical claim upon
which it relies turn out to be well founded.

If report cards have led surgeons to adopt defensive practices, are report cards therefore ethically unjustified?

Suppose there existed systematic evidence showing that the advent of cardiac
surgeon report cards has led to a general avoidance of high-risk patients by skilled
surgeons. Many who advance such an objection seem to regard such a consequence as a decisive reason to reject surgeon report cards. However, this is clearly
too hasty. The moral significance of a rise in defensive surgery must be weighed
against the moral considerations in favour of individual surgeon report cards.

An initial point to be made here is that one should not assume that *any*
avoidance by surgeons of high-risk patients demonstrates a problem with
surgeon report cards themselves. There is anecdotal evidence that many
surgeons have long avoided operating on high-risk patients, well before the
public release of surgeon-specific performance information was regarded as
being on the horizon.[14] There seem to be various reasons for this. Surgeons
often take pride in successful outcomes to their surgery, and they sometimes
feel that they have failed when a surgical procedure turns out badly. Also,
surgeons often attach considerable significance to their reputation in the
eyes of their peers, and are reluctant to 'buy trouble'. (Indeed, some surgeons
may well avoid high-risk patients even where performance data is collected for
internal reporting purposes only, within a given hospital, and yet a defensive
surgery reaction in this context could hardly be taken as a compelling reason
for abandoning internal reporting of surgeon outcomes;[15] so we might wonder
how a defensive surgery reaction could plausibly overturn the case for reporting surgeon outcomes externally, to the public.) So, it is clear that properly
substantiating the defensive surgery objection requires investigating the
extent to which the avoidance of high-risk patients *increases*, following the
public release of surgeon-specific performance information in a particular
region.

One way of dealing with the defensive surgery objection, without abandoning individual surgeon report cards, is by developing mechanisms for risk-
adjusting surgeons' performance data in ways that surgeons themselves have
confidence in, so as to minimize any incentives to avoid taking on high-
risk patients. For example, in a 'league table' report card format, the risk-
adjusted mortality rates shown beside each surgeon's CABG operations must
adequately factor in the particular mix of patients who underwent a CABG

procedure with the surgeon in question, so that the mortality rates for surgeons who take on relatively large numbers of high-risk patients do not become distorted and misleading as a result.[16] This is no easy task. The method used for risk adjustment in US states has undergone some refinements over the years, and work continues on improving approaches to risk adjustment in the UK. It does seem that some surgeons adopted defensive practices because they lacked confidence that the risk-adjustment processes used were adequate.[17] This underlines the importance of surgeon involvement in the development of adequate risk-adjustment processes. However, imperfect data should not be regarded as an absolute barrier to surgeon report cards – as Hannan (1998, p. 67) put it, it is important not to let 'perfect be the enemy of good'. It would, in any case, be premature at this stage to conclude that no mechanism of risk-adjustment can be developed that would prevent widespread avoidance by surgeons of high-risk patients.[18] One step taken in the UK, to try to discourage surgeons from avoiding high-risk patients, is to base a surgeon's mortality rate for CABG on patients who are not at high-risk in this procedure.[19] However, this step seems to deprive high-risk patients of information about risks of CABG which more closely approximates their situation, which creates ethical problems from the perspective of patient autonomy and informed consent (Clarke and Oakley, 2004).

Alongside adequate risk-adjustment mechanisms, careful thought about the context in which performance information is made available to patients (and to a surgeon's peers and other health professionals) may help avert defensive practices by surgeons, e.g. the context for the data; when it is made available to patients; who is available to help patients comprehend it; how much weight is put on this information (compared to other factors affecting the success of surgery), and so on. Also, surgeons could be educated in the ethical concerns (e.g. of justice) raised by reacting to report cards by avoiding high-risk patients.

Not all ethicists, of course, would regard the defensive surgery response to report cards as ethically unjustifiable. Utilitarians, for example, might argue that the avoidance of high-risk patients by surgeons may not necessarily be the overall harm that it is usually assumed to be, for the resources saved by not performing CABGs on high-risk patients might be better utilized elsewhere. (Indeed, this seemed to be one of the criticisms of hospitals moving more resources into cardiac care, when they knew they would be measured there: see Marshall et al., 2000.) This response should also be considered by non-utilitarians, as cost–benefits are regarded by most theorists as having some relevance to a just allocation of health care resources. However, this response may not be as plausible for non-cardiac (or less expensive) surgery, should report cards be introduced there, as justice in healthcare resource allocation would not necessarily seem to rule out, e.g. high-risk orthopaedic patients from accessing surgery, given that such surgery consumes less of the healthcare budget in the first place.

But in any case, the ethical justifiability of surgeon report cards is not settled by looking at what is the most efficient use of healthcare resources. For, independent of the effects that report cards may have on patient access to care, and on patient welfare overall, there is a strong autonomy-based argument for providing patients with access to performance information on individual surgeons. That is, the standard ethical requirements for informed consent by patients to medical procedures seem to entail that individual surgeon performance data be provided to patients who regard this information as material to their decision about surgery, since, after all, this is simply a further piece of information about the risks of surgery.[20] And this autonomy-based patient interest in obtaining surgeon-specific performance information would not necessarily be overridden by the need to safeguard high-risk patients from being disadvantaged by the existence of such information (where this need is to be met by abandoning surgeon report cards). Those who think otherwise would be advocating that patients generally should be denied access to material risk information, for the sake of preserving existing levels of access to surgical procedures by high-risk patients. But patients' autonomy-based interests in obtaining information about medical procedures are not thought justifiably sacrificed for the sake of broader social goals in the case of *other* sorts of currently available risk information (such as information about side-effects and complications of surgery), so why should it be any different when the risk information is about individual surgeons' mortality rates?

The above point about the relative weight of patients' autonomy-based interests compared with other considerations also highlights the importance of specifying precisely what it is that surgeons are worried about, which leads them to practise defensively. My reply above presupposes that surgeons are concerned about *patients* judging them harshly in light of their report card (and so avoiding them). But if it is their *peers'* disapproval and disesteem that surgeons are worried about[21], then this seems to carry little if any moral weight to begin with. For, if it is *peer* disapproval that surgeons are concerned about, the defensive surgery objection would amount to the claim that patients should be deprived of material risk information, so that surgeons' colleagues do not have attitudes of disapproval towards them. If this were the basis for surgeons' concerns about report cards, the most appropriate response would hardly be to abandon report cards, but rather, to teach one's colleagues not to jump to conclusions, and to consider a surgeon's report card in its proper context (which, after all, surgeons themselves are uniquely well-positioned to do).

Conclusions

I have argued that the available empirical evidence does not establish that surgeon report cards lead to a general avoidance of high-risk patients by surgeons. I also argued that, even if this sort of defensive surgery claim were supported by stronger evidence, the moral significance of such a response by surgeons would not be sufficient to outweigh the moral considerations in favour of publishing surgeon-specific performance information. The defensive surgery objection is therefore not a decisive reason to reject surgeon report cards.

Notes

1. Thanks to Richard Ashcroft, Steve Clarke, Tim Locke, Steve Matthews, Graham McLean, Yujin Nagasawa, and Mark Sheehan for valuable comments, and to audiences at Imperial College London, Charles Sturt University Wagga Wagga, and the University of Melbourne, where earlier versions of this chapter were presented. This research was supported by National Health and Medical Research Council Project Grant 236877.
2. This is in *relative* terms. Those for whom cardiac surgery would carry the *highest* risks are usually not operated on at all (as I discuss later).
3. Surgeon report cards have also been claimed to prompt another reaction (which may occur separately from or together with defensive surgery): that is, attempts by surgeons to 'game' the system by reclassifying a given procedure, manipulating risk factors, or altering patient data, in order to artificially reduce their mortality rate for a certain procedure (see Green and Wintfeld, 1995; Fine *et al.*, 2003).
4. Note an apparent inconsistency in this argument: surgeons often comment that most patients would not use this data (preferring to go on such factors as a surgeon's 'bedside manner'), yet surgeons are afraid of losing patients if their report card looks bad. Perhaps what worries surgeons here is looking bad in the eyes of their colleagues. (There is some evidence that this is already a factor.) But, wouldn't a surgeon's colleagues be above all those best positioned to understand the quirks of performance statistics, and so be least likely to jump to conclusions?
5. See Schneider and Epstein (1996). Also, a subsequent survey, by the same authors, of patients undergoing cardiac surgery found that 'one-third of patients said they would definitely switch surgeons if they found that their surgeon had a higher than expected mortality rate' (Schneider and Epstein, 1998, p. 1641).
6. Burack *et al.* (1999) state that their survey showed that 'most surgeons refused to operate on at least one high-risk coronary artery bypass patient over the prior year, primarily because of public reporting'. But, given that only two-thirds of New York cardiac surgeons responded to the survey, the study actually found that less than half (i.e. 43 per cent) of the 150 cardiac surgeons practising in New York State said that they had turned away at least one high-risk cardiac patient because of public reporting. (Whether cardiac surgeons who did not respond to the survey avoided high-risk patients due to public reporting is a matter for speculation.)
7. Of course, whether or not high-risk patients, as a group, would be better off once low-volume higher-risk surgeons cease performing CABG procedures, also depends on how many of such patients are able to find a surgeon to take them on in a timely manner.
8. Chassin (2002) describes how a Dr E, who had a high risk-adjusted mortality rate for cardiac surgery at Carson Memorial Hospital (in Rochester NY), ceased performing

such surgery, after the introduction of report cards. Chassin explains that Dr E had been trained only in vascular surgery, and not in cardiac surgery.

9. Indeed, Burack *et al.*'s (1999) survey of New York cardiac surgeons found that high-risk patients were more commonly avoided by the less experienced cardiac surgeons than by the more experienced cardiac surgeons. While a more experienced surgeon does not necessarily have greater skill than a less experienced surgeon, this survey fails to establish a general claim that high-risk patients cannot find a skilled surgeon to operate upon them.

10. See author's interview with Professor Mark Chassin, 13 February 2004.

11. A comprehensive book-length study of empirical research on cardiac surgeon report cards in the US concluded that there was little systematic empirical evidence to support the claim that report cards lead surgeons generally to avoid high-risk patients (see Marshall *et al.*, 2000).

12. A recent Queensland Government Commission of Inquiry found that 13 patients died and many others suffered adverse outcomes due to the negligence of surgeon Dr Jayant Patel. See *Queensland Public Hospitals Commission of Inquiry – Report* (Chaired by Geoffrey Davies), November 2005.

13. This was expressed in the focus group discussions conducted with Melbourne cardiac surgeons during 2004–2005, as part of the NHMRC-funded project on *An ethical analysis of the disclosure of surgeons' performance data to patients within the informed consent process* (Project Grant 236877: Chief Investigator: Dr Justin Oakley).

14. This emerged in focus group discussions conducted with Melbourne cardiac surgeons during 2004–2005, as part of the NHMRC-funded project on *An ethical analysis of the disclosure of surgeons' performance data to patients within the informed consent process.*

15. Some surgeon-specific outcome data has been collected by Australian cardiac surgeons and hospitals for internal reporting purposes for a number of years (see Hughes and Bearham, 2005). Many UK and US hospitals also collect some surgeon outcome data for internal purposes.

16. In their 2005 article (a revised version of which is published in this volume) surveying empirical studies on the impact of surgeon and other healthcare report cards in the US, Rachel Werner and David Asch also argue that worries about surgeons avoiding high-risk patients due to concerns about public reporting should be addressed through refining current risk-adjustment processes (see Werner and Asch, this volume). Yujin Nagasawa (this volume) also suggests improving methods of risk-adjustment as a way of dealing with defensive surgery.

17. Some UK cardiac surgeons are particularly sceptical about the capacity for existing risk-adjustment mechanisms to adequately adjust for risk in very high-risk patients (see author's interview with Sir Bruce Keogh, 29 October 2003). See also Neil *et al.* (2004). Also, there is some evidence that the EuroSCORE model for risk-adjustment would be a poor predictor of CABG outcomes in an Australian context: see Yap *et al.* (2005).

18. Along with developing a risk-adjustment process that surgeons themselves have confidence in, it is also important to encourage surgeons to respond rationally to report cards, as there may often be an element of irrationality in surgeons' responses to public report cards. (Thanks to Graham McLean for this point.)

19. See Bridgewater *et al.* (2003); Keogh *et al.* (2004). Another step is to build into a surgeon report card some kind of extra 'loading' for taking on high-risk patients. (Thanks to Steve Matthews for this point.) This is similar to what is done with the risk-adjustment process in New York State.
20. See Clarke and Oakley (2004).
21. There is evidence that fear of peer disapproval can be a powerful motivator for some surgeons. See the focus group discussions conducted with Melbourne cardiac surgeons during 2004–2005, as part of the NHMRC-funded project on *An ethical analysis of the disclosure of surgeons' performance data to patients within the informed consent process.*

References

Bridgewater, B., Grayson, A. D., Jackson, M. *et al.* (2003). Surgeon specific mortality in adult cardiac surgery: comparison between crude and risk stratified data. *British Medical Journal*, **327**, 13–17.

Burack, J. H., Impellizzeri, P., Homel, P. and Cunningham, J. N. (1999). Public reporting of surgical mortality: a survey of New York State cardiothoracic surgeons. *Annals of Thoracic Surgery*, **68**, 1195–200.

Chassin, M. R. (2002). Achieving and sustaining improved quality: Lessons from New York State and cardiac surgery. *Health Affairs*, **21**, 40–51.

Chassin, M. R., Hannan, E. L. and DeBuono, B. A. (1996). Benefits and hazards of reporting medical outcomes publicly. *New England Journal of Medicine*, **334**, 394–8.

Clarke, S. and Oakley, J. (2004). Informed consent and surgeons' performance. *Journal of Medicine and Philosophy*, **29**, 11–35.

Fine, L. G., Keogh, B. E., Cretin, S., Orlando, M. and Gould, M. M. (2003). How to evaluate and improve the quality and credibility of an outcomes database: validation and feedback study on the UK cardiac surgery experience. *British Medical Journal*, **326**, 25–8.

Green, J. and Wintfeld, N. (1995). Report cards on cardiac surgeons – assessing New York State's approach. *New England Journal of Medicine*, **332**, 1229–33.

Hannan, E. L. (1998). Measuring hospital outcomes: don't make perfect the enemy of good! *Journal of Health Services Research and Policy*, **3**, 67–9.

Hannan, E. L., Siu, A. L., Kumar, D., Kilburn, H. and Chassin, M. R. (1995). The decline in coronary artery bypass graft mortality in New York State. *Journal of the American Medical Association*, **273**, 209–13.

Hannan, E. L., Siu, A. L., Kumar, D., Racz, M., Pryor, D. B. and Chassin, M. R. (1997). Assessment of coronary artery bypass graft surgery performance in New York: is there a bias against taking high-risk patients? *Medical Care*, **35**, 49–56.

Hughes, C. F. and Bearham, G. (2005). Surgeon-specific report cards. *Australian and New Zealand Journal of Surgery*, **75**, 927–8.

Keogh, B. and Kinsman, R. (2002). *National Adult Cardiac Surgical Database Report 2000–2001*. London: Society of Cardiothoracic Surgeons of Great Britain and Ireland.

Keogh, B., Spiegelhalter, D., Bailey, A., Roxburgh, J., Magee, P. and Hilton, C. (2004). The legacy of Bristol: public disclosure of individual surgeons' results. *British Medical Journal*, **329**, 450–4.

Marshall, M. N., Shekelle, P. G., Brook, R. H. and Leatherman, S. (2000). Dying to know: Public release of information about quality of health care. RAND Corporation/Nuffield Trust. Available at: www.rand.org/publications/MR/MR1255/.

Neil, D., Clarke, S. and Oakley, J. (2004). Public reporting of individual surgeon performance information: United Kingdom developments and Australian issues. *Medical Journal of Australia*, **181**, 266–8.

Omoigui, N., Annan, K., Brown, K. *et al.* (1996). Potential explanation for decreased CABG related mortality in New York State: Outmigration to Ohio. *Circulation*, **93**, 27–33.

Peterson, E. D., De Long, E. R., Jollis, J. G., Muhlbaier, L. H. and Mark, D. B. (1998). The effects of New York's bypass surgery provider profiling on access to care and patient outcomes in the elderly. *Journal of the American College of Cardiology*, **32**, 993–9.

Schneider, E. C. and Epstein, A. M. (1996). Influence of cardiac-surgery performance reports on referral practices and access to care – a survey of cardiovascular specialists. *New England Journal of Medicine*, **335**, 251–6.

Schneider, E. C. and Epstein, A. M. (1998). Use of public performance reports: a survey of patients undergoing cardiac surgery. *Journal of the American Medical Association*, **279**, 1638–42.

Vass, A. (2002). Performance of individual surgeons to be published. *British Medical Journal*, **324**, 189.

Yap, C-H., Mohajeri, M., Ihle, B. U., Wilson, A. C., Goyal, S. and Yii, M. (2005). Validation of EuroSCORE model in an Australian patient population. *Australian and New Zealand Journal of Surgery*, **75**, 508–12.

17

Surgeon report cards and the concept of defensive medicine

Yujin Nagasawa

The University of Birmingham, UK and The Australian National University

Introduction

The performance records of cardiac surgeons have been disclosed publicly in several states in the USA, for example New York and Pennsylvania, since the early 1990s. In response to the growing interest in the quality of healthcare, such records have also begun to be disclosed in the UK, starting in 2004. Various studies seem to show that disclosure has, indeed, contributed to the improvement of the quality of healthcare.[1] However, at the same time, disclosure does have its critics.[2]

In this paper, I discuss what I call the 'defensive medicine objection' to the disclosure of performance data; that disclosure is not justified because it could cause surgeons to experience high levels of anxiety[3], which might eventually lead to the practice of defensive medicine. Although this objection is often mentioned by ethicists and medical professionals,[4] it has never been carefully analysed or evaluated. The aim of this chapter is to consider it in detail. I argue in favour of the objection; disclosure could, indeed, lead to the practice of defensive medicine if it is not conducted properly.[5]

Surgeons' anxiety

There are two main arguments for justifying the disclosure of performance data. According to the first, which might be called the 'rights-based argument', patients have the right to know the skill of their surgeons. This argument seems to be underpinned by the doctrine of informed consent, which aims mainly at protecting patients' right to autonomy. According to the second, which might be called the 'utility-based argument', disclosure is necessary because it is beneficial to patients. Providing information about the risk involved in surgeries is certainly beneficial to patients and surgeons' performance data could

Informed Consent and Clinician Accountability: The Ethics of Report Cards on Surgeon Performance.
Steve Clarke and Justin Oakley (eds.). Published by Cambridge University Press. © Cambridge University Press 2007.

be part of such information. In this chapter I focus mainly on the utility-based argument.

Critics argue that the truth about the disclosure of performance data is diametrically opposed to that which is claimed by proponents of the utility-based argument. In the long run, they claim, the disclosure of performance data causes unnecessary anxiety among surgeons and encourages them to practise defensive medicine, which is surely *un*beneficial, or even harmful, to patients.

That surgeons experience anxiety regarding the disclosure of performance data is widely recognised. For instance, Vass quotes from Bruce Keogh, the secretary of the Society of Cardiothoracic Surgeons of Great Britain and Ireland, as follows:

[S]urgeons were 'not comfortable' with publishing individual performance results but accepted it as inevitable. 'We have been collecting data on death rates for four years already, and acting upon it, but are concerned that publishing data could lead to the practice of defensive surgery . . .' (Vass, 2002, p. 189)

Surgeons' anxiety seems widespread also in the USA, where disclosure has already been practised for many years. Keogh *et al.* (2004) describe the phenomenon as follows:

[T]here is a feeling in the US cardiac surgery community that an unintended negative consequence of public disclosure is that surgeons may be protecting their results by avoiding higher risk cases if they feel that their results are drifting into a range that might attract unnecessary yet easily avoidable scrutiny. (p. 451)

Surgeons' anxiety is not harmful *per se*. It is harmful because, as the above quotations show, it could motivate surgeons to practise in ways that are harmful to patients. Schneider and Epstein (1996) surveyed a randomly selected sample of 50 per cent of Pennsylvania cardiologists and cardiac surgeons. 59 per cent of the cardiologists expressed increased difficulty, since the advent of surgeon report cards, in finding surgeons willing to perform coronary-artery bypass graft surgery in severely ill patients who required it. This difficulty is supported by the fact that 63 per cent of the cardiac surgeons reported that they were less willing to operate on such patients after report cards were introduced. According to Hannan *et al.* (1994), between 1989 and 1992 the risk-adjusted mortality rate for coronary artery bypass surgery in New York declined by 41 per cent, from 4.17 per cent to 2.45 per cent. Omoigui *et al.* (1996) hypothesize that this decrease is due to the fact that some high-risk patients are obliged to migrate out of New York for surgery.[6] While Peterson *et al.* (1998) criticizes this hypothesis, it is undeniable that the disclosure of performance data has been causing a number of surgeons to experience significant levels of anxiety, both in the US and the UK.

Traditional definition of defensive medicine

In order to determine whether or not the disclosure of performance data really motivates doctors to practise defensive medicine in a significant way, we need to understand the nature of defensive medicine. De Ville (1998) defines it as follows:

Defensive medicine: A clinical decision or action motivated in whole or in part by the desire to protect oneself from a malpractice suit or to serve as a reliable defence if such a suit occurs. (p. 570)

As this definition suggests, the practice of defensive medicine has been traditionally construed as an unwelcomed consequence of the increase in the number of medical malpractice suits. Here, the logic of physicians who practise defensive medicine is straightforward: they want to avoid being sued by their patients, so they simply prioritise their liability over other appropriate considerations.

It is widely recognized that there are two kinds of defensive medicine: positive defensive medicine and negative defensive medicine.

Positive defensive medicine

The unnecessary use of medical procedures in order to reduce physicians' exposure to malpractice risk.

The practice of positive defensive medicine involves an unnecessary use of additional medical procedures, such as diagnostic tests and X-rays. The term 'positive' refers to additional healthcare utilisation. Positive defensive medicine is problematic because it imposes additional time and financial costs on patients.

The practice of negative defensive medicine is often more harmful than that of positive defensive medicine.

Negative defensive medicine

The avoidance of high-risk patients or procedures in order to reduce physicians' exposure to malpractice risk.

The practice of negative defensive medicine involves an avoidance of high-risk patients or an avoidance of medical procedures primarily, but not solely, out of concern for malpractice liability. The term 'negative' refers to a reduction in healthcare utilisation. Negative defensive medicine is often more harmful than positive defensive medicine. A reduction in the use of medical procedures might initially appear to reduce time and financial cost. However, since the conditions are left untreated, there could be much greater costs in the long run. Moreover, it could impose significant physical and psychological risks on patients. It is not entirely obvious, however, that the practice of defensive medicine is *always* harmful to patients. Some claim that surgeons' avoidance of high-risk patients could even be *beneficial* for patients in certain situations. I discuss this point in the next section.

New definition of defensive medicine

As I explained above, defensive medicine has traditionally been defined in terms of physicians' attempts to avoid medical malpractice suits. However, the debate on the disclosure of performance data suggests that there is a new form of defensive medicine, one which arises from a different source: surgeons' anxiety regarding disclosure. In order to cover this new form, we need to revise the traditional definition of defensive medicine in the previous section as follows:

Defensive medicine

A clinical decision or action that is motivated in whole or in part by the desire (i) to protect oneself from a malpractice suit, or (ii) to serve as a reliable defence if such a suit occurs or (iii) to sustain or improve performance data accessible to others.

(iii) concerns the desire of surgeons to defend themselves against any unfavourable consequences of the disclosure of their performance data, which is independent of the increase in medical malpractice suits. Surgeons may have such a desire because if they practise normal medicine, their performance data might drift into a range that threatens their reputation regarding their surgical skills. Just as with their desire to avoid malpractice suits, their desire to sustain or improve that portion of their performance data that is accessible to others could lead to both positive and negative defensive medicine. Given that surgeons' performance data are collected continually, surgeons could well come to view every single act of surgery they perform as having the potential to either improve or worsen their performance data.

As I noted earlier, it is not obvious that the practice of defensive medicine is *always* harmful to patients. Some argue that it could not only be harmless, but even *beneficial* to patients.[7] Consider cases in which procedures envisaged by patients are unfamiliar to their surgeons, or in which patients' conditions are so poor that they are likely to be harmed by their inexperienced surgeons. In these cases, patients would benefit if these surgeons avoid their patients out of anxiety and the procedures are carried out by better-performing surgeons instead.[8]

These cases seem to show convincingly that it is a mistake to think that the practice of defensive medicine is *always* harmful to patients. However, that does not entail immediately that the defensive medicine objection is unsound. First of all, it has not been shown that in these kinds of cases patients normally find better-performing surgeons. Given their critical conditions, some patients might not have enough time to find better surgeons. In such situations, undergoing prompt surgery carried out by a less-experienced surgeon might be better than having belated surgery carried out by a better-performing surgeon or no surgery at all. Secondly, even if it has been shown that in these cases patients normally find better-performing surgeons, it is not clear that these cases are so common that they outweigh harms caused by defensive medicine in other cases.

Is surgeons' anxiety groundless?

The defensive medicine objection that I have discussed can be presented as an argument with the following structure.
1. The disclosure of performance data causes surgeons to experience significant levels of anxiety.
2. The anxiety that those surgeons experience encourages them to practise defensive medicine.
   Therefore,
3. The disclosure of performance data encourages the practice of defensive medicine.

The argument is obviously valid. I assume, for the sake of argument, that both premises (1) and (2) are, as a matter of fact, true. However, in the following, I examine whether or not (1) *should* be true; that is, whether or not surgeons should really be anxious about disclosure. Suppose that the anxiety experienced by surgeons is groundless. It is then easy for us to eliminate the force of the argument; all we need to do is to persuade surgeons that they have, in fact, no need to be anxious. If we are successful in persuading them, then the truth-value of (1) changes from true to false and the argument turns out to be unsound.

Various empirical studies suggest that surgeons' anxiety, which could lead to the practice of defensive medicine, is often derived from their misunderstanding of relevant facts. According to some studies, for instance, surgeons' anxiety is caused by their false belief that medical malpractice suits are very common these days. Localio *et al.* (1991) performed research to determine the relationship between adverse events caused by negligence and medical malpractice claims against physicians and hospitals. They estimate, based on the records of more than 30 000 patients, that the ratio of adverse events caused by negligence to malpractice claims in New York is 7.6 to 1, which seems relatively small. They claim, moreover, that even this infrequency overstates the chances that a negligent adverse event will produce a claim, because most of the events for which claims were made in the sample did not meet their definition of adverse events due to negligence. They conclude, therefore, that patients' injuries caused by medical negligence are only infrequently compensated by medical malpractice suits.

De Ville (1998) explains a number of neglected reasons why many patients do not recognize the outcomes of medical malpractice as potential cause for bringing malpractice suits against the surgeons (pp. 572–3). Firstly, patients who have been suffering from a pre-existing injury or illness often cannot distinguish the natural outcome of their injury or illness from those caused by medical malpractice. That is, many victims of medical malpractice do not initiate a malpractice suit simply because they do not recognize that they *are* victims in the first place. Secondly, even if they are aware of injury or illness caused by medical malpractice, many of them still do not initiate lawsuits because they do not possess sufficient knowledge of the legal system. That is, even if they are disposed to sue their physicians or hospitals they do not know how to do it. Thirdly, even if they are aware of injury or illness caused by medical malpractice and even if they do possess sufficient knowledge of the legal system, many of them still do not pursue legal remedies. For example, some patients have a religious or cultural commitment to avoid medical malpractice suits; or, to take another example, some patients live in rural communities that generally discourage personal injury suits.[9]

These observations seem to show that the practice of defensive medicine is often caused by physicians' excessive, irrational anxiety about being sued by their patients. However, unfortunately, this does not undermine the claim that *the disclosure of performance data* could lead to the practice of defensive medicine. For, as I explained above, a form of defensive medicine motivated by surgeons' anxiety about the disclosure is distinct from their anxiety about medical malpractice suits.

I have explained that both the increase of medical malpractice suits and the disclosure of performance data could result in surgeons' experiencing anxiety. However, the nature of disclosure is fundamentally different from that of medical malpractice suits. On the one hand, medical malpractice suits are always made by patients. Most patients are not medical professionals and, as I explained above, often they are not even aware of the existence of malpractice. On the other hand, however, surgeons' performance data are tracked constantly and professionally. As long as the tracking system is in order, surgeons' failures are always reflected in their record. In this sense, the disclosure of performance data could be a much more persistent source of anxiety in surgeons.

In the next section I consider another possible, and more promising, strategy to show that (1) need not be true, which is to disclose performance data with risk adjustments so that surgeons would not be motivated to practise defensive medicine.

Necessity of risk adjustments

Consider two surgeons, X and Y, the former of whom is the more skilled. Y constantly avoids high-risk patients because he worries that his mortality rate will drift into a range that threatens his reputation regarding his surgical skills. Thanks to his avoidance of high-risk patients, Y maintains a fairly good performance record. By contrast, X accepts high-risk patients. Since X is skilful, she saves a number of high-risk patients whom surgeons like Y avoid on purpose. However, of course, X cannot save all of her patients. Given that X constantly operates on high-risk patients and that Y operates mainly on risk-free patients, X's performance record appears less impressive than Y's.

Obviously, this is not fair to X. Given that X is more skilful than Y, her performance data should look better than Y's. In the above situation, Y's performance record looks better merely because he adopts the most effective strategy in this system. In order to solve this problem, we need to adopt a more appropriate way of presenting performance data.

There are two ways to present performance data: (1) present it without making any adjustments, and (2) present it with adjustments appropriate to the risks involved in particular cases. The USA adopts the latter. The UK adopted the former initially, but since April 2006 it has published surgeon-specific data, at least some of which are risk adjusted.

In the UK, performance data for cardiac surgeons have been collected for quite a long time, even though the data were not publicly accessible until 2004. From 2004 to 2006, the Society for Cardiothoracic Surgeons of Great Britain and Ireland (SCTS) released *unadjusted* mortality rates for isolated coronary artery bypass surgery and aortic valve surgery for all units in the UK on its website and in its 2000–2001 annual report. Fine *et al.* (2003) explain why the data were not risk adjusted: 'While expressing reservations over the value of reporting unadjusted or inadequately adjusted outcomes, the [SCTS] felt unable to proceed to full risk adjustment because of concerns about the quality and completeness of data on each patient within its national database' (p. 25).

The SCTS was right in thinking that the disclosure of incomplete or inadequately risk-adjusted data could be worse than that of unadjusted data. However, that does not mean that unadjusted data do not encourage surgeons to perform defensive medicine. The above example of Drs X and Y shows that unadjusted performance data represent surgeons' skills inaccurately and encourage surgeons to perform defensive medicine. In order to avoid this problem, we need to structure the system so that the skills of the surgeons are always reflected correctly in their record. That is, we need to adjust surgeons' performance data appropriately before disclosing them.

In contrast to the UK, performance data have been risk adjusted for a long time in the USA. Marshall *et al.* (2000) describe the system there as follows:

The New York cardiac surgery reporting system publishes hospital and surgeon specific risk-adjusted coronary artery bypass surgery (CABG) mortality data ... Clinical and administrative databases are used to collect information on age, sex, type of coronary artery disease, presence of myocardial ischaemia, level of ventricular function, presence of other diagnoses, severity of atherosclerotic process, previous heart operations, and the degree of emergency of the operation. These data are used to construct a multi-variate risk adjustment model to compare mortality rates among hospitals and individual surgeons ... Similar work has been done in Pennsylvania, and other states are following this example. (p. 54)

Although the process of disclosure in the USA is much more elaborate than that in the UK, many surgeons in the USA are still dissatisfied with it. According to a survey by Schneider and Epstein (1996) of a randomly selected sample of 50 per cent of Pennsylvania cardiologists and cardiac surgeons, 82 per cent of the cardiologists and all the cardiac surgeons were aware of the disclosure of performance data. Many of them said that the most important limitations of the disclosure were the absence of indicators of quality other than mortality (cited by 78 per cent), inadequate risk adjustment (cited by 79 per cent), and the unreliability of data provided by hospitals and surgeons (cited by 53 per cent). As this study suggests, there are two kinds of potential inaccuracy in performance data. The first is the absence of important factors that affect outcomes in medical practice. As Dranove *et al.* (2002) says, given the complexity of healthcare, many of the essential factors are known predominantly by healthcare providers, like surgeons themselves. Hence, there are a number of important factors that are not reflected in the performance data. The second is the presence of inadequate or unreliable information. As Keogh *et al.* (2004) remark, 'The improvement in mortality is easy to show. The avoidance of high-risk surgery is less easy to show because of the subjective and immeasurable nature of the clinical decision making process in these complex patients' (p. 451). In order not to encourage surgeons to perform unbeneficial defensive medicine, we need to disclose their performance data in such a way that the data correctly show important relevant factors in healthcare and eliminate inadequate and unreliable information.

I do not, here, make any attempt to state exactly how disclosure should be conducted. The issue of what sort of data collection and risk-adjustment increases or reduces the anxiety experienced by surgeons is a purely empirical matter. However, I hope to have shown convincingly that, contrary to what many people think, the disclosure of performance data could be harmful to patients in the long run. Of course it is impossible, and unnecessary, to satisfy *all* surgeons when we disclose their performance data. Nevertheless, it is important to conduct disclosure in such a way that it maximizes both the number of doctors who are comfortable with it and the number of patients who find it beneficial.

Conclusions

I have argued mainly for three things in this chapter. Firstly, the disclosure of surgeons' performance data could lead to a new form of defensive medicine, one that is not captured by the traditional definition of defensive medicine. Secondly, this new form of defensive medicine is more persistent than the traditional form that arises from physicians' anxiety regarding medical malpractice suits. Thirdly, in order to avoid defensive medicine, it is necessary to make risk adjustments on surgeons' performance records, although exactly how the adjustments should be made requires further empirical studies.

Many people think that the disclosure of performance data can be justified easily, on the grounds that it is obviously beneficial to patients. Given the complexities of medical practice, however, defending disclosure is not as easy as they think.[10]

Notes

1. Bentley and Nash (1998); Longo *et al.* (1997); Marshall and Brook (2002); Rainwater *et al.* (1998); Rosenthal *et al.* (1998).
2. For discussions of various objections to the disclosure of performance data, see Marshall *et al.* (2000); Clarke and Oakley (2004).
3. In this chapter, for the sake of simplicity, I take it that it is anxiety that motivates surgeons to practise defensive medicine. However, anxiety might not be the only possible motivation. For instance, some surgeons might be motivated to practise defensive medicine because of their *ambition* to decrease their mortality rates in their performance record, rather than their being anxious to increase them.
4. Dranove *et al.* (2002); Neil *et al.* (2004); Marshall *et al.* (2000); Keogh *et al.* (2004); Vass (2002).
5. Notice that this is a conditional claim that, if the disclosure is not conducted properly, then it could lead to the practice of defensive medicine. This does not entail that, if it is conducted properly, then it would not lead to the practice of defensive medicine; there might be many other factors that could encourage surgeons to practise defensive medicine.
6. How to explain the decline in the adjusted mortality rate remains controversial. Schneider and Epstein (1996) and Jollis and Romano (1998) argue that the decline is due to the inadequacy of risk adjustment. Ziegenfuss (1996) argues, on the other hand, that the decline is simply caused by the poor quality of the data.
7. See Chassin (2002) and Oakley (this volume).
8. Thanks to Steve Clarke, Justin Oakley and an anonymous referee on this point.

9. It is also often said that many patients decide to initiate malpractice suits only because their physicians do not admit their faults.
10. I would like to thank all the participants of the workshop on this topic at the University of Melbourne in 2004. I am particularly grateful to Steve Clarke, Neil Levy, David Neil, Justin Oakley and an anonymous referee for helpful comments and constructive suggestions.

References

Bentley, J. M. and Nash, D. B. (1998). How Pennsylvania hospitals have responded to publicly released reports on coronary artery bypass graft surgery. *Joint Commission Journal for Quality Improvement*, **24**, 40–9.

Chassin, M. (2002). Achieving and sustaining improved quality: lessons from New York State and cardiac surgery. *Health Affairs*, **21**, 40–51.

Clarke, S. and Oakley, J. (2004). Informed consent and surgeons' performance. *Journal of Medicine and Philosophy*, **29**, 11–35.

De Ville, K. (1998). Act first and look up the law afterward?: medical malpractice and the ethics of defensive medicine. *Theoretical Medicine and Bioethics*, **19**, 569–89.

Dranove, D., Kessler, D., McClellan, M. and Satterthwaite, M. (2002). Is more information better?: The effects of 'report cards' on health care providers. NBER Working Paper Series, 8697. http://www.nber.org/papers/w8697/.

Fine, L. G., Keogh, B. E., Cretin, S., Orlando, M. and Gould, M. M. for the Nuffield-Rand Cardiac Surgery Demonstration Project Group (2003). How to evaluate and improve the quality and credibility of an outcomes database: validation and feedback study on the UK cardiac surgery experience. *British Medical Journal*, **326**, 25–8.

Hannan, E. L., Kilburn, H., Jr, Racz, M., Shields, E. and Chassin, M. R. (1994). Improving the outcomes of coronary artery bypass surgery in New York State. *Journal of the American Medical Association*, **271**, 761–6.

Jollis, J. G. and Romano, P. S. (1998). Pennsylvania's focus on heart attack: grading the scorecard. *New England Journal of Medicine*, **338**, 983–7.

Keogh, B., Spiegelhalter, D., Bailey, A., Roxburgh, J., Magee, P. and Hilton, C. (2004). The legacy of Bristol: public disclosure of individual surgeons' results. *British Medical Journal*, **329**, 450–4.

Localio, A. R., Lawthers, A. G., Brennan, T. A. *et al.* (1991). Relation between malpractice claims and adverse events due to negligence: results of the Harvard medical practice study III. *New England Journal of Medicine*, **325**, 245–51.

Longo, D. R., Land, G., Schramm, W., Fraas, J., Hoskins, B. and Howell, V. (1997). Consumer reports in health care: do they make a difference in patient care? *Journal of the American Medical Association*, **278**, 1579–84.

Marshall, M. N. and Brook, R. H. (2002). Public reporting of comparative information about the quality of healthcare. *Medical Journal of Australia*, **176**, 205–6.

Marshall, M. N., Shekelle, P. G., Leatherman, S. and Brook, R. H. (2000). Public disclosure of performance data: learning from the US experience. *Quality in Health Care*, **9**, 53–7.

Neil, D., Clarke, S. and Oakley, J. G. (2004). Public reporting of individual surgeon performance information: UK developments and Australian issues. *Medical Journal of Australia*, **181**, 266–8.

Omoigui, N. A., Miller, D. P., Brown, K. J. *et al.* (1996). Outmigration for coronary bypass surgery in an era of public dissemination of clinical outcomes. *Circulation*, **93**, 27–33.

Peterson, E. D., Delong, E. R., Jollis, J. G., Muhlbaier, L. H. and Mark, D. B. I. (1998). The effects of New York's bypass surgery profiling on access to care and patient outcomes in the elderly. *Journal of the American College of Cardiology*, **32**, 993–9.

Rainwater, J. A., Romano, P. S. and Antonius, D. M. (1998). The California hospital outcomes project: how useful is California's report card for quality improvement? *Joint Commission Journal of Quality Improvement*, **24**, 31–9.

Rosenthal, G. E., Hammar, P. J., Way, L. E. *et al.* (1998). Using hospital performance data in quality improvement: the Cleveland health quality choice experience. *Joint Commission Journal on Quality Improvement*, **24**, 347–60.

Schneider, E. C. and Epstein, A. M. (1996). Influence of cardiac-surgery performance reports on referral practices and access to care: a survey of cardiovascular specialists. *New England Journal of Medicine*, **355**, 251–6.

Vass, A. (2002). Performance of individual surgeons to be published. *British Medical Journal*, **324**, 189.

Ziegenfuss, J. T., Jr. (1996). Health care quality report cards receive grade-incomplete. *American Journal of Medical Quality*, **11**, 55–6.

18

Training, innovation and surgeons' report cards

Tony Eyers

The Royal Prince Alfred Hospital, Sydney, Australia

The community stands in awe of cardiac surgeons, who daily stop and restart the beating heart, symbolic of life itself. The community also has a high regard for neurosurgeons who, somewhat less dramatically, not only save lives, but may in addition be able to prevent a life of paralysis or dementia. Other surgeons occupy lesser positions on the pedestal, depending on their work. So avid is the public for surgical stories, it could be argued, that the term 'the wonders of modern surgery' has become hackneyed; wearied by a string of TV shows from *Ben Casey* to *ER*, *House* and *Grey's Anatomy*, not to mention countless numbers of newspaper articles, magazine features and books on the subject.

But all surgeons stand on the shoulders of their predecessors. The current state is the product of a process, gradual at first, which has followed an exponential path over about a 150 years since the discovery of anaesthesia let the ethereal genie out of the bottle. Many more than three wishes have been granted, and perhaps surgical success has become so trite that some fundamental truths are overlooked.

- The progress from which we now benefit can only have been achieved by a process of trial and error involving human subjects. It seems singularly unlikely that the necessary experimentation was always conducted in a way that would satisfy modern ethical standards, yet we incorporate the knowledge in our current practice anyway.
- The individual cardiac, neuro- and other surgeons that we so admire have not arrived at the height of their powers by some form of transmutation, but rather by means of a very human process of learning, involving, as it always does, trial and error. For surgeons, the trial and error involves – and adversely affects – human subjects.

The learning curve

Atul Gawande (2002) put it succinctly when he wrote, 'there is still no avoiding those first few unsteady times a young physician tries to put in a central line,

Informed Consent and Clinician Accountability: The Ethics of Report Cards on Surgeon Performance. Steve Clarke and Justin Oakley (eds.). Published by Cambridge University Press. © Cambridge University Press 2007.

remove a breast cancer, or sew together two segments of colon. No matter how many protections are in place, on average these cases go less well with the novice than with someone experienced' (p. 24). He was, of course, referring to a 'learning curve'; that there are increased risks associated with being the subject of an invasive procedure when it is performed by someone who is learning how to do it. And, although most pertinent in surgery, learning curves apply to all 'invasive' procedures, including those performed in non-surgical branches of medicine such as anaesthetics, cardiology, gastroenterology and radiology, and non-medical areas such as nursing, physiotherapy and chiropractic.

Julian Dussek, the President of the Society of Cardiothoracic Surgeons of Great Britain and Ireland at the time, included the following statement in his submission to the Bristol Royal Infirmary Inquiry (Learning from Bristol, 1995, Annex A, ch. 14, para 80): 'The inference to be drawn from the phrase "learning curve" in the context of cardio-thoracic surgery is that there is an expected and acceptable excess of patients who will die or be harmed in the early experience of a learner but who would have fared better if they were operated upon by a surgeon who is on the plateau of experience.' We might take exception to the inclusion of 'acceptable' in his definition – we might prefer to introduce measures so as to avert the expected – but his underlying meaning is clear.

The learning curve applies to trainee surgeons attempting procedures with which they are inexperienced and also to trained surgeons attempting something new. The concept is not restricted to cardiothoracic surgery, although the result of a slip-up might be more immediate and dramatic in that specialty, particularly when the patients are children, as they were in Bristol. In the former case we rely on someone more experienced supervising the surgeons in training to protect their patients from harm, and in both cases clinical governance has still to devise appropriate forms of oversight.

There has been surprisingly little research performed to assess how effective supervision by a senior colleague is in protecting patients on whom surgery is being learned. We know that, with close supervision, trainees can operate safely at least some of the time. Turton et al. (1997) showed this was the case when consultants planned the surgical procedures for varicose veins that were subsequently performed by trainees. Bockler et al. (1999) showed that laparoscopic cholecystectomy performed by trainees under supervision was equivalent in outcome to operations performed by trained surgeons, although the surgery was significantly slower. There is, however, reason to question whether the level of supervision across a given healthcare system is sufficient to guarantee results similar to these, which have been reported from circumstances that might reasonably be expected to have been favourable. A recent survey of Australasian surgical trainees (Thomson et al., 2001) found that, while 70 per cent of general surgical trainees reported that they had a 'very adequate' level of supervision by their consultants at trauma operations, only 46 per cent of orthopaedic trainees felt the same. Another study from the United Kingdom involving large numbers of orthopaedic patients (Marston *et al.*, 1996) showed that the trainee surgeons had higher complication rates than the consultants who were training them. Recently, the Walker Inquiry (2004) into allegations of malpractice at Campbelltown and Camden Hospitals in Western Sydney, identified an association between resource allocation and adverse events, finding that junior doctors were sometimes required to work beyond their levels of competence and with inadequate senior supervision.

Also pertinent to supervision of trainee surgeons is an appreciation that some surgical procedures are inherently much easier to supervise than others. Procedures performed in the open where a supervisor can watch every move a trainee makes are very different from those where the trainee must be relied upon to perform a manoeuvre in the depths of a wound or where the supervisor's view is otherwise obscured. Other surgical techniques, despite being able to be watched, depend on tactile signals, felt only by the operator, that are subject to misinterpretation during the learning process. None of these issues have been well researched.

Thus there are grounds to wonder whether relying on supervision to protect patients from injury at the hands of trainee surgeons is sufficient, particularly in healthcare systems where surgeons-in-training are expected to perform some surgery unsupervised, or supervised by other surgeons-in-training, as is the case in Australia. There is an apparent need for levels of supervision to be stipulated and monitored. There is also an apparent need for research that addresses the efficacy of systems as a whole, rather than particular experiences, reported, one might well suspect, because of their favourable results.

Perhaps in recognition of the problem, a great deal of money is currently being invested throughout the western world in skills laboratories for trainee surgeons, so that at least some of the skills they require can be acquired away from either operating rooms or their patients' bedsides. But investigators (Paisley *et al.*, 2001) who tested all of the then-available surgical simulations, found no correlation between performance in any of them and the trainees' training stage or their surgical ability as judged by their mentors.

Needed and welcomed as skills centres might be, even their fiercest supporters agree that they will not correct the entire problem in the light of the contention (which is almost certainly justified) that all-round competence in performing an invasive procedure can only be learned as a result of experience with real patients. At some stage in their training, surgeons will always need to step up from the simulator to the operating table and to the live human patient lying on it. Similarly, trainees who have experienced a high level of supervision throughout their training will eventually have to 'go it alone' in the operating room.

While the library cupboard is relatively bare with regard to research on trainees, there has been plenty of research into what happens when trained surgeons undertake new procedures. One study (Lau *et al.*, 2002) found that it took 80 procedures for trained general surgeons to achieve a plateau of performance when they were learning how to repair inguinal hernias using a new (keyhole) technique. Another (Watson *et al.*, 1996) reported that the complication, re-operation and keyhole-to-open conversion rates were higher in the first 50 keyhole fundoplication cases performed by their overall group, and in the first 20 cases performed by each individual surgeon in the group. The adverse outcomes were even higher in the group's first 20 cases and in each individual's first five. They also observed that the group's experience provided some protection when surgeons commenced their individual learning after the group as a whole had passed beyond its learning curve, but the protection was by no means complete; adverse events still occurred more often in the hands of the learners. The documentation of recently introduced procedures, which tends to be better than the more traditional surgical techniques, leaves little room for doubt that patients receiving innovative treatments are more at risk than those receiving the same treatments later on, when the treatments have become routine.

What is usually left unanswered is whether the new treatment, albeit delivered less than optimally, gives better outcomes than the traditional therapy it seeks to replace. It is reasonable to conclude that some new treatments will be immediately superior, that some will be shown to be better only after being 'run-in', and that some will never be better. The first of these scenarios would not lead to 'equipoise' – the position where experts in a given field are unsure as to whether a proposed new treatment will be better than its traditional alternative. Without therapeutic equipoise, there is usually no justification for a randomized clinical trial, and innovations with sufficient theoretical promise to warrant their use in humans can immediately result in such an obvious benefit that no formal scientific comparison with the predecessor treatment is ever required. There has never been a formal trial of the efficacy of parachutes in preventing death when people jump from high-flying aircraft.

Recent progress in healthcare delivery has been dramatic. The last 30 years have seen the introduction of computers into medicine, with computerized tomography (CT), magnetic resonance imaging (MRI) and positron emission tomography (PET) scans, automated test results and digital X-ray images the result. Interventional radiology has been invented, and with it, coronary artery stents and endoluminal aneurysm repair. Amazing progress has been made with surgical procedures in every specialty. Personally I have been involved in the introduction of hepatic transplantation (Sheil *et al.*, 1987), isolated limb perfusion for regional chemotherapy (Thompson *et al.*, 2001), ileoanal pouch reconstruction after proctocolectomy (Young *et al.*, 1999), laparoscopic rectoplexy (Solomon and Eyers, 1996; Solomon *et al.*, 2002) and dynamic graciloplasty (Chapman *et al.*, 2002) into clinical practice.

Justification

In years gone by, the decisions that put patients at risk in the name of training and innovation were taken to be justified on the basis of the profession's responsibility to ensure continuance and progress. But medicine's professionalism, and its ability to self-regulate, have been brought sharply into question in recent years. There can be no denying a recent coming of age of the ethical framework in which the actions of medical professionals are judged. Clinical governance, credentialing for individual procedures, incident monitoring systems and surgeons' report cards are all being implemented in response to the community's need for some form of oversight of surgeons' activities other than their own internal processes. These developments have occurred *pari passu* with an appreciation of the importance of individual patient autonomy in medical decision-making.

The shift, while no doubt solving some old problems, has presented us with a new one. On the one hand, we aspire to error-free healthcare accessed by fully autonomous clients. On the other, we have to acknowledge that a process of trial and error involving patients is required in the 'blooding' of future surgeons and in surgical innovation. There is a double standard in our teaching hospitals, and those involved (particularly the trainers and administrators) have a conflict of interests in continuing with the status quo.

Surgeons who supervise training are held responsible for the outcomes of the patients on whom they allow their trainees to operate; something that they understand and accept. Levels of supervision vary, but the reality is that, as it stands, the healthcare delivery system in Australia relies on a certain amount of surgery being performed by trainees without 'in-house' supervision, and by junior trainees being supervised by more senior trainees. This tends to happen more often after hours and at the growing edge of the system where resources are most often stretched, as demonstrated by the Camden and Campbelltown Hospitals Affair mentioned previously (Walker, 2004).

It might come as surprise to those on the outside to learn that surgeons who supervise training in the current system have only a limited ability to deny their trainees access to patients for teaching. The degree to which each teacher delegates is closely scrutinized, and the continuing accreditation of each of the teaching positions depends on the trainees in them achieving an adequate number of teaching cases. Loss of accreditation is interpreted as a failure in a teaching hospital and affects reappointment and the quality of the junior staff that can be recruited to work there, so numbers have to be maintained. Atul Gawande (2002) asked,

Do we ever tell patients that, because we are still new at something, their risks will inevitably be higher, and that they'd likely do better with doctors who are more experienced? Do we ever say that we need them to agree to it anyway? I've never seen it. Given the stakes, who in his right mind would agree to be practiced upon?

Many dispute this assumption. 'Look, most people understand what it is to be a doctor', a health policy expert insisted, when I visited him in his office not long ago. 'We have to stop lying to our patients. Can people take on choices for societal benefit?' He paused and then answered his own question. 'Yes', he said firmly.

It would certainly be a graceful and happy solution. We'd ask patients – honestly, openly – and they'd say yes. Hard to imagine, though. I noticed on the expert's desk a picture of his child, born just a few months before, and a completely unfair question popped into my mind.

'So did you let the resident deliver?' I asked. There was silence for a moment. 'No,' he admitted. 'We didn't even allow residents in the room.' (pp. 30–1)

It is not hard to understand how we came to be in the position in which we find ourselves. A century ago, when our public hospital system was being developed, access to doctors was a prerogative of the rich. A flourishing private sector existed, but those who could not afford it had precious little to guarantee the standards or competence of those whose care they were forced to seek. In this context a public institution staffed by 'house surgeons' who had acquired a modicum of procedural training from senior surgeons probably had something really beneficial to offer. Thus a culture grew whereby the work of the 'house surgeons' was periodically checked in person by senior surgeons acting in an honorary capacity. What better circumstance could there be to train the next generation of surgeons and 'have a go' at potential innovations? In Australia these arrangements were in place until the late 1960s, when a gradual dismantling started, thanks to major contributions from the Gorton,[1] Whitlam[2] and Hawke[3] Governments.

These senior surgeons were not simply acting in the paternalist sense of 'father knows best' – of taking an autocratic, but essentially benevolent, decision. Instead, they were deciding to take a course likely to be detrimental to some individuals in the overall interests of a broader group to whom they felt some professional responsibility. How they weighed the future interests of their paying patients against the immediate interests of their indigent ones remains moot. Today, there might be situations where decisions of this kind would be justified (they are commonly made in politics), but they seem even more problematic in medicine than conventional paternalistic decisions because issues of justice are implicated as well as autonomy. However, Clarke and Oakley (2004) have acknowledged there might be some role that professional autonomy might legitimately play in limiting the promotion of patient autonomy (p. 19).

Caplan (1988) has argued that, as all members of society stand to benefit from the results of clinical research, membership of society should imply an obligation to participate in the research. Clarke and Oakley (2004) have considered whether Caplan's principle can plausibly be extended to participation in surgical training: 'Because each of us has been or is likely to be the beneficiary of a practitioner's skills at some stage in our lives, there is a reciprocal (*prima facie*) moral obligation upon each of us to accept a trainee surgeon, on some occasion, when we need surgery ... [Perhaps a preparedness] to accept the benefits [of a skilled surgeon at some stage in our lives] ... without being prepared to make comparable sacrifices, could be acting as a "free rider"' (pp. 28–9).

Because it is not simply the skill of trained surgeons from which we benefit, but also the sophistication of the procedures at their disposal, it can be similarly argued that, because each of us has been or is likely at some stage in our lives to be the beneficiary of progress in surgery, there is a reciprocal (*prima facie*) moral obligation upon each of us to accept an innovative procedure, on some occasion, when we need surgery. Comparable charges of being a 'free rider' can also be made.

Distribution and coercion

But even if we can reasonably justify exposing patients to the risks of surgical teaching and innovation, we are left with two further difficulties. The first is that the burden of the moral obligation identified by Caplan is not fairly distributed in the Australian community. Our trainees' operative experience is obtained almost exclusively on patients whose care is funded directly by the government – those who are unable, or unwilling, to pay for private health insurance or the cost of the particular hospitalisation. They bear the entire burden of any Caplan-like moral obligation to participate in surgical teaching. In terms of distributive justice little has changed despite the advances made since the 1960s.

Our public hospitals also tend to be the ones where innovative procedures are first introduced into clinical practice; perhaps because the academic environment means that they are more likely to be inventive, or influenced by developments occurring elsewhere. Perhaps there are also historical factors that parallel those applying to surgical training. The private sector appears to be less well adapted to innovation. Operations tend not to be done in private here until the responsible Government instrumentality, Medicare Australia, has included a so-called 'Item Number' in the Medical Benefits Schedule, which relates to the specific service provided. This listing is required before insurance arrangements involving both the patient and the hospital can take effect. In addition, there is an inherent conservatism in private surgical practice, which tends to value reliability more highly than progressiveness, although there are always entrepreneurs. All of the innovations in which I have personally been involved (see p. 269) have been pioneered in the public sector, despite my having access to both sectors.

Recently various governance mechanisms have been introduced in Australia that, while not exactly facilitating surgical innovation, do enable it. In New South Wales a 'Model policy for the safe introduction of new interventional procedures into clinical practice' was developed during 2003 and individual Area Health Services were required to have an appropriate mechanism of oversight in place by the end of September 2004 (NSW Health Department Circular 2003/84). The Australian Government Department of Health and Ageing, along with the Australian Health Ministers' Advisory Council, the Medical Services Advisory Committee, and the New Zealand Ministry of Health have established the Australian and New Zealand Horizon Scanning Network, to provide advance notice of significant new and emerging technologies to health departments in Australia and New Zealand. And there is the Australian Safety and Efficacy Register, New Intervention Procedures – Surgical (ASERNIP-S), an initiative of the Royal Australasian College of Surgeons, funded by the Commonwealth Department of Health and Ageing (see Chapman *et al.*, 2002).

Hopefully, these measures will reduce the inequities, but it remains the case today that those who are unable, or unwilling, to pay for private health insurance or the cost of the particular hospitalization also bear a disproportionate part of the burden of any Caplan-like moral obligation to participate in surgical innovation.

The second difficulty that remains after we have attempted to justify surgical training and innovation in our teaching hospitals is that the patients involved in training and innovation are not recruited as altruistic volunteers.

In comparison, research involving humans is tightly regulated. It is subject to an international agreement and administered in Australia by the National Health and Medical Research Council's National Statement (National Statement, 1999). The oversight is designed, among other things, to minimize participants' risks and to ensure that they are proportionate to the benefits that might be gained. It seeks to ensure that patient autonomy is respected, and that participation is voluntary, free of coercion and based on altruism.[4] Information statements for prospective participants in medical research make it clear that they have an option not to participate, with clauses such as, 'Participation in this study is entirely voluntary: You are in no way obliged to participate and – if you do participate – you can withdraw at any time. Whatever your decision, please be assured that it will not affect your medical treatment or your relationship with medical staff.'[5]

There is no corresponding process for surgical training involving humans. There is no international agreement and no National Statement. In Australia, we have a system that allows individuals who can afford it to opt out by paying privately for 'the doctor of their choice' – someone who is never a trainee.

But, because there is no convention that allows patients to opt out of having their operations performed by trainee surgeons, the patients who remain in the public system are not really altruistic volunteers. They have been selected for use in training by the healthcare delivery system, and are generally not given the option of whether or not they want to be involved. Moreover, at times the consent process can be contaminated by a sort of organized inattention to any additional risks that might be involved in being operated on by a surgical trainee.

The situation for innovative procedures tends to be rather better than training in terms of voluntary participation, and can be expected to improve further when the various governance measures mentioned earlier have been 'rolled out' across the system.

Report cards

Such is the context in which we must judge the implications of surgeons' report cards for surgical training and innovation, assuming that it is within our guile to devise report cards that provide meaningful measurements of surgical outcomes and safety. These cards would have the potential to further confound inequity within the Australian healthcare system. Alternatively they could help improve it. They would be confounding if they ignored any risks associated with surgical training and innovation, or the already-distorted distribution of the risks. They would improve the system if they led to better measurement of the risks and focused attention on the quality of care delivered during the processes.

A recent Australian High Court case (*Chappel v Hart*, 1998) provides some context for the dilemma that report cards pose. An ear, nose and throat surgeon was found negligent as a result of an operation that had affected the quality of his patient's voice. Any risk to her voice was material to her (she was a teacher) and surgeons are obliged to inform their patients of all material risks. She should have been told that there was a risk that the operation would affect her voice: she was not. What made the case a medico-legal precedent was that the finding of negligence made against the surgeon was based, not on the plaintiff convincing the court that she would not have gone ahead with the surgery had she known of the risk, but rather that she would have found a more experienced surgeon to do her operation.

Unfortunately, the decision implies that there is a direct correlation between experience and surgical excellence or safety: the majority of the judges concluded that the risk would have been lower had a more experienced surgeon performed the operation. But more experienced surgeons may well not be any safer than less experienced ones, provided they have all climbed beyond their learning curve, and ultimately the most experienced will become less safe unless they are wise enough to retire before their skills decline. Julian Dussek's concept of a learning curve leading to a 'plateau of experience' seems a better way to understand surgical prowess. A plateau has an up-slope and a down-slope and varies in altitude.

Report cards should provide a better measurement of surgical excellence or safety than the raw numbers assumed in the *Chappel v Hart* decision. Had they been in place, they might have been used by the defendant to counter the more experienced expert witness who testified against him. Perhaps they could have been used to reassure the plaintiff and thus prevent the litigation in the first place. Arguably, they could also have allowed the plaintiff to choose her ENT surgeon from a list of those available according to their individual track records and how much she was prepared to pay, because report cards have the capacity to be used to justify high surgical fees for those with the best records.

In Australia, there is no restriction on how much a surgeon can charge for an operation performed in the private sector. Once they are trained, our surgeons have no further obligation to the public sector and are able, if they wish, to restrict their practices to the private sector. It can be forgotten that their skills were originally acquired at the expense of those who can no longer afford to use these surgeons. Report cards might mean that high fees come to be based more firmly on performance than chutzpah and rhetoric, but there is a danger that they will worsen the inequities we already have between the public and private sectors.

Despite the risk they pose to distributive justice, enabling consumers to select a better surgeon on the basis of measured outcomes and safety remains a powerful motivation to introduce report cards. But the idea that report cards could identify a continuum of surgical excellence, one that would enable all participating surgeons to be placed in ranked order, is both misguided and unnecessary. And it is the continuum that poses the greatest danger to distributive justice, by fuelling competition for the 'top dollar'.

It is misguided because the practical difficulties involved in defining exactly what to measure in order to produce a rank order must devalue the ultimate ranking obtained. The possibilities include practice volumes, outcome measures, survival ratios, complication rates and patient satisfaction. There would be a need to stratify the measurements for the sickness, complexity and difficulty of the cases undertaken by the surgeons and of the standard of the resources available to them. Any result of this complex calculation must involve measurements that are, at least in part, subjective and weightings that are themselves dependent on value judgements.

Fortunately, there is no need to rank surgeons in this way. What the community really requires is a measure of competence. It needs to be able to identify surgeons who have never achieved competence in the procedures they opt to perform. It needs to identify those who are past their prime. It needs to find those whose performance fluctuates into inadequacy from time to time, perhaps because of drug or psychological problems. This would be best accomplished not by attempting to use the report cards to produce an order of ranking, but rather to document an agreed level of adequate performance, which can be followed over time.

Adequacy data should be kept for both individual surgeons and for surgical Units, enabling like to be compared with like. Teaching environments should be compared with one another rather than with the private sector, and individual surgeons' data should recognize whether or not individual cases were used in teaching or innovation. The data should also be used to identify 'outliers'. Those who appear to be underachieving can then be investigated, allowing remedial action to be taken if appropriate. Those who appear to be overachieving may be able to provide insights that could help advance surgery further.

Used in this way, report cards should have a positive impact on surgical training and innovation. Recognizing that teaching and innovation are occurring is fundamental to any potential benefit. Ignoring it would serve to keep the issue underground and make surgeons reluctant to engage in training. It puts trainees in an impossible position if they are expected suddenly to be the equal of fully trained surgeons. Training occurs in Units that have all been formally accredited for the purpose. Innovation in surgery is subject to an increasingly sophisticated level of governance and volunteerism. There can be no argument that an adequate standard of care needs to be delivered, despite the presence of either teaching or innovation. The prospect of being compared with peer Units and found to be an outlier would be a powerful incentive to optimize supervision and case-selection for trainees. Identifying the cases that have been involved in teaching and innovation in the card dataset will also improve our ability to accurately measure the risks incurred by the patients involved.

I am reminded of a favourite aphorism of one of my surgical mentors (Jerome DeCosse, personal communication, 1982). Whenever anyone suggested using some new-fangled piece of equipment in surgery, he would remind us that 'A fool with a tool is still a fool.' Surgeons' report cards need to be used wisely.

Notes

1. The Gorton Government (1968–71) introduced a schedule of doctors' fees on which health insurance arrangements are based. The schedule applied only to services provided in hospitals and thus contained mostly surgical services. Originally based on the Australian Medical Association's list of recommended fees, it was taken over by the Federal Government, and health insurance companies' rebates were set so as to return all but a small 'gap' that remained the responsibility of the patient to pay.

Adherence to the schedule resulted in a gap of no more than 5 dollars initially. But surgeons were still able to charge more than the listed fee, resulting when they did in a bigger gap than 5 dollars. Access to public hospitals as non-chargeable patients was subject to a means test and senior doctors in the public hospitals provided their services on an honorary basis.

2. The Whitlam Government (1972–75) introduced Medibank. With this change, the Federal Government of Australia started to pay the majority of most doctors' fees. The payments included general practitioner services provided outside hospitals, where the government paid 85 per cent of the scheduled fee. Doctors could bill their patients 'up front' (the patients were subsequently reimbursed the 85 per cent), or they could choose to 'bulk bill' the patients, charging the 85 per cent of the scheduled fee directly to the Government and waiving the remainder. The government reimbursed patients 75 per cent of the scheduled fee for services provided in hospitals and health insurance providers reimbursed the remainder. Charges over the schedule resulted in a gap for which the patient was responsible. Access to public hospitals as non-chargeable patients remained subject to a means test. Senior doctors in the public hospitals were paid an hourly rate for services that had previously been provided on an honorary basis.

3. The Hawke Government (1983–91) introduced Medicare. It allowed all Australians to access public hospitals as non-chargeable patients irrespective of their means. An assumption that senior doctors would provide services to these patients at the hourly rates that had applied under Medibank led to much industrial unrest (The Doctors' Dispute), and ultimately revised payment schedules were developed for senior doctors treating non-chargeable patients in public hospitals that were accepted by the doctors.

4. However it can still be argued that many individuals who participate in research that involves risk (as opposed to inconvenience) do so mostly in the hope that they might personally be helped by the intervention that is being tried. The same cannot be said of the risks associated with learner surgery.

5. Sydney South Western Area Health Service Ethics Review Committee (Central Zone) has an on-line application form template with advice to applicants that includes the statement quoted above as a suggestion for inclusion in the Participant Information Statement.

References

Bockler, D., Geoghan, J., Kleni, M. *et al.* (1999). Implications of laparoscopic cholecystectomy for surgical residency training. *Journal of the Society of Laparoendoscopic Surgeons*, **3**, 19–22.

Caplan, A. L. (1988). Is there an obligation to participate in biomedical research? In *The Use of Human Beings in Research, with Special Reference to Clinical Trial*, ed. S. F. Spicker, I. Alon, A. de Vries and H. T. Engelhardt. Dordrecht: Kluwer, pp. 229–48.

Chapman, A. E., Geerdes, B., Hewett, P. *et al.* (2002). Systematic review of dynamic graciloplasty in the treatment of faecal incontinence. *British Journal of Surgery*, **89**, 138–53.

Chappel v Hart (1998) HCA 55.

Clarke, S. and Oakley, J. (2004). Informed consent and surgeons' performance. *Journal of Medicine and Philosophy*, **29**, 11–35.

Gawande, A. (2002). Education of a knife. In *Complications: A Surgeon's Notes on an Imperfect Science*. London: Profile Books, pp. 11–34.

Lau, H., Patil, N. G., Yuen, W. K. and Lee, F. (2002). Learning curve for unilateral endoscopic totally extraperitoneal (TEP) inguinal hernioplasty. *Surgical Endoscopy*, **16**, 1724–8.

Learning from Bristol: the report of the public inquiry into children's heart surgery at the Bristol Royal Infirmary, 1984–1995 (1995). Command Paper: CM 5207 http://www.bristol-inquiry.org.uk/evidence/index.htm.

Marston, R. A., Cobb, A. G. and Bentley, G. J. (1996). Stanmore compared with Charnley total hip replacement: A prospective study of 413 arthroplasties. *Journal of Bone and Joint Surgery (British Volume)*, **78**, 178–84.

National Statement on Ethical Conduct in Research Involving Humans (1999). Issued by the National Health and Medical Research Council (NHMRC) in accordance with the NHMRC Act (1992). Commonwealth of Australia.

Paisley, A. M., Baldwin, P. J. and Paterson-Brown, S. (2001). Validity of surgical simulation for the assessment of operative skill. *British Journal of Surgery*, **88**, 1525–32.

Sheil, A. G., Thompson, J. F., Gallagher, N. D. *et al.* (1987). Initial report of the Australian National Pilot Liver Transplantation Programme. *Medical Journal of Australia*, **147**, 372–80.

Solomon, M. J. and Eyers, A. A. (1996). Laparoscopic rectopexy using mesh fixation with a spiked chromium staple. *Diseases of the Colon and Rectum*, **39**, 279–84.

Solomon, M. J., Young, C. J., Eyers, A. A. and Roberts, R. A. (2002). Randomized clinical trial of laparoscopic versus open abdominal rectopexy for rectal prolapse. *British Journal of Surgery*, **89**, 35–9.

Thompson, J. F. and de Wilt, J. H. (2001). Isolated limb perfusion in the management of patients with recurrent limb melanoma: an important but limited role [comment]. *Annals of Surgical Oncology*, **8**, 564–5.

Thomson, B. N., Civil, I. D., Danne, P. D. *et al.* (2001). Trauma training in Australia and New Zealand: results of a survey of advanced surgical trainees. *Australian and New Zealand Journal of Surgery*, **71**, 83–8.

Turton, E. P., McKenzie, S., Weston, M. J. *et al.* (1997). Optimising a varicose vein service to reduce recurrence. *Annals of the Royal College of Surgeons of England*, **79**, 451–4.

Walker, B. (2004). Special Commission of Inquiry into Campbelltown and Camden Hospitals. Final Report. www.lawlink.nsw.gov.au/special_commission.

Watson, D. A., Baigrie, R. J. and Jamieson, G. G. (1996). A learning curve for laparoscopic fundoplication. Definable, avoidable or a waste of time? *Annals of Surgery*, **224**, 198–203.

Young, C. J., Solomon, M. J., Eyers, A. A. *et al.* (1999). Evolution of the pelvic pouch procedure at one institution: the first 100 cases. *Australian and New Zealand Journal of Surgery*, **69**, 438–42.

19

Doctors' report cards: a legal perspective

Ian Freckelton

Crockett Chambers, Melbourne; University of Sydney, and
Monash University, Melbourne, Australia

Introduction

The concept of report cards for doctors is one aspect of accountability for medical practitioners' conduct, success rates, efficiency and effectiveness in communication. Report cards for doctors and for health institutions at this stage have no formal legal status, although, like a variety of other documents, they have the potential to be utilized in an evidentiary sense as a yardstick for delineating acceptable from actionable conduct. In the past, ethical codes of conduct and practice, guidelines and protocols have all been used by both the civil courts and disciplinary tribunals as indicia of whether medical practitioners who have not complied fully with them have breached their duty of care to patients. An important question for the future is whether doctors' report cards can, or should, fulfil a similar function. If so, a secondary question is how they can be framed so as to minimize the potential for misuse.

The impetus toward enhanced professional accountability has been generated and facilitated by the law for two decades. It has become a core characteristic of latter-day tort law and disciplinary law, in particular, as the informed consent revolution continues to redefine what is required of medical practitioners' interactions with their patients.

This chapter contextualizes the phenomenon of doctors' report cards within the impetus toward greater accountability by health service providers. It contends that doctors' report cards are an inevitable development, against which doctors' performance to some extent will be measured, but that care needs to be taken in developing such report cards so that expectations are reasonable, so that the contents of report cards achieve their objectives and so that they do not have counter-productive consequences. In particular, it is contended that report cards should be framed in such a way and contain sufficient disclaimers for it to be unlikely that courts and tribunals will utilize them uncritically as the ultimate measuring point for the work of medical practitioners.

Informed Consent and Clinician Accountability: The Ethics of Report Cards on Surgeon Performance.
Steve Clarke and Justin Oakley (eds.). Published by Cambridge University Press. © Cambridge
University Press 2007.

The changing culture

Many have remarked upon the shift in countries such as the United States, Canada, Australia and to a lesser degree the United Kingdom, away from deference to the medical profession towards an insistence on provision of relevant information so as to enable the exercise of patient choices. This is part of the demand that professional paternalism and elitism be abandoned in favour of participatory decision-making between health professionals and patients, wherever possible.

The United States

The affirmative duty to disclose medical risks was first imposed upon the medical profession by the decision of the United States Court of Appeals for the District of Columbia in *Canterbury v Spence*, 464 F 2d 772 at 784 (DC Cir 1972) in which Robinson J. held that 'Respect for the patient's right of self-determination on particular therapy demands a standard set by law for physicians rather than one which physicians may or may not impose upon themselves.' However, proof of negligence and of its consequences for a given patient is far from straightforward. A case which has prompted considerable controversy in this regard has been that of *Johnson v Kokemoor* 199 Wis 2d 615, 545 NW 2d 495 (1996). Ms Johnson sued Dr Kokemoor for failing to inform her adequately of the risks associated with surgery to remove a brain aneurysm. A jury returned a verdict in Ms Johnson's favour, finding that 'a reasonable person in the plaintiff's position would have refused to consent to surgery by the defendant if she had been fully informed of its attendant risks and advantages' (at 620–1). On appeal, Dr Kokemoor argued that the trial court erred by admitting evidence of his limited experience in performing the particular type of operation, which he had failed to disclose fully, and a comparison of the 'morbidity and mortality rates for this type of surgery among experienced surgeons and inexperienced surgeons like himself' (at 621). Specifically, Dr Kokemoor had reassured Ms Johnson that the 'risks associated with her surgery were comparable to the risks attending a tonsillectomy, appendectomy or gall bladder operation', namely around 2 per cent. However, this significantly understated the risks; the medical studies he had relied on 'reported morbidity and mortality rates of fifteen [15] per cent' for even the most accomplished surgeons, and other evidence fixed the rate at 30 per cent when the surgery was performed by a doctor of Dr Kokemoor's limited experience (at 644).

The Wisconsin Supreme Court upheld the admissibility of evidence concerning Kokemoor's limited experience and the relative risks of morbidity and mortality. Cautioning that informed consent cases are necessarily 'fact-driven and context-specific', the court stopped short of 'always requir[ing] physicians to give patients comparative risk evidence in statistical terms to obtain informed consent'. Nonetheless, it held that '[t]he fundamental issue in an informed consent case is less a question of how a physician chooses to explain the panoply of treatment options and risks necessary to a patient's informed consent than a question of assessing whether a patient has been advised that such options and risks exist' (at 646–7). It found that, as Dr Kokemoor had elected to explain the risks confronting the plaintiff in statistical terms, he could not complain when the plaintiff demonstrated that Dr Kokemoor had 'dramatically understated' those risks by also using statistical evidence (at 647).

Canada

In 1980 the Canadian Supreme Court also recognized an obligation on the part of medical practitioners to provide substantial information to patients, although it was cautious in its usage of the expression 'informed consent' (*Reibl v Hughes* [1980] 2 SCR 880; see also *Hopp v Lepp* [1980] 2 SCR 192 at 210).

In *Ciarlariello v Schacter* [1993] 2 SCR 119 the Supreme Court was asked again to consider the provision of patient consent, on this occasion in the context of testing for a cerebral aneurysm and where consent may have been withdrawn. It held that every patient's right to bodily integrity encompasses the right to determine what medical procedures will be accepted and the extent to which they will be accepted. It emphasized that the right to decide what is to be done to one's own body is based on the principle of autonomy and includes the right to be free from medical treatment to which a person does not consent.

The Supreme Court of Canada was invited to reconsider its position in *Reibl* 17 years later in *Arndt v Smith* [1997] 2 SCR 539, a case in which Ms Arndt sued Dr Smith for costs associated with rearing her daughter, who was congenitally injured by chickenpox that Ms Arndt contracted during her pregnancy. She contended that had Dr Smith properly advised her of the risk of injury to her foetus, she would have terminated the pregnancy and avoided the costs she had instead incurred. The majority in the Supreme Court held that, when determining whether the loss claimed by Ms Arndt was caused by Mr Smith's failure to advise of the risk, the court should adopt the test set out in *Reibl v Hughes*, observing that the test relies on a combination of objective and subjective factors in order to determine whether the failure to disclose actually caused the harm of which the plaintiff complains. The test requires that the court consider what the reasonable patient in the plaintiff's circumstances would have done if faced with the same situation. The trier of fact must take into consideration any 'particular concerns' of the patient and any 'special considerations affecting the particular patient' in determining whether the patient would have refused treatment if given all the information about the possible risks.

The majority held that it was appropriate to infer from the evidence in the particular case that a reasonable person in the plaintiff's position would not have decided to terminate her pregnancy in the face of the very small increased risk to the foetus posed by her exposure to the virus which causes chickenpox. While Ms Arndt did make a very general inquiry concerning the risks associated with maternal chickenpox, the majority found that there was nothing to indicate to the doctor that she had a particular concern in this regard. It upheld the finding of the trial judge that the failure to disclose some of the risks to the foetus associated with maternal chickenpox did not affect Ms Arndt's decision to continue the pregnancy to term. It followed that the failure to disclose did not cause the financial losses for which she sought compensation.

The United Kingdom

In the United Kingdom the *Bolam* test (*Bolam v Friern Hospital Management Committee* [1957] 1 WLR 582 at 586–7) as reformulated in *Sidaway v Governors of Bethlem Royal Hospital* [1985] AC 871 at 881 has been the law for in the order of 40 years: '[A] doctor is not negligent if he acts in accordance with a practice accepted at the time as proper by a responsible body of medical opinion even though other doctors adopt a different practice.' Lord Diplock in *Sidaway* (at 895) held that the Bolam test extended to the provision of information by doctors to patients about risk. As he put it, to decide what risks the existence of which a patient should be warned about and the terms of such a warning is as much an exercise of professional skill and judgement as any other part of a doctor's comprehensive duty of care to a patient. However, the majority in *Sidaway* declined to apply the doctrine in *Canterbury v Spence* (see above).

The *Bolam* test was moderated to some extent by the House of Lords in 1997 in *Bolitho v City and Hackney Health Authority* (1997) UKHL 46; (1998) AC 232 where it was held that 'in cases of diagnosis and treatment there are cases where, despite a body of professional opinion sanctioning the defendant's conduct, the defendant can properly be held liable for negligence [on the basis that] . . . . it cannot be demonstrated . . . that the body of opinion relied upon is reasonable or responsible.' The evolving position in the United Kingdom was pushed to the next step by the House of Lords in the specific context of failure to warn of risks in *Chester v Afshar* [2004] UKHL 41. A surgeon had operated on a patient's back and did not warn her of the small (1 per cent–2 per cent) but unavoidable risk that the operation might have a seriously adverse result, known as cauda equina syndrome. This is what ensued for the patient, although it was in no way the result of procedural negligence by the surgeon. The patient sued, alleging not that she would never have had the operation if she had been given advice about the risks but that she would not have consented to the surgery on the day and would have consulted with others about whether to submit to the surgery.

The scenario divided the House of Lords 3:2. At first instance, the trial judge found the surgeon liable in damages. The House of Lords by a bare majority affirmed the trial judge's decision, all members emphasizing the contemporary significance of warnings about risk. For the purposes of this chapter, the approach to obligatory warnings by a medical practitioner is the most important aspect of the decision. Many of the statements by the Law Lords are indicative of an increasing international convergence of judicial (and community views) about patient entitlements. It is significant too, that much of the rhetoric from the Law Lords was in terms of patient 'rights', and that they expressed themselves in unequivocal language.

Lord Bingham, for instance, stressed that the obligation of the surgeon to advise the patient of the risks of cauda equina syndrome 'is not in doubt. Nor is its rationale: to enable adult patients of sound mind to make for themselves decisions intimately affecting their own lives and bodies' (at [5]). Lord Steyn was more expansive, holding that what he termed 'the correlative rights and duties of the patient and the surgeon' must be kept in mind:

The starting point is that every individual of adult years and sound mind has a right to decide what may or may not be done with his or her body. Individuals have a right to make important medical decisions affecting their lives for themselves: they have the right to make decisions which doctors regard as ill advised. Surgery performed without the informed consent of the patient is unlawful (at [14]).

He emphasized that a surgeon owes a legal duty to a patient to warn him or her in general terms of possible serious risks involved in the procedure, the only exception being where it would be contrary to the best interests of the patient. Lord Steyn commented, 'In modern law medical paternalism no longer rules and a patient has a prima facie right to be informed by a surgeon of a small, but well established, risk of serious injury as a result of surgery' (at [16]). By way of rationale, he identified that a rule requiring a doctor to abstain from performing an operation without the informed consent of a patient serves two purposes: it tends to avoid the occurrence of the particular physical injury the risk of which a patient is not prepared to accept, and it ensures that due respect is given to the autonomy and dignity of each patient (at [18]).

It was with this philosophical background that the House of Lords approached the issue of whether causation was established sufficiently for the plaintiff to be awarded compensatory damages. By majority it found that there was causation, as a matter of public policy, in spite of the fact that the plaintiff had not proved that, had it not been for the surgeon's failure to provide her with information about risks, she would not have submitted to the operation.

Australia

In 1992 the Australian High Court followed to some degree in the United States tradition in *Rogers v Whitaker* (1992) 175 CLR 479. In the context of a woman particularly anxious about the possible results of an operation upon her vision, it rejected the United Kingdom *Bolam* test and in its place changed the yardstick, following the North American example, and focusing upon the needs of patients for information. It did so in the context of advice to a patient of the risk of succumbing to a remote risk (1:14 000) of ophthalmic surgery and contracting sympathetic ophthalmia, thereby losing sight in both eyes. The patient had expressed anxiety about risks to her vision and had been reassured by the surgeon.

The High Court held that the law imposes on a medical practitioner a duty to exercise reasonable care and skill in the provision of professional advice and treatment. It classified the duty as a 'single comprehensive duty covering all the ways in which a doctor is called upon to exercise his skill and judgement' and endorsed the view to this effect of Lord Diplock in *Sidaway*, finding that the duty extends to the examination, diagnosis and treatment of the patient, as well as the provision of information in an appropriate case. The Court held that medical practitioners must advise patients of what it termed 'material risks' inherent in proposed treatment. It held that a risk is material if 'in the circumstances of the particular case, a reasonable person in the patient's position, if warned of the risk, would be likely to attach significance to it or if the medical practitioner is or should reasonably be aware that the particular patient, if warned of the risk, would be likely to attach significance to it' (at 490). It expressed this responsibility to be subject to the doctrine of therapeutic privilege, under which in certain limited circumstances doctors remain free to withhold information from patients on the basis of the significant countertherapeutic effects that provision of the information would be likely to have. The court grappled with the question of causation. McHugh, Kirby and Gummow JJ specifically endorsed the English 'subjective approach', and found that the question to be asked is what the particular patient would have done in terms of treatment or a procedure, if given the proper warning by the medical practitioner.

After just under a decade, the High Court in *Rosenberg v Percival* [2001] 205 CLR 434; was urged to reconsider its 'material risks' test in light of the many criticisms that had been made of its ruling in *Rogers v Whitaker* (see e.g. Kerridge and Mitchell, 1994; Robertson, 1991; Schuck, 1994; Olbourne, 1998; Mendelson, 1998; McInness, 1998; Girgis, Thomson and Ward, 2000). It declined to do so, emphatically endorsing its previous approach. Justice Kirby wrote the most extensive judgment. He held that reasons of both principle and policy supported the stringency of the *Rogers v Whitaker* approach: 'the rule is a recognition of individual autonomy that is to be viewed in the wider context of an emerging appreciation of basic human rights and human dignity. There is no reason to diminish the law's insistence, to the greatest extent possible, upon prior, informed agreement to invasive treatment, save for that which is required in an emergency or otherwise out of necessity' (at [145]). He held that it is desirable to recognize that defects in communication demand the imposition of minimum legal obligations, so that 'even those providers who are in a hurry, or who may have comparatively less skill or inclination for communication, are obliged to pause and provide warnings of the kind that *Rogers* mandates' (at [145]). He observed that the collateral advantages of such an approach include redressing to some degree the risks of conflicts of interest and duty which a provider may sometimes face in favouring one healthcare procedure over another, and to redress the inherent power inequality between the professional provider and a vulnerable patient (at [145]).

However, the obligation to provide information sufficient to enable patient decision-making is only part of the guidance given latterly to health practitioners by the High Court. In the important decision of *Chappel v Hart* (1998) 195 CLR 232, a different aspect of the advice required to be given to patients was the focus of the litigation. The patient required a Dohlman's Pouch procedure to address a blockage in her throat. As in *Rogers v Whitaker*, the patient was concerned about the risks of the procedure and asked about whether there was a specific adverse result that could ensue from the operation. This meant that, like Mrs Whitaker, she fell into the category of patients for the purpose of provision of information about 'material risks' for whom extra information needs to be supplied because of their especial anxieties or concerns (see too the patient in *Chester v Afshar*). The surgeon simply reassured her. Ultimately, it was conceded that the surgeon should have warned her that there was a possibility that the patient's oesophagus could be punctured, that if certain bacteria should be present, then mediastinitis could ensue, that in such circumstances she could suffer damage to her laryngeal nerve, and thus that her voice could be affected (see Bennett and Freckelton, 2006).

As in the later English case of *Chester v Afshar*, the more difficult question to be decided in *Chappel v Hart* was whether this was all the information that should have been provided by the surgeon. The alternative in *Chappel v Hart* was that the surgeon might also have communicated to her that he had performed only a modest number of such procedures, and that a surgeon who had performed many more would carry a lower risk of setting in train the events that could lead to an adverse impact on her voice – namely, puncturing her oesophagus. The other question that the High Court considered was whether the failure to provide her with information about risks brought about any harm, given that the procedure in this instance was not elective, as it was in *Rogers*, but had to be performed to avoid the patient dying.

By majority, the Court held that the patient had suffered harm by reason of the failure of the surgeon to respond adequately to his patient's inquiry. It held that she was deprived of the chance of having the operation performed by a more experienced surgeon who would have run a lower risk of the adverse results. The patient at trial testified under oath that had she been told of the risks of the operation she would have sought out the most experienced surgeon available so as to minimise the risks that she was running. Justice Gaudron was the strongest on the point, holding that it was the surgeon's duty to inform the patient that there were more experienced surgeons practising in the field. Justice Kirby inclined to a similar effect, commenting that 'intuition and common sense suggest that the greater the skill and more frequent the performance, the less the risk of perforation' (at [97]). The court also endorsed the position that where a person suffers an injury in the immediate aftermath of a tortious act, there is a rebuttable presumption that the tort has caused the injury.

Many aspects of the decision have proved controversial. At one level the analysis of Gaudron J., in particular, has much to commend it in terms of obligating doctors to supply to patients a category of information likely to make a difference as to whether or not they provide consent to a surgical or other form of health intervention. The information required by a patient, after all, extends beyond just the actuarial risks applicable to a particular procedure. There are other factors that bear upon the predictable outcome. Included among these are the proficiency of the practitioner (including his or her experience in the procedure), and the conditions obtaining at the particular healthcare facility. However, it has been pointed out that there is also a significant downside to a common law or legislated obligation to provide information about levels of proficiency and experience which could potentially impact on the risks run by a particular patient in submitting to the procedure at the hands of the particular practitioner (see, e.g. Freckelton, 1999).

Under the formulation of the duty expressed by Gaudron J., if the healthcare practitioner knows that another (more experienced or more skilful) practitioner may run a lower risk in a procedure, in particular a surgical procedure, the practitioner must tell the patient because that knowledge could make a difference to the patient's provision of consent.

The environment within which report cards are emerging

A fact-finding dilemma for curial and disciplinary decision-makers is to gauge whether what has been done by a medical practitioner in a particular instance is in conformity with accepted practice, common conduct or whether the doctor is an outlier, unrepresentative of the community of views about orthodox or at least minimum standards of practice. Doctors' report cards are coming into being in a legal environment in which both tort and disciplinary law regularly seek yardsticks against which to measure treatment outcomes and doctors' conduct. Doctors' report cards are just one of the yardsticks. They sit alongside:

- codes of ethics;
- codes of practice;
- clinical guidelines;

- hospital protocols and regulations;
- statistical analyses of levels and types of service;
- legal decisions of the courts and tribunals; and
- disciplinary body advisories.

Part of the new culture in which report cards take their place is that in the early part of the twenty-first century, dramatically increasing amounts of information are being made available to consumers in order to enable them to make more informed evaluations of whether they wish to have procedures undertaken on them, by which doctor, when, in what circumstances, and at which facility. Examples of such information are the material made available by the National Health Service in the United Kingdom about 'primary care trusts' and about hospitals, as well as by the Society of Cardiothoracic Surgeons in relation to mortality rates for coronary artery bypass surgery from the fewer than 200 United Kingdom cardiac surgeons. Controversy continues to attach to the data made available and the uses to which both the public and those working in institutions can put the information (see Marshall, Mohammed and Rouse, 2004). As of April 2006, the United Kingdom Healthcare Commission published the risk-adjusted survival rates for cardiac surgery, reported both in terms of cardiac units and individual surgeons (http://heartsurgery. healthcare commission.org.uk/Survival.aspx). The new system is further discussed in the introduction to this volume.

In a number of areas it has already become the norm for medical practitioners to make available information as to the apparent success of procedures, the incidence of rehospitalisations, the incidence of relapses and the rates of death in the aftermath of surgery. There is a background to the provision of such information in respect of cardiac surgery in both the United States and now the United Kingdom (see, e.g. Green and Wintfeld, 1992; Neil, Clarke and Oakley, 2004), although in North America such documentation has been generated in relation to fields of medicine as diverse as caesarean section cases (see, e.g. Pennsylvania Cost Care Containment Council, 1999) and diabetes treatment (see, e.g. Bavley, 2006). In the United Kingdom an impetus toward provision of individual practitioner data was given by the revelations flowing from the Bristol Royal Infirmary Inquiry of 2001 and the government's commitment, first announced in 2004, to publish additional information about individual consultant outcomes (Bristol Royal Infirmary Inquiry, 2001; Milburn, 2002). For the United States report cards have been regarded by some as an incident of managed care (see, e.g. Coile, 1999; Kaplan, 1998), and praised or reviled accordingly.

Part and parcel of the increased access to consumer information is the making available to patients and potential patients of information about conditions placed upon doctors' registration or licensure status, as well as information about civil actions successfully undertaken against them. Thus, for instance, in respect of Californian medical practitioners, from 1 January

1998, malpractice judgments and awards of any amount are disclosed by the Californian Medical Board (see *http://www.medbd.ca.gov/*). However, the policy issues relating to making publicly accessible all issues pertinent to the registered status of medical practitioners are far from straightforward. Many a patient would want to know about whether a doctor's substance dependency, bipolar disorder, sexual behaviours, cognitive decline or physical illness had led to a condition, limitation or restriction being placed upon their registration: whether by voluntary act on the part of the doctor or by order of a regulatory authority. However, doing so discloses the practitioner's personal health information and is likely in the information age to devastate their capacity to reintegrate into the practising community. It can preclude rehabilitation and discourage doctors from seeking the medical assistance that they require for conditions impairing their capacity to practise safely and competently.

The legal status of report cards

As yet there is little by way of authority about the likely impact of doctors' report cards on civil actions for negligence or upon disciplinary hearings. However, by analogy with the other kinds of reference points mentioned above, what can be said is that report cards will constitute a further information source against which doctors will be measured. When a doctor's results from, say, cardiac surgery, are below that which is statistically 'normal', the doctor is likely to be required to explain why this is so. An onus will shift, in an evidentiary sense, to justify why performance is substandard from a statistical perspective. On occasions, this will be a straightforward task – on the basis of their patient profiles, for instance – but on other occasions the statistics have the potential to bear eloquent witness to a pattern of unacceptably poor performance.

Two particular parallels can be identified. In Australia it is common for professional service review committees to be called upon to hear allegations of overservicing against medical practitioners (see Bell, 2005). Such allegations derive from statistical review of doctors' consultation or prescription patterns (see, e.g. *Yung v Adams* (197) 80 FCR 453; *Oreb v Willcock* [2004] FCA 1520; *Hutcher v Cohn* [2004] FCA 1548) when they deviate significantly from the mean. On occasions, by reason for instance of their particular form of practice, doctors are able to justify 'by exceptional circumstances' their levels of service and prescribing; on other occasions the statistics reveal aberrant and problematic forms of practice.

Another yardstick that has been utilized on occasions is clinical guidelines. In a number of decisions in the United Kingdom and Australia, for instance, reference has been made by courts to clinical guidelines to ascertain accepted and conventional approaches to dealing with presenting symptomatology (see Freckelton, 2002). Thus, in an English case where the standards of the cervical screening program had not been complied with, slides having been labelled 'negative' for no satisfactory reason, the Court of Appeal declined to interfere with the trial judge's decision which utilized the standards as a yardstick for competent practice (*Penney, Palmer and Cannon v East Kent Health Authority* [2000] Lloyd's Rep Med 41). In the important decision of *Airedale NHS Trust v Bland* [1993] AC 789, the House of Lords considered guidelines produced by the Medical Ethics Committee of the British Medical Association in relation to the discontinuance of artificial nutrition and hydration for patients in a permanent vegetative state. Lord Goff stated that a doctor acting in conformity with the guidelines would be acting in accord with a responsible and competent body of relevant professional opinion. The importance of clinical guidelines, including in the legal context, has led the National Health Service (1996) to issue guidance upon the assessment of guidelines, recommending that they should be technically valid, reproducible, reliable, cost-effective, representative, clinically applicable, flexible, clear, reviewable, clearly documented and amenable to clinical audit.

Forms and terms of report cards

It is apparent though, that it is simplistic to speak in terms of doctors' report cards generally – there are many forms. An example is that to which reference has previously been made – information about the disciplinary history of a medical practitioner. However, there are many others. Some report cards contain little by way of quantitative data. They are principally qualitative and dependent upon doctors' self-reports or patient satisfaction reports (see, e.g. Lowe, 2005). By contrast, some report cards deal in raw numbers and focus upon the incidence of adverse outcomes in the aftermath of particular procedures. Some enable ready comparison of practitioners' data against those of others. Some are framed explicitly against averages and include risk-adjustments (e.g. the United Kingdom Healthcare Commission's data in relation to cardiac surgery – see above); others do not.

An issue for the legal system relates to the advantages perceived by medical practitioners in generating such information (voluntarily or by compliance) and in portraying such information in a particular way. The motives can vary significantly. Zuger (2005) has commented:

Past efforts to grade doctors have been clumsy at best. The names on all the 'Best Doctor' lists tend to reflect old boys' networks rather than actual merit. Internet sites posting doctors' credentials let consumers weed out true miscreants, but not evaluate the remaining multitudes. But far more precise rankings lie just over the horizon, with doctors publicly graded and paid by the good results they achieve. Medicare announced the first such program this winter: a pilot 'pay for performance initiative' will reward large group practices with bonuses for keeping their elderly patients vaccinated, their cardiac patients properly medicated and their diabetics well controlled. It is only a matter of time before individual doctors are similarly ranked and paid.

What has become apparent is that report cards pose at least six major risks:
- They can be utilized by individuals and institutions in an attempt to obtain a perceived competitive advantage over professional rivals;
- They may result in employment pressures for 'under-rating' doctors;
- Comparative data may be deceptive by failing to include relevant information or by being skewed in order to present unreliable impressions;
- They may lead to the practice of defensive medicine;
- They may lead to patients with a risky profile or who may worsen the statistics being excluded from procedures; and
- They may be misunderstood by courts and tribunals, and so become reified as the gold standard against which doctors' performance and outcomes in all circumstances should be compared.

Regulatory issues have emerged in relation to some doctors' probity in respect of provision of performance data, and also in respect of misleading claims based upon proffered data. Another difficulty in an increasingly competitive environment for provision of medical services is for practitioners to act counter-therapeutically in an effort to enhance their report cards artificially. There is a risk of doctors avoiding patients with high risk profiles – such as advanced age, difficult clinical conditions or risk factors such as previous treatment failure, relapse, or a history of smoking (see e.g. Moscucci *et al.*, 2005; Fiscella and Franks, 1999). Furthermore, there is a danger that the most experienced, best resourced and most expensive practitioners will be in a position to load their success rates, while those working in less advantaged conditions may appear by comparison to have impoverished skill levels by reason of artefacts in figures and factors that will adversely impact upon their apparent rates of success and proficiency.

An aspect of the risks of inaccurate perception is that doctors' 'success rates' are affected by many factors. They extend beyond the actuarial calculation of success and relapse rates for certain procedures. They include the functionality of particular teams within units, hygiene practices and infection rates at particular institutions, as well as factors as elusive as morale, resource prioritisation and workplace satisfaction amongst practitioners and those working with them.

In addition, there are many factors that, in principle, require fine-grained analysis of medical practitioners' safety and performance. While by a certain age surgeons' performance will drop away, it does not follow that with experience necessarily come higher levels of performance and lower rates of error. Suboptimal performance can be caused by multifarious factors such as: the emotional or psychological condition of the practitioner; the state of freshness or exhaustion or stress of the practitioner; the recent drinking habits of the practitioner; the level of work satisfaction or morale of the practitioner; the quality of peer review engaged in by the practitioner; the level of supervision exercised over the practitioner; and the extent of ongoing medical education engaged in by the practitioner.

Naturally, such personal information cannot be made publicly available, even if it could be collated. In short, while coarse-grained information such as actuarial data on procedures' success rates and even practitioners' success rates in respect of a particular procedure are helpful data, the concerned patient would profit from much in the way of additional information indicating trends and other factors. Even sophisticated data such as those of the United Kingdom Healthcare Commission in respect of cardiac surgery are obfusc in respect of the adjustments caused by particular risk factors. This means that their utility for a given patient with a particular risk factor or constellation of risk factors is limited.

In 1998 Epstein (p. 1691) argued that 'Most of all, we need to find better ways to use quality reporting to empower purchasers and consumers and improve quality of care.' The situation has changed little, with the succeeding years bringing an avalanche of publicly available information about diverse procedures, individual medical practitioners and specific healthcare facilities.

From both the perspective of effectively providing information to members of the public (the ostensible reason for report cards) and minimizing the risks of report cards being misunderstood in courts and tribunals, there is a need for sophisticated presentation of cocktails of relevant information. As such information will be utilized in civil litigation and disciplinary forums whenever there is deviation from or adherence to norms within such data, the way in which the data are presented will be vital.

There is a need for co-ordinated efforts to construct report cards in such a way that they do not discourage practitioners from procedures that are in the public interest, but which meaningfully assist patients in important decision-making, and provide a level of assistance to courts and tribunals in need of measures against which to assess the conduct and performance of medical practitioners. As advised by the National Health System Guidelines on Guidelines (see above), the framing of report cards needs to be done in such a way as to ensure flexibility and to communicate effectively the limits of the information contained in them. What follows, amongst other things, is that such data must neither be too prescriptive nor framed in such a way as too readily to permit the interpretation that adverse inferences or assumptions should necessarily be made in respect of outliers or low/high scorers. If this objective is not achieved, the risk is that the legal system will inadvertently misuse and misunderstand the information in report cards. The challenge is genuinely to enhance patient decision-making (without generating alarm or complacency) and to avoid medicine by statistics and uncritical trial by numbers.

References

Bavley, A. (2006). Diabetes report cards: care makes strides. *Kansas City Star*, 8 February.

Bell, A. (2005). Protecting medicare services: trials of a peer review scheme. *Journal of Law and Medicine*, **13**, 29–105.

Bennett, B. and Freckelton, I. (2006). Life after the Ipp reforms: medical negligence law. In *Disputes and Dilemmas in Health Law*, eds. I. Freckelton and K. Petersen. Sydney: The Federation Press.

Bristol Royal Infirmary Inquiry (2001). *Learning From Bristol: the Report of the Public Inquiry into Children's Heart Surgery at the Bristol Royal Infirmary 1984–1995*. Cmnd 5207.

Coile, R. C. (1999). Challenges for physician executives in the millennium marketplace. *Physician Executive*, **25**, 8.

Department of Human Services, Victoria (2003). *Regulation of the Health Professions in Victoria*. http://www.dhs.vic.gov.au/pdpd/workforce/downloads/regulation_health_professions_vic.pdf, visited 5 March 2006.

Duckett, S., Hunter, L. and Rassaby, A. (1999). *Health Services Policy Review. Discussion Paper*, Melbourne: Victorian Government Department of Human Services.

Epstein, A. M. (1998). Rolling down the runway: the challenge ahead for quality report cards. *Journal of the American Medical Association*, **279**, 1691.

Fiscella, K. and Franks, P. (1999). Patients' education and doctors' report cards. *Annals of Internal Medicine*, **131**, 745–51.

Freckelton, I. (1999). Materiality of risk and proficiency assessment: the onset of health care report cards? *Journal of Law and Medicine*, **6**, 313–18.

Freckelton, I. (2001). Rogers v Whitaker Reconsidered. *Journal of Law and Medicine*, **9**, 5–11.

Freckelton, I. (2002). Clinical practice guidelines: legal repercussions. *Journal of Law and Medicine*, **10**, 5–9.

Gaffney, K. (2005). Health report card fears make doctors forgo potential life-saving heart treatment. http://www.eurekalert.org/pub_releases/2005–01/uorm-hrf010705.php, visited 5 March 2006.

Girgis, S. T., Thomson, C. and Ward, J. (2000). The courts expect the impossible: medico-legal issues as perceived by New South Wales General Practitioners. *Journal of Law and Medicine*, **7**, 273–80.

Green, J. and Wintfield, N. (1992). Report cards on cardiac surgeons – assessing New York State's approach. *New England Journal of Medicine*, **332**, 1229–32.

Herkutanto, H. and Freckelton, I. (2006). Indonesian health practitioner regulation. *Law in Context*, **23**, 229–40.

Kaplan, J. G. (1998). Report cards – part II: physicians rating MCOs. *Managed Care Interface*, **11**, 60.

Kerridge, I. H. and Mitchell, K. R. (1994). Missing the point: Rogers v Whitaker and the ethical ideal of informed and shared decision-making. *Journal of Law and Medicine*, **1**, 239–244.

Lowe, K. (2005). Doctors report cards not always clear when comparing care. *Johns Hopkins Gazette*, March 7. http://www.jhu.edu/~gazette/2005/07mar05/07report.html, visited 5 March 2006.

Marshall, T., Mohammed, M. A. and Rouse, A. (2004). A randomized controlled trial of league tables and control charts as aids to health service decision-making. *International Journal for Quality in Health Care*, **16**, 309.

McInnes, M. (1998). Failure to warn in medical negligence – a cautionary note from Canada: *Arndt v Smith, Torts Law Journal*, **6**, 135–43.

Mendelson, D. (1998). The breach of the medical duty to warn and causation: *Chappel v Hart* and the necessity to reconsider some aspects of *Rogers v Whitaker*. *Journal of Law and Medicine*, **5**, 312–19.

Milburn, A. (2002). Secretary of State's Speech to Parliament Announcing the Government's Reponse to the Bristol Royal Infirmary Report, United Kingdom House of Commons: Hansard, 17 January.

Moscucci, M., Eagle, K. A., Share, D. *et al.* (2005). Public reporting and case Selection for Percutaneous Coronary Interventions: an analysis from two large multicenter Percutaneous Coronary Intervention databases. *Journal of the American College of Cardiology*, **45**, 1759–65.

National Health Service Executive (1996). *Good Practice Booklet on Clinical Guidelines*, London: Department of Health.

Neil, D. A., Clarke, S. and Oakley, J. G. (2004). Public reporting of individual surgeon performance information: United Kingdom developments and Australian issues. *Medical Journal of Australia*, **181**, 266–8.

Olbourne, N. (1998). The Influence of Rogers v Whitaker on the Practice of Cosmetic Plastic Surgery. *Journal of Law and Medicine*, **5**, 334–47.

Pennsylvania Cost Care Containment Council (1999). *C-section Deliveries in Pennsylvania*. http://www.phc4.org/csection/, visited 5 March 2006.

Robertson, G. (1991). Informed consent ten years later: the impact of *Reibl v Hughes*, *Canadian Bar Review*, **70**, 423.

Schuck, P. M. (1994). Rethinking Informed Consent. *Yale Law Journal*, **103**, 899.

Zuger, A. (2005). Report Cards for Doctors? Grades Are Likely to Be A, B, C . . . and I. *New York Times*, 1 March. http://plaza.snu.ac.kr/~premed/The%20New%20York% 20Times%20%20Health%20%20Health%20Care%20Policy%20%20Essay%20Report% 20Cards%20for%20Doctors%20Grades%20Are%20Likely%20to%20Be%20 A,% 20B,%20C%20_%20_%20_%20and%20I.htm, visited 5 June 2006.

Index